An Introduction to Clinical Governance and Patient Safety

Edited by

Elizabeth Haxby

David Hunter

Siân Jaggar

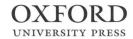

OXFORD

UNIVERSITY PRESS

D0916451

OXFORD
UNIVERSITY PRESS

Great Clarendon Street, Oxford OX2 6DP

Oxford University Press is a department of the University of Oxford.
It furthers the University's objective of excellence in research, scholarship,
and education by publishing worldwide in

Oxford New York

Auckland Cape Town Dar es Salaam Hong Kong Karachi
Kuala Lumpur Madrid Melbourne Mexico City Nairobi
New Delhi Shanghai Taipei Toronto

With offices in

Argentina Austria Brazil Chile Czech Republic France Greece
Guatemala Hungary Italy Japan Poland Portugal Singapore
South Korea Switzerland Thailand Turkey Ukraine Vietnam

Oxford is a registered trade mark of Oxford University Press
in the UK and in certain other countries

Published in the United States
by Oxford University Press Inc., New York

© Oxford University Press 2010

British Library Cataloguing in Publication Data
Data available

Library of Congress Cataloging in Publication Data
Data available

Typeset in Minion by Glyph International, Bangalore, India
Printed in the UK
on acid-free paper by
CPI Antony Rowe, Chippenham, Wiltshire

ISBN 978–0–19–955861–2

10 9 8 7 6 5 4 3 2 1

Foreword

Professor Sir Bruce Keogh

In England we have taken the view that good clinical quality is derived from the three domains of clinical effectiveness, patient safety, and patient experience.

Improvements in clinical effectiveness are driven by the relentless advance of medical science and technology, but improvements in patient safety and a focus on patient experience have lagged behind. This imbalance needs to be addressed and as a result patient safety has become a top priority in the National Health Service.

When patients seek help from a clinician, or engage a healthcare system, they understand that diseases and the associated treatments carry a certain amount of risk and they weigh up the relative pros and cons before embarking on a given therapeutic course. What they do not expect is to experience less effective treatment or to suffer adverse consequences as a result of poorly conducted treatment or badly organized care.

Clinical governance is the framework by which organizations seek to focus on clinical quality, including safety issues, through internal scrutiny coupled with organizational learning. This is an integral part of good healthcare delivery and all healthcare professionals, including doctors, should have a clear understanding of the basic principles and how to use them to benefit in their daily practice.

Traditionally medical training has focused on the acquisition of skills and knowledge related to diagnostic procedures and therapeutic intervention. It is now evident that there is a need to develop other aspects of clinical practice such as communication, team working and an understanding of the process of clinical judgement and human error.

This book aims to provide a simple overview of clinical governance in context. It highlights the important principles that need to be understood in order to function effectively as a clinician in the current complex and highly pressurized healthcare environment. It is compiled in short sections with examples taken directly from daily practice to illustrate the approaches that can be taken to common problems. The scenarios used have been sourced from all branches of medicine to ensure it is relevant to all medical trainees. It will assist in preparation for both consultant interviews and future practice. Contributions have been made by consultants, junior medical staff, and managers to ensure that issues are reflected from several different perspectives.

Professor Sir Bruce Keogh
NHS Medical Director

Contents

Section 8 **Fundamental principles**

Contributors

Murray Anderson-Wallace
Managing Director,
AWR Strategic Communications

Jilla Bond
works in patient and public
involvement in the NHS

Edwin Borman
Consultant Anaesthetist and
Clinical Director,
University Hospital,
Coventry and Warwickshire NHS Trust

Lesley Bromley
Consultant Anaesthetist UCLH NHS
Foundation Trust

Maria Cabrelli
Director of Estates & Facilities,
Kingston Hospital NHS Trust, Surrey

Eve Cartwright
PALS Manager,
Royal Brompton and Harefield NHS
Foundation Trust

Nick Coleman
Non-executive Director,
Royal Brompton and Harefield NHS
Foundation Trust

Chris Connell
Implementation Consultant,
National Institute for Health and
Clinical Excellence

Richard Connett
Assistant Director (Head of Performance),
Royal Brompton & Harefield Hospital
NHS Foundation Trust

Robert Craig
Director of Operations,
Royal Brompton & Harefield Hospital
NHS Foundation Trust

Peta Jane Eastland
Senior Lecturer,
Northumbria University

Paul Farquhar-Smith
Consultant in Pain, Anaesthetics
and Intensive Care,
Royal Marsden NHS
Foundation Trust

Catriona Ferguson
Consultant Anaesthetist &
Royal College of Anaesthetists
college tutor,
Royal Nose Throat & Ear Hospital,
Grey Inn Road, London

Simon Finney
Consultant Anaesthetist,
Royal Brompton & Harefield Hospital
NHS Foundation Trust

Les Gemmell
Consultant Anaesthetist / Intensivist,
Betsi Cadwaladr University
Health Board

Allan Goldman
Paediatric Intensivist,
Great Ormond St Hospital, London

Gareth Goodier
Chief Executive Cambridge University
Hospitals NHS Foundation Trust

Helen Goodman
Project Manager,
Royal Brompton and Harefield
NHS Foundation Trust

David Greaves
Consultant Anaesthetist, Newcastle
Hospitals NHS Foundation Trust

Sarah Hammond
Specialist Registrar in Anaesthetics,
London

Richard Hartopp
Anaesthetic Specialist Registrar,
London

Elizabeth J Haxby
Lead Clinician in Clinical Risk,
Royal Brompton Hospital

Guy Hirst
Director, Atrainability Limited

Judith Hulf
Clinical Lead for
Revalidation Academy of
Medical Royal Colleges

Nicholas Hunt
Director of Service Development,
Royal Brompton and Harefield NHS
Foundation Trust

David Hunter
Consultant Anaesthetist
and Intensivist,
Royal Brompton Hospital London

Siân Jaggar
Consultant Anaesthetist &
Royal College of Anaesthetists
college tutor,
Royal Brompton & Harefield Hospital
NHS Foundation Trust

David James
Consultant Anaesthetist & Clinical
Director of Peri-operative Care,
Critical Care & Pain, GSTT,
London

Carol Johnson
Director of Human Resources,
Royal Brompton & Harefield Hospital
NHS Foundation Trust

Mel Johnson
Calderdale and Huddersfield NHS
Foundation Trust

Mary Lane
Consultant Anaesthetist,
Royal Brompton and Harefield NHS
Foundation Trust

Gillian C Leng
Deputy Chief Executive,
National Institute for Health and
Clinical Excellence

Peter Littlejohns
Clinical and Public Health Director,
National Institute for Health and
Clinical Excellence

Carole M Longson
Director, Centre for Health
Technology Evaluation,
National Institute for Health and
Clinical Excellence

Alison Lovatt
Calderdale and Huddersfield NHS
Foundation Trust

Tom Magill
works in patient and public
involvement in the NHS

Mirella Marlow
Programme Director – Devices and
Diagnostic Systems,
National Institute for Health
and Clinical Excellence

Rachel Matthews
Programme Lead for Patient and
Public Involvement,
National Institute for Health
Research (NIHR),
Collaboration for Leadership in
Applied Health Research and Care
(CLAHRC) for Northwest
London

Henry McQuay
Nuffield Professor of Clinical
Anaesthetics,
Nuffield Department of Anaesthetics,
University of Oxford,
Oxford

Jeremy Mitchell
Consultant Anaesthetist & Lead
Clinician in Clinical Risk,
Harefield Hospital Royal
Brompton and Harefield NHS
Foundation Trust

Augustine J Pereira
Consultant in Public Health Medicine

Nelson Phillips
Professor of Strategy and
Organizational Behaviour,
Imperial College Business School,
London

Gaynor Pickavance
DNV Healthcare UK,
providing risk management services on
behalf of the NHS Litigation Authority

Claire Read
Editorial Manager,
The Learning Clinic,
London

Ruth Robertson
Senior Researcher,
The King's Fund

Andrew Rochford
Honorary Clinical Lecturer & SpR in
Gastroenterology,
Newham University Hospital
NHS Trust

Ian Runcie
Consultant Radiologist,
Princess Royal Hospital,
Haywards Heath, Sussex

Kirstyn Shaw
Revalidation Policy & Programme
Manager at Academy of Medical
Royal Colleges

Heather Shearer
Senior Fellow, Improvement Faculty,
NHS Institute for Innovation and
Improvement

Stephen Squire
Director of Equipment Management,
Royal Brompton & Harefield Hospital
NHS Foundation Trust

Kieran Sweeney
Formerly Honorary Professor of
General Practice,
Peninsula College of Medicine and
Dentistry

Ruth Symons
National Health Service Litigation
Authority

Deborah Trenchard
Life Coach

Angela Walsh
Network Manager,
North West London Critical
Care Network

Mike D Williams
Former CEO, Radcliffe Infirmary,
Oxford and Musgrove Park Hospital,
Taunton; Research Fellow,
University of Exeter Business School;
Associate Lecturer,
Peninsula College of Medicine
and Dentistry

Paul Williams OBE
Chief Executive, NHS Wales

Suzette Woodward
Director of Patient Safety,
National Patient Safety Agency

Alison Wright
Manager of near-real time
feedback services,
Picker Institute Europe,
Oxford

Chapter 1

Clinical governance and patient safety: An overview

Sarah Hammond

Key points

- Clinical governance was introduced in the late 1990s to provide a quality framework for the National Health Service (NHS).
- Clinical governance aims to set clear standards, monitor implementation, and publish results with periodic inspection by regulatory bodies.
- All healthcare organizations must have a clinical governance strategy and a quality improvement programme.
- Clinical governance was originally based on a 'seven pillars approach' and has evolved to include fundamental principles of leadership, systems awareness, teamwork, communication, and ownership.
- A focus on improving patient safety and reducing harm is provided through the Chief Medical Officer reports, work of the NHS Institute for Innovation and Improvement, and the Patient Safety First Campaign.

Definition of clinical governance

A framework through which NHS organisations are accountable for continually improving the quality of their services and safeguarding high standards of care by creating an environment in which excellence in clinical care will flourish (Scally and Donaldson 1998)

What does clinical governance mean?

The key components of clinical governance in the current NHS are

- ensuring patient safety,
- learning from mistakes,
- encouraging openness,
- sharing and maintaining good practice, and
- continuing professional education and development.

It is about ensuring the health service is patient-centred. The NHS Clinical Governance Support Team, now obsolete, described clinical governance through the seven pillars model. There are seven pillars to which five fundamental principles were later added with the goal being an effective patient–professional partnership.

The seven pillars are the following:

1. *Clinical effectiveness*: The extent to which healthcare interventions and treatments work.

2. *Risk management effectiveness*: Minimizing risk to patients, staff, and organizations.

3. *Patient experience*: Ensuring services are centred around needs of patients.

4. *Communication effectiveness*: Communication channels for adequate information exchange with patients, public, and throughout the organization.

5. *Resource effectiveness*: Utilization of resources including staff, equipment, and facilities for optimal benefit for patients.

6. *Strategic effectiveness*: Planning, delivery, and development of services, which reflect local and national requirements.

7. *Learning effectiveness*: Continuing professional development of all staff.

The five fundamental principles are as follows:

1. *Systems awareness*: The NHS is a national organization providing healthcare at local primary care level and up to regional, specialized quarternary care. The complex network of systems within this arrangement frequently results in failures for patients and staff. Improved system delivery of healthcare, which is patient focused, must be evidence-based.

2. *Teamwork*: Effective teams perform better and produce better results. A greater emphasis on development of team resource management leads to improved patient outcome.

3. *Communication*: This is a fundamental component of all functioning healthcare: between patient and professional; between professional groups; between clinicians and managers and between the trust and outside organizations. Communication must be effective, timely, and through appropriate means. Ineffective communication is the most common contributing factor to system errors and failures in patient safety.

4. *Ownership*: Staff within organizations must be empowered to take responsibility, solve problems, and bring about change.

5. *Leadership*: Effective leaders are required at all levels within the management and clinical structure of healthcare organizations. Successful leaders must have appropriate experience and skills to be highly effective.

Origins of clinical governance and key documents

The key to appreciating the importance of clinical governance in current clinical practice is understanding its conception and progression with the development of the NHS.

The NHS was established in 1948 and had no agenda for quality of care; in 1983 the Griffiths report described a lack of accountability for quality at local level, which led to the appointment of managers to lead healthcare units. Medical staff became involved in management teams, which introduced clinical responsibility for service quality. The year 1997 saw the first government white paper 'The New NHS, Modern, Dependable' to address issues of quality and effectiveness. Two national organizations to improve efficiency and effectiveness were announced:

- National Institute for Clinical Excellence (NICE) [now called the National Institute for Health and Clinical Effectiveness] to promote high-quality national guidelines for treatments based on up to date clinical evidence.

- The Commission for Health Improvement, renamed the Healthcare Commission (HCC) in 2004 and the Care Quality Commission from April 2009, would ensure the NHS established and maintained high standards of quality and safety for patients and staff.

In 1998, 'A First Class Service: Quality in the New NHS' outlined the government's strategy to create a 'modern service that delivers high quality care for all'. This introduced the concept of clinical governance, which became a fundamental tool for NHS organizations to ensure high standards of care were achieved. The paper decribed its plans for staff to have lifelong learning to maintain professional standards and for the NHS to be 'more open and truly accountable to the public'.

In 1999, 'Clinical Governance in the New NHS' provided guidance for NHS Trusts on the implementation of clinical governance. It stated that by April 1999, lead clinicians should be identified and appropriate structures set up for overseeing clinical governance within each NHS Trust.

Alongside this, 'Supporting Doctors, Protecting Patients' provided proposals for professional regulation and set out minimum standards for controls assurance.

The 'NHS Plan: a Plan for Investment, a Plan for Reform' was published in 2000 to 'reform the NHS of the 1940s to one fit for the 21st century centred around the patient'. Extra income would improve NHS facilities by

- recruiting significant numbers of new doctors and nurses,

- provision of extra hospital beds,

- building new hospitals,

- providing up to date information technology services, and

- ensuring clean wards and better hospital food.

Good Medical Practice, produced by the General Medical Council (GMC), provides guidance for all doctors on the provision of good clinical care and covers all aspects of clinical practice. It highlights continuing professional development as a means of maintaining and improving performance and encouraging openness and honesty in relationships with patients, especially when things go wrong.

Three significant events and the subsequent inquiries influenced the clinical governance agenda and resulted in major changes to professional regulation, risk management practices, and processes:

1. In 1999, The Royal Liverpool Children's Inquiry investigated retention and disposal of human organs and tissue removed at post mortem. The inquiry found inadequate

consent processes, poor communication with parents, and a disorganized set up. Key recommendations included consent for post-mortem examination to be obtained by the clinician responsible and the appointment of clinicians to management roles with appropriate experience.

2. In 2001 the results of *The Bristol Royal Infirmary Inquiry* into paediatric cardiac surgery services were published. The report stated a third of children received less than adequate care during the period 1984–1995 due to lack of teamwork, leadership, and an environment in which problems were not adequately identified or addressed. Recommendations were made to learn from the mistakes and implement change.

3. In 2006 '*Good Doctors, Safer Patients*' was produced in response to the Harold Shipman Enquiry with the purpose of promoting and assuring good medical practice. Recommendations included introduction of regular assessment and appraisal of doctors' practice. It also aimed to reduce the blame culture associated with poor performance and the need to formalize medical education as part of medical regulation. Further information regarding the revalidation process for health professionals was detailed in 'Trust, Assurance and Safety – The Regulation of Health Professionals in the 21st Century'.

'*High Quality Care for all: NHS Next Stage Review Final Report 2008*' was compiled by Lord Darzi, Parliamentary Under Secretary of State, in consultation with 2000 clinicians and allied health professionals from all over the country. His report published in early 2009 outlined improvements to the NHS to ensure high quality care for all. He recommended greater patient choice and guaranteed access to the most clinically and cost-effective drugs and treatments. Lord Darzi stated 'to ensure quality is at the heart of the NHS there needs to be an emphasis on patient safety and published data on the quality of care'. As a result, new assessment processes will be developed focussing on quality of care, safety, and patient experience. Each Trust will be required to have a 'Quality Account' published annually with a range of indicators agreed both locally with commissioners and nationally with the new Care Quality Commission.

Assessment of clinical governance

To ensure the NHS is implementing recommendations and continually improving quality and safety, assessments and inspections are undertaken by regulatory bodies.

The Healthcare Commission

The HCC had responsibility for evaluating clinical governance procedures and processes within NHS Trusts. Its purpose was to promote continual improvement in England's healthcare services with a focus on issues of public interest. This was achieved by a process of assessment and investigation and the findings were published in a report which was accessible to the public called the Annual Health Check. This assessment of performance against core standards was carried out annually for all trusts within England including all acute trusts, primary care trusts, mental health trusts, and ambulance services. Whilst each organization undertook a self-assessment to determine its level of compliance, the HCC periodically inspected Trusts to ensure declarations were reflected in practice.

The ratings were divided into two areas:

- Quality of Services accounted for seven domains:
  - Patient safety
  - Clinical and cost effectiveness
  - Clinical governance
  - Patient focus
  - Accessible and responsive care
  - Care environments, amenities, and public health
  - Performance against national targets
- Use of resources was an assessment of how trusts managed resources, financial reporting, and value for money.

The scores for the two areas were rated excellent, good, fair, or weak.

Additional aims of the HCC included safeguarding the public by acting promptly on complaints and failings and providing authoritative independent and relevant information on the quality of healthcare.

Care Quality Commission

This organization was established in April 2009 as a single, integrated regulator for health and adult social care to replace the three bodies, which had this role previously: The Healthcare Commission, The Mental Health Act Commission, and the Commission for Social Care Inspection. It will ensure regulation and inspection activity across health and adult social care is coordinated and managed to ensure better outcomes. For the first time, NHS and social care providers will be required to register with the new regulator in order to provide services. The regulatory system will provide a clearer framework of requirements which NHS organizations must meet in order to provide services.

Commissioning for Quality and Innovation

In 'High Quality Care for All' Lord Darzi included a commitment to make a proportion of providers' income conditional on quality of service provision and innovation through the Commissioning for Quality and Innnovation (CQUIN) payment framework. For the acute sector, payment will be linked to locally determined goals. His vision is 'an NHS where teams consistently measure what they do, improve the care they provide and compare themselves against others'. The framework encourages improvement for all providers whatever the starting point using financial incentives.

Patient safety

Definition: 'Protection of patients against harm that results from the efforts or lack of efforts of the healthcare system'.

Patient safety is now a worldwide issue, which is central to the clinical governance framework. Evidence suggests 10% of in-patients in NHS hospitals suffer an adverse event, which negatively impacts on their outcome, and 50% of these are preventable. The recognition that many patients are harmed by their healthcare has led to national and international initiatives to improve safety and quality of care. Within the NHS a number of organizations have a specific remit to promote patient safety and improve care.

'Organisation with a Memory' published in 2000, chaired by the Chief Medical Officer (CMO), reported on learning from adverse events in the NHS. It stated many adverse incidents were avoidable if lessons had been learned, for example, the repeated accidental administration of intrathecal vincristine resulting in paralysis and death. The report describes combinations of unsafe, unpredictable acts by staff, and organizational conditions, which result in weak systems. The group highlighted the need to develop a safety culture within the NHS, which encouraged staff to report all adverse incidents including 'near misses'. This strategy has proven effective in many other high-risk industries including aviation.

National Patient Safety Agency (NPSA)

The NPSA, an arm's length body of the Department of Health, was established in response to the recommendations of 'Organisation with a Memory'. The aim was to make improving patient safety a priority in the NHS through informing, supporting, and influencing organizations through incident reporting, analysis, and sharing safety lessons.

In 2004 the NPSA produced 'Seven Steps to Patient Safety', which provided an overview of patient safety tools and effective incident reporting as follows:

1. build a safety culture, one which is open and fair;
2. lead and support your staff: establish clear and strong focus on patient safety within the organization;
3. integrate risk management: develop systems to manage risk and identify what could go wrong;
4. promote reporting: ensure ease of reporting for staff;
5. involve patients and the public: listen to patients and develop open communication;
6. learn and share safety lessons: encourage staff to use root cause analysis to investigate why things go wrong and share the lessons with others; and
7. implement solutions to prevent harm: embed lessons through changes to practices, processes or systems.

In 2007, the CMO produced 'Safety First', which described progress made in improving patient safety. Although commending some changes which had occurred, the CMO commented the pace of change was too slow. He provided recommendations on 'how to reaffirm patient safety at the heart of the healthcare agenda'. The four key themes were as follows:

1. Implementation of systems and interventions, which actively reduce harm to patients.

2. More effective methods of addressing issues raised from patient safety incidents.

3. Creation of an environment which motivates and inspires NHS staff to provide patient care, which is as safe as possible.

4. Provision of strong leadership regarding patient safety within NHS organizations to ensure its priority.

This was followed by the NPSA publication 'Five actions to improve patient safety reporting' in 2008. This reported that Trusts with high levels of patient safety incident reporting had stronger organizational cultures of safety. Key actions included raising awareness of the incident reporting process, its potential value for improving care, and its relevance to all staff.

NHS Institute for Innovation and Improvement

The NHS III supports the NHS in transforming healthcare for patients by developing new ways of working, new technology, and world class leadership. It is working with healthcare organizations to improve training, practice schemes and programmes to build a high-quality, reliable, and safe NHS.

It is focused on four areas:

1. Improving systems and processes to provide safer care

2. Accelerating improvement in commissioning

3. Improving clinical and service quality and controlling costs

4. Quality and value: providing practical frameworks for raising standards

The Leading Improvement in Patient Safety Programme (LIPS), developed by the NHS III, supports this work by helping Trusts to develop the capacity and capability to make patient safety the highest priority. It provides training and tools on

◆ approaches to quality improvement,

◆ leadership,

◆ engaging clinicians,

◆ human factors in healthcare,

◆ communication, and

◆ team work.

These measures can be introduced into primary and secondary care organizations quickly and simply.

Patient Safety First Campaign

The Patient Safety First Campaign was launched within the NHS in England in 2008 to make the safety of patients the highest priority and make all avoidable death and harm unacceptable. The campaign is led by frontline clinicians and managers and requires active participation by organizations and their staff. It initially focused on the application of five interventions to reduce avoidable risks and harm associated with healthcare in the acute sector. In addition to a quest to improve leadership, there are four clinical interventions relating to known major sources of harm in hospitals.

- *Safety for leadership*: to ensure a leadership culture at Board level, which promotes quality and patient safety and an environment where continuous improvement in harm reduction becomes routine.
- *Reducing harm from deterioration*: reduce in-hospital cardiac arrest and mortality rate through earlier recognition and treatment of the deteriorating patient.
- *Reducing harm in critical care*: improve critical care through the reliable application of care bundles.
- *Reducing harm in perioperative care*: improve care for adult patients undergoing elective surgical procedures in the hospital setting (prevention of surgical site infection and World Health Organization's Safe Surgery Checklist).
- *Reducing harm from high-risk medicines* (anticoagulants, injectable sedatives, opiates, and insulin).

Similar campaigns have been highly successful in the United States, Denmark, and Canada with clear evidence of lives saved and reduction in harm. The campaign will be extended to include evidence-based interventions in primary care, mental health, and ambulance services.

Recommended further reading

www.dh.gov.uk
www.cqc.org.uk
www.institute.nhs.uk
www.npsa.nhs.uk
www.patientsafetyfirst.nhs.uk

Section 1

Risk management

Effective risk management is fundamental to governance in any organization including healthcare, which is more complex than most. Clinicians tend to focus on immediate risks posed to patients by particular procedures. At an organizational level, a much wider perspective must be taken encompassing operational, financial, clinical, and reputational risks, and their control. This section explains the elements of risk management starting with a general awareness of healthcare as a risky activity (*Risk awareness*). Risks can be identified from internal sources including safety incidents, as well as external sources, such as safety alerts and confidential enquiries (*Risk identification*). An estimate of the magnitude of any particular risk is required since this shapes the response in terms of investment and resources (*Risk assessment*). The Board is responsible for ensuring that all risks are minimized and mitigated as far as reasonably practicable. It requires assurance through the committee structure that this is the case (*Risk control*). In healthcare it is not possible to eradicate risk, but being aware of the risky nature of healthcare, and by taking a stepwise approach to risk identification, assessment and control, a fluctuating profile of risk can be established as identified risks are controlled and new risks identified (*Risk assurance*). Important sources of information about risks include *Complaints and claims*, each of which has clearly defined protocols for management and response. Trusts are also subject to external assessment of their risk management structures and processes by the National Health Service Litigation Authority (*Risk Management Standards*).

Chapter 2

Risk awareness

Suzette Woodward

Key points

- Risk awareness is understanding risk-prone situations and the ability to anticipate or predict hazards, risks, and incidents and minimize the resultant personal and organizational risk.
- Key factors which support risk awareness are an open and fair culture, an understanding that errors can and will occur and that there is potential for harm in all aspects of healthcare.
- Barriers to developing risk awareness include the presence of a blame culture and failure to understand human factors such as bystander apathy, fixation errors, groupthink, and involuntary automaticity.
- Tools which can promote risk awareness include safety briefings and debriefings, safety leadership walkrounds, and foresight training.

Introduction

Risk awareness is the recognition of the potential for hazards, risks and incidents that occur within the healthcare environment and result in patient harm. It is also referred to as mindfulness, attentiveness, anticipation, or foresight. Being risk aware means that individuals and organizations are potentially able to prevent error and subsequent harm to patients by putting plans and contingencies in place. Within organizations an effective patient safety culture is said to exist when there is high awareness of safety issues at all levels from Trust Board to Ward. This requires the Board to be aware of key risks and safety issues, which is in turn dependent upon an open and fair culture in which the staff are encouraged to speak up about their concerns and to report them appropriately. For example, the Board needs to know about hospital-acquired infection rates, mortality and morbidity, and falls and drug errors so that they can devise and support strategies for improvement, monitor their implementation, and ensure resources are available and that the facilities are fit for the purpose. In order to achieve this culture of safety, awareness of potential problems must be part of daily life, 24 hours a day, 7 days a week for managerial, administrative, and clinical staff.

Frontline staff are key people who need to understand about the potential for risk, and to be proactive and respond to hazards and risks before they become incidents involving patients. They need to be able to stand back and review the environment and systems in place to work out what could go wrong, e.g. briefing at the start of an operating theatre session. It is important:

◆ to ensure the right patient is present,

◆ all relevant information is accessible,

◆ all the necessary equipment is available, and

◆ that team members are clear about their roles and responsibilities and have been introduced.

Equally, debriefing at the end of the theatre session helps the team to talk through the risks and any issues of concern that happened during the session, together with any improvements they can make for the future.

Factors which help improve risk awareness

1. *An open and fair culture.* This is an environment in which the staff can speak out if they are concerned about a risk and are supported when they do so no matter where they are in the organizational hierarchy. For example, a junior doctor feeling able to challenge a consultant or a member of the nursing staff in order to prevent the administration of the wrong drug to a patient.

2. *An understanding of the potential for error, risk, and harm.* This involves increasing understanding of risk-prone situations and the ability to anticipate or predict hazards, risks, and incidents, which could affect the safety of patients. A wider understanding can be gained by reviewing all sources of risk and harm through case note reviews, incident reports, complaints, and litigation claims. Daily safety briefings and debriefings for teams to discuss the potential risks for that shift or session are also excellent ways in which risk awareness can be significantly increased, e.g. identifying patients with the same name on a ward.

3. *An acceptance that errors can and will occur and that they can never be eliminated.* A risk-free system is not a practical reality and is rarely desirable. In most cases, it could only be achieved by halting the hazardous activity altogether, resulting in the loss of the benefits which the activity brings. For example, administering chemotherapy to a patient with cancer has an effect on eliminating cancer cells but at the same time has a high likelihood of affecting good cells. However, the benefit of receiving chemotherapy (a potential cure) outweighs the risks (e.g. reduced immune system, hair loss, vomiting). Accepting that errors can and will occur would mean that individuals will be more vigilant to the potential safety gaps in the system they are working in and will look for ways to trap errors.

4. *The ability to minimize risk.* This is often referred to as mitigation or risk reduction in terms of likelihood and effect. For example, by ensuring that drugs which look and sound alike are not stored next to one another in a resuscitation trolley or drug cupboard. This reduces the chances of picking up the wrong drug. Similarly, limiting the number of formulations of the same drug available can contribute to reducing the chance of an overdose.

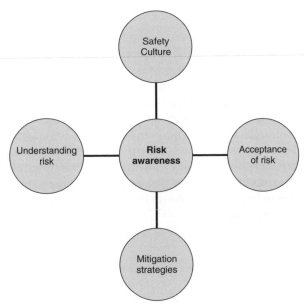

Fig. 2.1 Factors which improve risk awareness.

Barriers to effective action

Even when awareness of risk is heightened, it may be difficult for frontline staff to act appropriately to manage or reduce the risk. The following are examples of things that can inhibit individuals from acting safely in a risky situation.

1 *Blame culture*

Few people are willing to come forward and discuss risks if they fear disciplinary action. A punitive blame culture is a major inhibitory factor to speaking up about what could go or has gone wrong. To raise awareness of risks it is vital to promote a culture in which individuals are willing to come forward in the interests of patient safety. This is not a 'blame-free' system, but one which has a 'just culture' where openness, fairness, accountability, and responsibility are key.

2 *Bystander apathy*

Bystander apathy refers to a phenomenon whereby people are less likely to take action as the number of other people involved increases. People are less likely to take responsibility for a task if they assume someone else will do it, or that other people are more qualified to take charge. For example, when transferring patients from one area to another, such as from a ward to intensive care or from an operating theatre to ward or even just from one care setting to another, steps can get missed or forgotten because someone thinks someone else is doing it. Checklists can be very helpful in this context to avoid missing key steps or information being forgotten; for example, using the surgical safety checklist developed by the World Health Organization (WHO) can help to avoid errors.

3 *Fixation*

Fixation is said to be present when errors occur because a person becomes so convinced that their first interpretation is correct that they do not seek evidence that would challenge their assumption. For example, an initial diagnosis is made and despite information which challenges this, the team continues to treat the patient according to the initial diagnosis; e.g. a patient could be admitted to a surgical ward for an inguinal hernia repair and whilst in the ward the patient exhibits some of the symptoms of myocardial infarction, including chest pain and sweatiness. However, staff are fixated on the surgical problems and attribute all the symptoms to the inguinal hernia. Therefore, they do not recognize the symptoms of the myocardial infarction or their severity because their mindset was on preparing the patient for surgery. Healthcare staff must learn to review the situation frequently to ensure that new information is considered in context.

4 *Groupthink*

Most times the 'wisdom of the crown' enhances decision-making, however occasionally there is a downside to large groups. This is often referred to as 'groupthink'. This occurs when people within a group fixate on one way of doing things and gain strength from the collective view. No other options are considered and no one questions the strategy often to avoid confrontation and conflict. Without challenging ideas and actions, groups can allow or make decisions without considering concerns from individuals, which are not voiced through fear of upsetting the consensus of the group. For example, if a junior individual within an operating theatre can see that the surgeon is about to operate on the wrong organ or wrong limb. Because everyone else in the room, who are perceived as more experienced, do not seem to have noticed, the individual feels unable to speak out, questioning his or her own judgement against the collective judgement.

5 *Involuntary automaticity*

Similar to bystander apathy, sometimes errors are not identified because people are going through the motions of carrying out a check but are not consciously engaged in the checking process. For example, a nurse and a doctor checking the dosage of a drug. Each assumes the other has checked so the dose must be right. This can happen even with multiple checks. As each check is made, the error is compounded because an assumption is made that the previous check was correct. An example would be a patient in an acute ward prescribed hydralazine (for hypertension) instead of hydroxyzine (for itching). The chart may have been rewritten by a doctor with poor handwriting, who did not usually treat the patient. The prescription chart was faxed to a pharmacist who was busy because it was the Friday before a bank holiday weekend. The drug was dispensed and sent to the ward in a bottle labelled with the patient's name. The patient was given the wrong drug three times a day for five days before the error was recognized by another pharmacist, who was checking prescription charts in the ward. All the staff treating the patient had given him the drug over the five days but no one had noticed that it was the wrong drug.

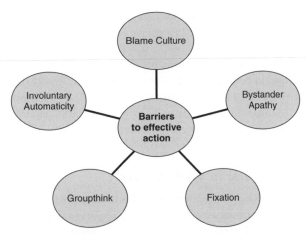

Fig. 2.2 Barriers to effective action.

Tools which help improve risk awareness

Training and education of healthcare staff at the outset of the journey to becoming future doctors and nurses should involve the following:

- rates and types of patient safety incidents in healthcare,
- human error and human factors,
- improvement methodology and skills needed to recognize and deal with error,
- how to report risks and incidents, and
- mechanisms for learning from error such as root cause analysis.

Improved interpersonal and communication skills so that once individuals are aware of a risk they can speak up or challenge it in a way in which they will be heard.

Safety briefings and debriefings

Safety briefings and debriefings are a simple, easy-to-use tool and can be utilized by frontline staff to share information about potential risks on a daily basis. Briefings involve a short meeting with everyone who is involved in the shift or session to talk about potential problems or risks. Safety briefings help staff to recognize and understand where they and the patients are most at risk and so plans can be made to mitigate the risks. Briefings can take place at the beginning or end of the day or session. They are used to

- help increase staff awareness of patient safety issues,
- create an environment in which staff share information freely, and
- integrate safety issues into daily work.

In January 2009 the National Patient Safety Agency (NPSA) launched the WHO Safe Surgery Checklist in England, following the publication of a study in *New England Journal of Medicine* which demonstrated a dramatic reduction in mortality and complications in patients for whom the checklist had been used before, during, and after the procedure. The checklist ensures that staff work as a team to carry out a safety briefing pre-operatively and that they are prepared for the case and any problems that may arise.

Debriefings are often used after an incident. This helps staff to understand what went wrong and why, and to develop strategies to prevent the recurrence of mistakes in the future. Staff are encouraged to identify issues of concern and to present their ideas for improvement. Briefings and debriefings require both the leadership and the team working to function effectively. Leaders must establish the briefings and make it clear that everyone has a voice, and the team members must respect each other and listen.

Executive or leadership walkrounds

Leadership walkrounds help to create awareness of risks across an organization.

These are visits to clinical areas conducted regularly by senior staff including executives and Board members. The aim is to bring senior managers and frontline staff together to discuss safety issues directly. Specific questions are asked, such as 'what are the things you are worried about today?' or 'what risks did you deal with yesterday?' The walkrounds are followed by a debriefing where the leaders think about changes that can be made and help to implement them. The benefits are an increased awareness both at the frontline and at leadership level of safety issues, a visible demonstration of senior leadership, and a promotion of an open and fair culture. Fundamentally they are about obtaining and acting upon risks and safety problems before they become significant events. Walkrounds can also provide an opportunity for junior doctors and nurses to shadow an executive member of their organization.

Foresight programme

The foresight programme developed by the NPSA uses risk assessment tools to help support situational awareness. Professor James Reason, in 2004, provided clinical staff with a simple mental model for raising awareness which he calls the three-bucket model. Building on this model, the NPSA developed a 'foresight training resource pack' to support clinical staff working in all care settings to improve awareness of the factors that combine to increase the likelihood of patient safety incidents.

Foresight is the ability to identify, respond to, and recover from the initial indications that a patient safety incident could take place. The pack contains a range of training scenarios, both paper- and video-based, and supporting materials for use by the trainers. The scenarios prompt participants to think of the factors that can lead to patient safety incidents, and encourage discussion and learning.

This self-review tool asks each individual (it could also apply to teams) to score themselves in relation to three factors: self, context, and the task or tasks being carried out. They score themselves as follows for each factor:

- 1 for low risk
- 2 for medium
- 3 for high risk

The three factors are taken into account in the following ways.

Self: The self bucket relates to the current state of the individual involved, for example, lack of knowledge, fatigue, negative life events, inexperience, feeling under the weather. Consider the following situation.

> A healthcare professional working at night is more likely to be affected by the consequences of shift work, such as fatigue (score 1), and there may be factors outside work, e.g. a divorce, which will impact on their performance (score 2) and in addition they may not be familiar with a particular patient (score 3).

Context: The context bucket reflects on the nature of the work environment, for example distractions, interruptions, shift handovers, lack of time, lack of resources, poor equipment, risks within the environment, skill mix, team factors, number of changes, levels of authority, hierarchy, and team interactions. For example, an agency nurse misses handover (score 1), and is not familiar with an infusion device she needs to use (score 2), and does not know who to ask for help (score 3).

Task: The task bucket depends on the error potential of the task, for example leaving out steps in a task (more likely to happen near the end of a task), suggest doing steps in the wrong order or undertaking multiple tasks simultaneously. It also includes levels of experience, resources, equipment, knowledge, and complacency. Specific issues in relation to individual patients are also included, such as complexity, vulnerability, or even infectious status. A junior doctor is giving multiple drugs to a sick patient (score 1) who is isolated in a side room, and the doctor has left the drug chart in the treatment room (score 2) and has not labelled the syringes (score 3).

The three factors are then added together. Depending on the total score, the individual's 'buckets' are potentially full and they should therefore be aware that they are more likely to do something wrong. At this point, they should metaphorically 'press the pause button', step back, and decide whether there is anything they could do to reduce the risks. For example, delaying a procedure until the conditions are right. A low score of 3 does not mean that the individual or team is at its safest, and the highest score of 9 does not mean that they are at their riskiest. The self-review simply helps individuals become more aware of how safe they potentially are at that point in time and they can adjust their actions accordingly. This can be described as error wisdom or self-vigilance.

Summary

Risk awareness is vital for organizations, teams and individual healthcare staff. Understanding how risks to patient care are generated and accepting that risk is always present within the complexity of a hospital, ward, or operating theatre helps to reduce the chance that something will go wrong and cause harm. Many barriers to developing a safety culture exist, but there are tools, including training and education, the use of safety briefings and checklists along with developing foresight, that can help engender a proactive approach. Bringing executives and frontline staff together to discuss risks and safety at every level is fundamental to building safer systems in healthcare.

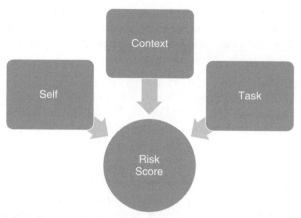

Fig. 2.3 Personal risk assessment model.

Further reading

National Patient Safety Agency. Foresight Training Programme. Available at: www.npsa.nhs. uk/nrls/improvingpatientsafety/humanfactors/foresight/.

Reason, J. (2000). Human error: models and management. *British Medical Journal* **320**, 768–770.

Sexton, J.B., Thomas, E.J., and Helmreich, R.L. (2000). Error, stress, and teamwork in medicine and aviation: cross sectional surveys. *British Medical Journal* **320**, 745–749.

Toft, B. (2005). Involuntary automaticity: a work-system induced risk to safe healthcare. *Health Services Management Research* **18**, 211–216.

Vincent, C. (2006). *Patient Safety*. Edinburgh: Churchill Livingstone.

Chapter 3

Risk identification

Elizabeth Haxby and Richard Hartopp

Key points

- Risk identification is key to a comprehensive risk management program that will include clinical, operational, and financial risks.
- Risk identification can be reactive or proactive.
- National Health Service (NHS) Trusts have an obligation to have risk identification procedures in place under both Health and Safety Legislation and the NHLSA Risk Management Standards for Acute Trusts.
- Risks can be identified from internal sources such as incidents, complaints, and claims as well as from external sources such as the NPSA, NCEPOD, and Healthcare Commission reviews.

Introduction

All NHS institutions are required by the National Health Service Litigation Authority (NHSLA) Risk management Standards for Acute Trusts to have a systematic approach to clinical risk management, since it is a fundamental part of the provision of safe, effective healthcare. Hazards and risks are features of all aspects of healthcare at every level and to manage them effectively, a robust approach to risk identification is needed.

Definitions

- Harm is any physical or psychological damage to an individual.
- A hazard is a situation that has potential to cause harm.
- Risk is a combination of the likelihood and consequence of that hazard being realized.

Risks are present in all areas of healthcare and in this chapter the focus is on clinical risks that can result in patient harm. However, consequences can have an impact beyond the patient and affect the financial and operational state of an organization, as well as its reputation, which may also be compromised. Risk identification follows risk awareness in the risk management process and is essential to frontline care as well as at Board level.

Clinical risks may be identified from many sources;

1. Clinical incident or patient safety incident (PSI) reporting
2. Complaints and claims

3. Clinical audit

4. Mortality and morbidity meetings

5. Executive safety walkrounds

6. Proactive risk assessment

7. National reports, e.g. NCEPOD, CEMACH

8. Patient safety alerts, e.g. National Patient Safety Agency (NPSA) and Medicines and Healthcare Products Regulatory Agency (MHRA) alerts.

1. Patient safety incident reporting

The concept of critical incident reporting arose from psychological studies in the U.S. Air Force during World War II. It has since been refined and used across other areas including civil aviation, nuclear power, and healthcare. The purpose of critical incident reporting (known as patient safety incidents in healthcare) is to learn from events or near misses, prevent their recurrence, and to reduce the threat of harm to patients. The National Patient Safety Agency (NPSA) defines a patient safety incident as follows:

> **Any incident which could have or did cause harm, loss or damage to a patient receiving care in the NHS.**

In 1995 the Clinical Negligence Scheme for Trusts (CNST) was established by the NHSLA and Trusts wishing to join the scheme had to adhere to a set of risk management standards. These included the necessity to having an effective patient safety incident reporting system in place. '**An Organisation with a Memory**' (DoH 2000) acknowledged that little had been learned from adverse events in the past and that medical error was a pervasive issue. Subsequently the government published plans for promoting patient safety in '**Building a Safer NHS**'. From these roots grew the NPSA and National Reporting and Learning System (NRLS).

The challenge to improve safety is substantial. In the period from June 2007 to July 2008 over 800,000 incident reports were sent to the NPSA:

- 65% resulted in no harm
- 6% resulted in moderate harm
- 1% resulted in severe harm.

Incident reporting structure

Every Trust has a local patient safety incident reporting system with relevant policies for both routine reporting and for the reporting of Serious Untoward Incidents (SUIs).

The key features of a reporting system are:

- Paper or electronic submission of reports – mandatory fields designed for all incidents clinical and non-clinical,
- Centralized reporting with incident data held in a database to assist analysis and linked to complaints, claims, and Patient Advice and Liaison Service (PALS) information,
- Confidential reporting,

- Ease of reporting,
- Clear indications what to report – a list of 'triggers' for reporting may be published to assist reporters.

  Reporters are required to provide key information, including

- details of who, what, when, where and how an incident occurred, and
- factual and objective information about what happened.

  To ensure prompt action reporting must

- be timely,
- be regarded as a positive action,
- be voluntary, and
- have different levels of response proportionate to severity of the incident.

In an effective reporting system, significant numbers of incidents will be reported and analysed for common trends. This helps to identify areas of risk, e.g. drug errors, which can be analysed further and can facilitate introduction of prevention strategies, for instance electronic prescribing has been shown to reduce prescribing errors by 70%.

Reportable incidents may not be clinical and include anything with potential to cause harm to patients or staff. It also includes risks to the organization itself – material, financial, or to its reputation. Incidents are graded for severity by a standard 'traffic light system' developed by the NPSA (see Box 3.1).

Every patient safety incident will be investigated at a local level in the clinical area in which it occurred or more severe incidents will involve the Risk Management team (see algorithm in Appendix 1). Clinical risk or patient safety committees should

Box 3.1 NPSA incident severity grading

Terms	Definition
No Harm (Green)	**Impact prevented** – Any adverse incident that had the potential to cause harm but was prevented resulting in no harm. **Impact not prevented** – Any adverse incident that ran to completion but no harm occurred.
Low (Yellow)	Any adverse incident that required extra observation or minor treatment and caused minimal harm to one or more persons
Moderate (Orange)	Any adverse incident that resulted in a moderate increase in treatment and which caused significant but not permanent harm to one or more persons
Severe (Red)	Any adverse incident that appears to have resulted in permanent harm to one or more persons
Death (Red)	Any adverse incident that directly resulted in the death of one or more patients

regularly review safety incident reports above a certain severity and also the corresponding investigation and root cause analysis (vide infra) in order to

◆ ensure appropriate action is taken,

◆ review action plans for previous events, and

◆ examine trends at individual or organizational level.

Where incidents happen which have the potential to occur across the organization, e.g. patient identification failures, these may require a Trust-wide response. Trust Boards receive regular reports on incident rates, types, and levels of harm and so can monitor trends. The NPSA receives copies of all incident reports via the NRLS, and will be instrumental in setting up the 'Patient Safety Direct' system, a single point of access for all healthcare personnel and ultimately patients to report incidents. This latter service was announced in Lord Darzi's 'Our NHS, Our Future' report (2007).

Fostering a safety culture

Patient safety incident reporting is essentially a reactive process and is prone to under-reporting. This may be due to a lack of appreciation of the importance of reporting (e.g. that the outcome of an incident did not warrant a report) or to other factors:

◆ Fear of recrimination or blame (litigation)

◆ Complexity of reporting

◆ No obvious response

◆ Lack of feedback

It is estimated that only 10–15% of all incidents are actually reported. Defining a list of incidents that must be reported may be helpful. This is particularly appropriate for a specific clinical setting such as a maternity unit. Events may recur, and event monitoring can be used to investigate these repeating patterns for a root cause.

Root cause analysis

A number of tools are available to assist in establishing the root cause of an incident and this helps to identify key areas of risk. Root cause analysis (RCA) can be undertaken in a number of ways using a variety of tools including

◆ the 5 whys technique,

◆ fishbone template,

◆ timelines,

◆ failure modes and effect analysis (FMEA), and

◆ barrier analysis.

[The details of all of these techniques are beyond the remit of this book but can be readily found on the NPSA website.]

The aim of RCA is to ensure a multidisciplinary approach to finding out what happened and why, so that robust preventive strategies can be put in place to reduce the risk of recurrence. The success of incident reporting depends on developing a culture in which staff are confident that they will not receive unfair blame for an event or near-miss episode and organizations must develop a 'just and fair blame' culture. To ensure patient safety is top priority, maintenance of a high profile for risk management through regular training days (e.g. on how to report incidents, how to perform RCA, and newsletters) is vital.

The global trigger tool

Voluntary reporting systems miss a considerable number of incidents. The Institute for Healthcare Improvement (IHI) in the United States has developed a trigger tool for reviewing clinical records as a more effective means of identifying harmful events. The global trigger tool (GTT) is used to quantify the degree and severity of harm and to select and test harm reduction strategies. The tool uses retrospective review of a random sample (e.g. 20 per month) of hospital notes using 'trigger' words to help identify possible harm events, e.g. returns to theatre for bleeding. If a trigger is identified, then a more detailed review is performed to assess if patient harm occurred. It is not designed to identify every patient safety incident in a single record and is time limited in order to produce a functional and practical approach to risk management. This tool was out as part of the 'Patient Safety First Campaign' in England (2008) to help healthcare organizations take a more proactive approach to identifying harm events and monitoring their progress in reducing risks consistently.

2. Claims and complaints

Claims and complaints databases can be examined to identify the specific events leading to unwanted outcomes for patients. Investigating clinical complaints can show up faults in

◆ organizations and systems of care delivery,
◆ patient pathways,
◆ the facilities in which care is provided, and
◆ individual practice.

Claims and complaints are an opportunity to see the consumer's view of the service, one that clinicians and managers cannot experience. The PALS service is also a route through which patient comments and complaints can be channelled into the risk management system to be systematically reviewed and hence lessons can be learned. Key areas of risk can be identified by taking an overview of incidents, complaints, and PALS issues if the aim is to learn from the experience. It is of course important that there is feedback to all concerned parties.

3. Clinical audit

Audit is entrenched within governance as a tool to guide best practise and can readily be used to examine risk. Audits may be at the local or the national level such as the National Audit Project (NAP) at the Royal College of Anaesthetists, which has published on a number of areas, e.g. major complications of central neuraxial blockade (NAP 3-2009), and major complications of airway management are currently being audited (NAP 4).

4. Morbidity and mortality meetings

These departmental meetings are an opportunity for clinicians to examine undesirable patient outcomes. If necessary, changes to service provision or systems of care can be made. They are an obligatory part of governance.

5. Executive safety walkrounds

The Institute for Healthcare Improvement (IHI) in the United States developed the concept of Patient Safety Executive Walkrounds during which a ward or clinical area is visited by a member of the executive team to discuss patient safety issues. The aim is to ensure that staff have an opportunity to raise their concerns, board members get first hand accounts of day-to-day problems in care delivery, and together they look for solutions. This can ensure that support and resources are directed appropriately. This concept formed part of the leadership intervention of the Patient Safety First Campaign in England and is a highly inclusive approach to identifying risks to patients and ensuring that they are addressed promptly.

6. Proactive risk assessment

Not all risk identification should be reactive. Proactive risk identification can help to identify potential problems before they occur. This may, for example, involve a group of experienced staff examining a new patient treatment protocol before its implementation, or the planned layout of a new theatre complex in order to identify areas of concern using their own experience.

The NPSA alert 20 from March 2007 on high-risk injectable medicines required a proactive approach and examined specific drugs with greater than usual potential for harm. A risk assessment matrix (Box 3.2) was circulated to assist healthcare organizations in identifying high-risk medications. All drugs in a particular clinical area, e.g. theatres, are risk-scored, risk reduction methods identified, and the risk re-calculated. Risk reduction strategies are mandatory for any drug being given a red score, for instance i.v. adrenaline infusions which require

+ more than one vial of concentrated solution,
+ complex calculations,
+ a syringe driver, and
+ present a therapeutic risk if used incorrectly.

Risk reduction might, for instance, include training in syringe drivers or providing written protocols for drug preparation.

7. National reports and surveys

Several reports have been published in which national surveys of incidents are reported and analysed to reduce harm. The most important are the National Confidential Enquiry into Maternal and Child Health (CEMACH) and the National Confidential Enquiry into Patient Outcome and Death (NCEPOD). These reviews now form part

Box 3.2 Risk assessment matrix for injectable medicines.

	Risk factors for drug
1	Therapeutic risk
2	Use of a concentrate
3	Complex calculation
4	Complex method
5	Reconstitution of powder in a vial
6	Use of a part vial or ampoule, or use of more than one vial or ampoule
7	Use of a pump or syringe driver
8	Use of non-standard giving set/device required

Six or more risk factors = high-risk product (Red). Risk reduction strategies are required to minimize these risks.

Three to five risk factors = moderate-risk product (Amber). Risk reduction strategies are recommended.

One or two risk factors = lower-risk product (Green). Risk reduction strategies should be considered.

of the remit of the NPSA. The national confidential enquiries are unique in their ability to collate reports of harmful incidents from a large number of institutions and distribute the results across the NHS. They have widespread influence on systems of work and are a vital means of identifying major risks.

CEMACH

The National Confidential Enquiry into Maternal Deaths made its first report in 1952 and is the most prestigious and longest running clinical audit in the world and considered to be the 'gold standard' on which all subsequent confidential enquiries have been based. CEMACH began in 2003 and incorporates the confidential enquiry into maternal deaths into a combined review with perinatal deaths and one on child health. CEMACH collects a standard dataset of all maternal and perinatal deaths for study and produces annual trends in mortality and a comprehensive triennial report. This enables monitoring of rates and causes of death. Topics requiring further review are noted and acted upon, in time-limited 'task and finish' projects using audit methodology to identify risks. Recommendations for improvements in service provision, staffing levels, and clinical standards are generated.

National Confidential Enquiry into Patient Outcome and Death

The Confidential Enquiry into Perioperative Deaths (CEPOD), a joint venture between anaesthetists and surgeons, grew to cover all specialities as NCEPOD. NCEPOD reviews the management of patients, conducts research and confidential surveys, and publishes the results.

Studies and reports include

◆ 'Who Operates When?' (WOW) (1997 and 2003)

◆ 'Trauma: Who Cares?' (2007)

◆ Deaths after first time coronary artery bypass (2008)

By analysing information from a large number of Trusts and units, NCEPOD provides a valuable source of risk information. For example, the WOW reports prompted an increase in senior attendance during surgical procedures and also demonstrated that few Trusts were adequately staffed for out-of-hours work. This made clear the need for further action at the local level.

8. Patient safety alerts

◆ National Reporting and Learning System (NRLS)

The NPSA regularly circulates Patient Safety Alerts based on analysis of incidents reported via the NRLS. Over the last eight years, repeated patient safety incidents have led to alerts that have significantly altered everyday clinical practice. Several deaths were reported due to an inadvertent administration of high concentration potassium chloride (KCl). The resulting Safety Alert led to the current practice that all KCl ampoules are locked in the Controlled Drug cupboard, which has resulted in a dramatic reduction of incidents of this type. Examples of some recent patient safety alerts are shown in Box 3.3.

The NPSA also produces Rapid Response Reports (RRR) that have been developed as part of a strategy to enable NHS organizations to report their most serious incidents and ensure rapid spread of the information. In this way, common and serious problems can be identified, and if appropriate education, warnings, and examples of local solutions and good practice are cascaded via Chief Executives of Trusts to the relevant departments. Recent RRRs have included highlighting the dangers of opioid drugs and the risks associated with chest drain insertion.

◆ The NHS Central Alerting System (CAS)

CAS combined the CMO's Public Health Link and the Safety Alert Broadcasting System (SABS) into one system for easy access. CAS produces

• safety alerts,
• drug alerts,

Box 3.3 Recent patient safety alerts

2009	WHO safe surgery checklist	Introduction of checklists for all surgical procedures
2004	Crash Call	National number '2222' created
2002	Potassium chloride	Potassium chloride concentrated solutions to be kept in locked cupboards to prevent inadvertent use

- emergency alerts, and
- medical device alerts

on behalf of the NPSA, the MHRA, and the DoH. The CAS website also includes links to these organizations. These national reports and surveys enable lessons to be shared widely where previously they may have been isolated to the institution involved.

Risk identification is fundamental to improving quality and safety in healthcare. It should be both reactive and proactive and occur at every level in an organization from Board to ward so that effective systems and processes are put in place to minimize the risk of harm to patients.

Further reading

Vincent, C. (2001), *Clinical Risk Management – Enhancing Patient Safety*, 2nd ed. BMJ Books: London.

Organisation with a Memory, DoH (2000). http://www.dh.gov.uk/en/Publicationsandstatistics/Publications/PublicationsPolicyAndGuidance/DH_4065083.

Seven Steps to Patient Safety, NPSA (2004). http://www.nrls.npsa.nhs.uk/resources/collections/seven-steps-to-patient-safety/?entryid45=59787.

The National Patient Safety Agency. www.npsa.nhs.uk.

The Institute for Healthcare Improvement. www.ihi.org.

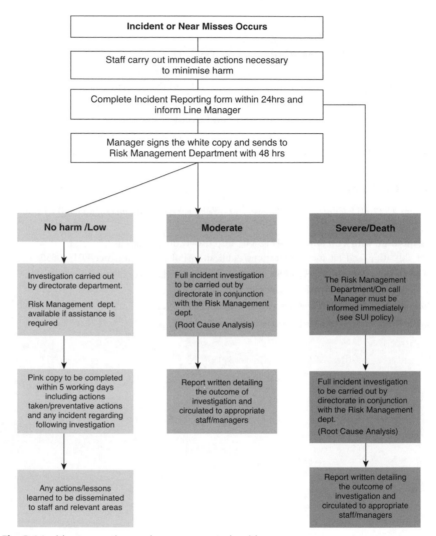

Fig. 3.1 Incident reporting and management algorithm.

Chapter 4

Risk assessment

Alison Lovatt and Mel Johnson

Key points

- Risk assessments are undertaken to estimate the consequences and likelihood of a particular risk being realized.
- They can aid and standardize complex decision-making processes.
- All risk assessment must be informed by evidence based practice and undertaken by appropriately trained staff.
- Effective risk assessment is a continuous process and must be repeated if circumstances alter or new risks are identified.
- Risk control strategies must be tested to ensure that actions prescribed have the desired outcomes.

Introduction

> An honest concern about quality, however genuine is not the same as methodical assessment based on reliable evidence.
>
> Maxwell R. (1984) Quality assessment in health
> *British Medical Journal* 288, 21470–2.

Assessing risk is something people all do instinctively; it aids daily decision-making (e.g. deciding when it's safe to cross the road or whether a house is affordable). Healthcare systems are very complex. This complexity brings risk and hence frameworks to aid in risk assessment are necessary as part of an effective risk management process. These processes help ensure that risks are properly assessed and actions taken lead to provision of the best and safest possible healthcare. To understand how truly integral risk assessment is in current healthcare practice, it is helpful to imagine working without it. Organizations need to ensure that services and facilities are safe and also understand their risk profile in relation to the local health economy, other providers, and the management of financial issues, e.g. the risk of losing a service such as elective orthopaedics to an independent provider could have significant organizational and financial impact on an acute trust. Clinical examples include: deciding who needs treatment most urgently in an accident and emergency department, or which patients in wards are most likely to fall or develop pressure ulcers.

Risk assessment in healthcare

Risk assessment exists at all levels of healthcare from guiding individual clinical decisions for an individual patient, e.g. difficult intubation up to Trust board making policy and strategy decision about service development. In various guises from simple to complex, risk assessments are used at all stages of the patient journey, for example

- Assisting decisions about priority and route of admission
- Helping to determine appropriate investigations and treatment
- Ensuring safe and effective discharge to another provider

Risk assessment is not a new concept, but following high-profile litigation cases and serious incidents, awareness of it at both organizational and systems levels within healthcare has increased dramatically recently. Risk assessment is a fundamental part of effective risk management of healthcare systems and is now integral to providing safe healthcare. In order to develop a formal structured approach to risk assessment, techniques and tools have been adapted from other industries and in particular from the Health and Safety executive. Many different risk assessment systems are in use and the approach will vary depending on the type and potential magnitude of the risk being assessed. Risk assessment is however necessary at all levels within healthcare by all professions and grades from those delivering direct patient care to those responsible for operational and financial decision making. Finally risk assessment is not a one-off process but rather a continuous one with constant reviews and updates.

The risk assessment process

Risk assessment can be both reactive and proactive.

- *Reactive assessment*: Carried out in response to a patient safety incident as part of the root cause analysis process to reduce the chance of re-occurrence, e.g. guidelines on how to perform a procedure such as chest drain insertion using ultrasound.

- *Proactive assessment*: Undertaken to prevent patient safety incidents by looking at pathways or systems of care to identify what could go wrong and what the consequences might be, e.g. a plan to send test results to patients by email rather than by post.

The NHSLA Clinical Negligence Scheme for Trusts (CNST) requires Trusts to carry out detailed organization-wide risk assessments against 50 criteria. This is aimed at ensuring that Trusts have a comprehensive record of all potential risks in key areas of practice, for example medicines management, clinical records, consent, trainee supervision, etc. The details of risk assessments are held centrally in a risk register (see Chapter 8) with details of actions required to control the risks and the person responsible for delivering the action plan with relevant timescales. Risks can be prioritized according to severity and should be regularly reviewed by the relevant departments, committees and managers to ensure that care is delivered as safely as possible within an appropriate environment by appropriately qualified staff.

Risk assessment can be undertaken for an individual patient, e.g. falls risk assessment, a clinical area such as ward, e.g. nurse led cardioversion or an entire hospital, e.g. risk of fire. The tool used in any particular instance will vary from very simple to more complex. Some examples are given in the following sections.

Assessing severity

Determining that a risk exists using the approach outlined in the previous chapter is just the first part of the process. There are tools and guidance available to help assess severity of risk too and determine the course of action or intervention to be taken. All healthcare organizations will have a Risk Management Strategy, which includes the details of the risk assessment processes to be used. A common framework used throughout the NHS for assessing risk balances the

♦ anticipated or actual consequences of the event, i.e. the severity and

♦ likelihood of the event happening again over a stated period or for a given activity.

Most organizations use a matrix to determine the severity. Although the details can vary across organizations, the most common type is a five by five matrix (see Fig. 4.1) showing consequence ranging from death (also termed catastrophic in some matrices) (5) to no harm (1) multiplied by likelihood of re-occurrence from certain (5) to rare (1).

By using the matrix to calculate the product of severity and likelihood, a risk rating is calculated. The colour coding in the matrix provides broad general categories of risk whereas the numbers allow risks to be ranked according to severity. The category of risk defines at what level within the organization the risk needs to be acknowledged, e.g. all red rated risks should be reviewed at Board level whereas yellow and green risks can be managed at departmental or divisional level. The risk rating determines how quickly action plans need to be developed and implemented. The risk assessment process will also aid in business and financial planning with the aim of ensuring that high rated risks get highest priority for investment and resources. As the action plan is implemented to control the risk the rating will fall and this is recorded in the risk register.

It is important to note that the risk rating may also be affected by

♦ the number of patients affected by a risk, e.g. a large number of patients may be affected by cervical screening failures,

♦ the possibility of major adverse publicity, e.g. an in-patient suicide, and

♦ the financial costs of a failure.

More sophisticated risk assessment processes have been designed and developed to identify where a potential error may occur in systems and processes as a whole rather than at constituent parts. Risk assessment techniques can be categorized as qualitative or quantitative. A detailed description of the various approaches is beyond the scope of this book but examples include the following:

Qualitative

♦ Structured 'what-if' technique (SWIFT) is a good technique for considering human and organizational factors within processes and procedures as well as equipment failure which may affect safety.

♦ Human error analysis (HEA) is a structured approach to identifying and assessing human errors originally developed in the aviation industry.

Death	= 5	5	10	15	20	25
Severe	= 4	4	8	12	16	20
Moderate	= 3	3	6	9	12	15
Low	= 2	2	4	6	8	10
No harm	= 1	1	2	3	4	5
Severity		Rare = 1	Unlikely = 2	Possible = 3	Likely = 4	Certain = 5
		Likelihood				

Description of the Likelihood Ratings

Likelihood Rating	Description
Certain	Will undoubtedly recur, possibly frequently
Likely	Will Probably but is not a persistent issue
Possible	May recur occasionally
Unlikely	Do not expect it to happen again but is possible
Rare	Can't believe that this will ever happen again

Description of the Severity Ratings

Severity	Description
Death	Any PSI that directly resulted in death
Severe	Any PSI that appears to have resulted in permanent harm
Moderate	Any PSI that resulted in a moderate increase in treatment and which caused significant but not permanent harm
Low	Any PSI that required extra observation or minor treatment and cause minimal harm
No Harm	Impact prevented - Any PSI that had the potential to cause harm but was prevented, resulting in no harm. Or Impact no prevented - Any PSI that ran to completion but no harm occurred

Fig. 4.1 5×5 Risk assessment matrix (Keele university/NPSA).
Based on Risk matrix in NPSA, *A risk matrix for risk managers*, 2008.

- Systematic human error reduction and prediction approach (SHERPA)is used to identify where errors occur in a process, e.g. drug administration and to suggest suitable design solutions to mitigate errors.
- Hazard and operability study (HAZOP) is a structured and systematic technique for identifying all possible deviations from the design intent using words such as 'more', 'less', 'no', and 'wrong' applied to attributes of a system. The HAZOP method is the basis for safety risk assessment approach used for 'Hospital at Night Solutions' (see www.npsa.nhs.uk).

- Failure modes and effects analysis (FMEA) is often used to detect weaknesses in automated safety systems and electronic systems. The *failure mode* refers to any flaw in a process or device that affects a patient (or an organization). The *effects analysis* refers to the examination of the outcome of such a failure. The system may be applied for instance to a new referral and diagnostic process for patients referred from primary to secondary care.

Quantitative

- Fault tree analysis uses a logic diagram approach to estimate the frequency of failures in complex systems by considering a combination of underlying faults or errors.
- Event tree analysis works in the opposite way and considers possible outcomes following an initial event and gives an estimate of the likelihood of each outcome. This is useful for analysing the consequences of failure, e.g. a monitor alarm does not work.
- Quantified risk assessment is a structured method used to quantify the level of risk. This is widely used in chemical and oil industries where there is a potential for major adverse events which may result in injuries, fatalities or environmental damage. Consequences and likelihood of each event are estimated using models.
- Cost benefit analysis is a formal discipline used to assess the case for a project or proposal.

The tools described above to facilitate risk assessment are generic and can be used in a variety of settings. It is important that within each organization there is a consistent approach to the risk assessment process so that different individuals carrying out risk assessments on the same problems will produce roughly the same rating although it is important to emphasize that there is a degree of subjectivity in the assessment process. This can be illustrated by the fact that different parts of a hospital may assign a different value to what may be the same apparent risk, e.g. the risk of patient falls in intensive care is likely to be lower than in a general ward since in the former, the patients are mostly confined to bed or mobilized only when supervised by a physiotherapist whereas in a general ward, patients will be mobilized independently in many cases.

In some circumstances, bespoke risk assessment tools can be developed and validated for specific risks. This is illustrated in the following case studies.

Case study: A risk assessment of bed safety rails

Bed rails were designed to prevent patients falling out of bed. However, a number of publications have highlighted the risks associated with their use including patient entrapment and this example demonstrates that risk assessment is a method of looking at all relevant risks and balancing these to arrive at a rational decision. The example is an individual nurse-to-patient risk assessment tool designed to aid nurses in deciding if the use of bed safety rails is appropriate. In this case, a risk rating may be arrived at after initial assessment and then reviewed after actions have been implemented to assess the new level of risk. This helps to ensure that the risk of a particular activity has not been increased by the intervention.

For example

◆ initial risk rating may be likely x moderate = Amber 15

◆ risk rating after implementing the tool and applying risk reduction measures unlikely x low = Green 4

The tool starts with an initial assessment of the patient's condition to decide if the patient is at risk of falling from the bed and if safety rails are required (see Fig. 4.2). If the answer is no, then no action is required outside of standard precautions, such as

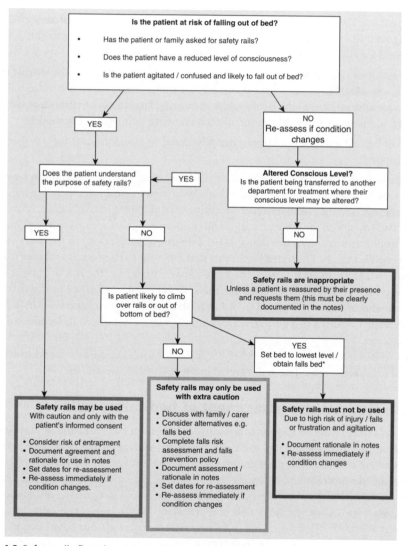

Fig 4.2 Safety rails flowchart: Assessment of immediate risk.
*A falls bed is an electric profiling bed that can be lowered to the floor to prevent injury should the patient fall out.

providing a call bell. If a risk of fall from the bed is identified, then the flowchart guides the nurse to decide on the best course of action depending on other risk factors such as agitation or altered consciousness. Even when a risk has been rated, the initial assessment may be subject to change, for example, if a patient's condition changes post-operatively. Over-reliance on risk assessment and severity rating following the suggested management plan can be dangerous unless regular prompts for review are built into the system. This is especially true when a risk is assessed immediately after a patient safety incident has occurred since the true consequence may not be immediately apparent. Over time, the assessment may change by either increasing or decreasing the severity and requiring adjustment of the associated intervention plan. The flowchart instructs the nurse to reassess the patient for possible changes to condition in several places. For this to be effective, it is not adequate to merely put the prompt into the tool. There also need to for prompts to be built into the patient care system reminding the nurses to revisit the assessment whenever necessary. For example, regular review, i.e. daily/weekly and a prompt that will remind staff of the need to reassess if the condition changes. This could be part of an integrated care pathway document (see Chapter 12).

Case study: Assessing risk in pregnancy as part of a pathway

In complex and potentially high-risk areas of care (e.g. pregnancy and childbirth) the assessment of risk has long been an established process. Pregnancy and childbirth is a normal physiological process, and the vast majority of pregnant women remain fit and healthy throughout. However, for some women, pregnancy induces risks, which may compromise their health or that of their unborn child. Certain factors are indicative of increased risk of maternal morbidity and mortality. A comprehensive risk assessment of a pregnant woman, which identifies such factors, is an essential part of a safe maternity service. Unfortunately, it is not possible to apply a simple one-dimensional risk assessment tool, but rather a series of assessments are built into various stages of the patient pathway. These rely on the knowledge base and judgement of the clinical staff making the assessment to determine the safest way to proceed following identification of any risk factors that must be managed appropriately.

Although the risk assessment in pregnancy is multi-factorial and complex, the principles remain the same as with any other in that the assessment identifies variations from normal parameters and suggests interventions for controlling or treating the risk. Clearly, in pregnancy, the risk assessment process is continuous throughout the ante-natal, delivery, and post-natal periods. Risk factors may change with the onset of particular complications, e.g. pre-eclampsia. The risk assessment tool should prompt awareness of parameters in a wide variety of areas.

- Existing status/social issues
- Existing medical conditions
- Previous pregnancy history
- Current pregnancy

Table 4.1 Risk assessment of social issues in a pregnant woman

Presenting factors that may raise alerts	Normal parameters (low risk)	Example of some associated risks	Potential interventions
Age < 19	Age 20–36	Pregnancy may be unplanned and young girl unsupported	Intense support from specialist midwife Consider referral to social services Consider child protection issues
Age > 37	Age 20–36	Increased risk: Foetal abnormalities Hypertension	Early tests and investigations (e.g. amniocentesis) May require consultant led care
Smoker	Non-smoker	Increased risk Sudden Infant Death Syndrome	Information to woman and referral to smoking cessation team
BMI > 35	BMI <35	Higher incidence of gestational diabetes	Unsuitable for midwife led care Birth needs to be in consultant led unit
Disclosed history of domestic violence	No history of domestic violence	Pregnancy increases incidence of violence. Higher incidence of miscarriage and stillbirth	Try to see woman alone Refer to woman's refuge if wanted Child protection issues

 ◆ Continuous factors
 ◆ Identification of deviation from normal parameters
 ◆ Provision of potential interventions to ameliorate risks

The assessment acts as a guide to the most appropriate investigations, interventions, and safest pathway of care at each stage from presentation to post-delivery, for example, whether the woman can remain under the care of a mid-wife or needs to be cared for by a consultant obstetrician, whether delivery can occur at home or if operative delivery will be required. One section of the risk assessment relating to social issues is demonstrated in Table 4.1.

Implementing successful risk assessment

The implementation plan must be based on best practice and any risk assessment tool used must be

 ◆ appropriate for the type and level of risk, e.g. quantitative or qualitative approach,
 ◆ thoroughly tested and validated, and
 ◆ monitored to ensure taking the designated action leads to the desired outcome.

The danger is that a tool that has not been thoroughly tested for effectiveness and reliability can give false assurance and in some cases can actually increase risk if actions taken on one part of the system have a detrimental effect on another part or on the system as a whole, e.g. changing the time of warfarin dosage to fit in with a junior doctor's shift patterns may cause problems if the laboratory cannot process the samples efficiently.

Underpinning safe and effective risk assessment is the level of knowledge and expertise necessary to apply any tools safely. The two tools illustrated are designed with specific professions in mind; they assume a level of understanding and skills commensurate with that particular professional group. It is unlikely that a general nurse would be able to apply the maternity tool effectively and visa versa. It is therefore necessary that the healthcare organization has structures in place to ensure that tools are used by the professional group they are designed for and that staff undergo relevant training and updates.

Summary

Risk assessment tools, which are fit for purpose, will lead to improved consistency in decision making and safer and more effective care. Risk assessment is relevant to clinical, organizational, and financial aspects of healthcare and should be a routine activity in any department or unit. Risk assessments allow organizations to understand their risk profile and develop treatment plans to reduce risk by prioritizing resources through effective business and financial planning. Risk assessment can be undertaken for individual patients, processes of care or whole departments using generic tools, or by developing more specific and bespoke tools for particular groups, e.g. pregnant women. The application of a systematic approach to risk assessment in an organization offers many advantages. It enhances safety by identifying what could go wrong and allowing appropriate controls to be put in place and may prevent future patient safety incidents by evaluating systems and processes and standardizing decision making.

Acknowledgements

Safety rails flow chart and Risk assessment of social issues in a pregnant woman table attributable to Calderdale and Huddersfield NHS Foundation Trust.

Further reading

Maxwell, R. (1984). Quality assessment in health. *British Medical Journal* **288**, 21470–21472.

Healthcare risk assessment made easy (March 2007). National Patient Safety Agency. Available at www.npsa.nhs.uk.

Risk assessment programme overview (November 2006). National Patient Safety Agency. Available at www.npsa.nhs.uk.

Chapter 5

Risk control options

Mary Lane

Key points

- Risk control, also known as risk treatment, is the cyclical process of selecting, implementing, and monitoring measures taken to modify risk.
- In healthcare, risks are an inevitable part of developing new treatments and therapies and the risk management infrastructure must support this by acknowledging that risks often cannot be eliminated completely.
- Risk control targets both elements of risk: reducing the probability of the risk occurring as well as limiting its impact on patients or organizations.
- Risk control measures can be considered to be any policies, activities, procedures, checks, and behaviours (human factors) that are used by organizations to contain risks.
- Any residual risk generated by risk treatment should be reviewed and monitored along with risk treatment.

Introduction

The aim of risk management is to ensure that effective controls are in place to mitigate identified risks. Previous chapters have identified the preliminary stages of the risk management process including risk awareness, identification, and assessment. Controlling risk is the next phase of ensuring delivery of safe high-quality care. Risk controls, also sometimes known as treatments, can take many forms depending on the location and nature of the risk.

The approach to risk control will vary depending on the level of risk of an activity. For example, where the potential outcome is catastrophic, e.g. incompatible blood transfusion, controls will be multiple and require strict implementation and continuous review to ensure they are functioning effectively.

Where the outcome is less catastrophic, e.g. wound infection, then the aim is to increase the reliability of the system as far as reasonably practicable for instance by ensuring that all patients are bathed before surgery. Failure in this case is undesirable but the outcome is unlikely to be catastrophic since there are other measures in place to reduce the likelihood of post-operative infection.

Risk control options

There are five commonly recognized options for risk control:

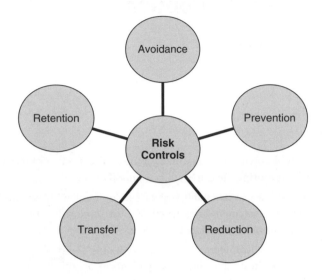

Fig. 5.1

1. **Risk avoidance**

Also known as risk removal, this involves:

◆ eliminating the risk by avoiding it or

◆ changing the conditions so that the risk will not arise.

Avoidance is the control measure used for risks that will have an unacceptably high negative impact and cannot be reduced to a suitable level, or where the potential benefits are not enough to justify the risk. Avoiding the risk therefore means making an informed decision to do things completely differently or not engage in the risk activity at all. This may not always be a practical solution as some risk is inevitable in most aspects of healthcare. For example, there may be circumstances where specialist institutions have to use different risk control options for risks they are capable of dealing with when compared to other institutions where the risk is best avoided, e.g. management of rare conditions such as cystic fibrosis is best undertaken in tertiary or quaternary specialist centres and the related risks will need to be controlled. Secondary centres will refer all patients with CF to tertiary centres and thus avoid the risks associated with managing these patients. The same may be applied within the same organization. As an example, many drugs come in multiple concentrations packaged in a similar way. Gentamicin, a potentially toxic aminoglycoside antibiotic, comes in at least four different formulations. It is easy to envisage the wrong strength being selected by someone in a hurry or under stress. The resulting overdose could result in nephrotoxicity amongst other side effects. A simple solution is to stock only one strength so that all staff become familiar with just a single formulation and the risk of mis-selection is effectively avoided. This, however, may not be appropriate in a paediatric intensive care unit and alternative control measures, such as reducing the risk with double checking, will need to be put in place in that area.

2. **Risk prevention**

This option can be used for both elements of risk.

- To prevent the risk from occurring or
- To prevent any negative impact from the risk should it occur.

Prevention is a risk control treatment that puts in place measures (such as procedures, policies, activities and checks) to stop the risk being realized and/or prevent any negative impact arising when the risk occurs.

In this case, an example might be having a policy, which requires staff to carry out pregnancy tests on all women of childbearing age prior to any procedure that involves a significant dose of radiation. In this way, potential risk of harm to a developing foetus is prevented. Clearly, there are circumstances when it is necessary to proceed with an investigation in a pregnant woman who has some concomitant disease or problem in which case a radio-opaque shield is placed over the pelvis to reduce the radiation dose.

3. **Risk reduction**

This is a common method of risk control in healthcare organizations and aims to target both elements of risk:

- reducing the likelihood of the risk being realized and
- reducing the impact or effects of risk ie mitigating the negative consequences

When considering risk reduction measures, the degree of desired risk reduction must be commensurate with the cost of such a reduction. This applies not only to the cost of a negative outcome for the patient and organization but also to the reduction in potential benefits as well. Any residual risk must then be acceptable to the organization or dealt with via another form of control such as a contingency plan. Examples of risk reduction control measures in healthcare include:

- policies,
- protocols,
- guidelines,
- provision of training,
- ensuring adequate supervision, and
- ongoing audit of services provided.

Carrying out surgery on the wrong side or limb is catastrophic for the patient concerned. Evidence indicates that such failures are often the result of human factors such as poor communication in teams. It is therefore vital to ensure that systems are in place to reduce this risk as far as possible. Most trusts will have a 'correct site surgery' policy in place, which requires staff to mark the surgical site pre-operatively whilst the patient is conscious and able to confirm the site. Following this there will be pre-procedure checks to ensure that the site is marked and the consent form corresponds appropriately as does as any imaging. The NPSA has recently issued an alert requiring all Trusts to introduce the 'WHO Safe Surgery Checklist' (NPSA, January 2009), which includes these checks. It requires a member of the theatre team after discussion with other team members to sign that all appropriate checks have been carried out to ensure they have the correct patient, undergoing the correct procedure on the correct side. Enhancing team working through training can help to ensure that more junior or inexperienced members of the team can speak up if they are uncertain about something or of they feel the checks have not been completed properly. Evidence suggests that simple processes like this can significantly reduce the risk of error.

4. Risk transfer

This involves transferring or sharing the risk and/or its impact with a third party. Unfortunately, it does not predictably reduce the likelihood or consequences of risk. The process of transferring the risk may indeed create further problems. The nature of the risk may be altered and actually result in increased risk to the patient. New risks may also develop related to the transfer process and these are often due to communication failures. This is not a common method of risk control in healthcare since the risk, with its potential negative impact, still exists, and the transferring organization will usually still retain a duty of care to the patient.

A clinical example of risk transfer might be programmes in which post-operative patients are planned for early discharge for care in the community. In this case, the risk of certain post-procedure complications are essentially transferred into the community, e.g. wound infections, DVT, etc. Whilst the hospital rates for infection or DVT may be reduced accordingly, the risk of readmission is increased and patient safety compromised unless the early discharge programme is adequately staffed and monitored. At the organizational level, insurance programmes such as the Clinical Negligence Scheme for Trusts hosted by the National Health Service Litigation Authority (see Chapter 8) is an example of transferring risk in relation to liability for the costs of medical negligence claims. In all cases when setting up risk control systems, it is vital to look at the balancing issues, i.e. what is the potential negative impact of altering the system at one point since this may well outweigh the benefits of the planned changes by introducing new risks elsewhere in the patient pathway.

5. Risk retention

This control option accepts the risk as is, both its impact and likelihood. It is not a common risk control method in naturally risk-averse healthcare organizations unless the potential benefits are deemed worthy or the likelihood and impact of the risk are extremely low. Ideally this method of risk control should be combined with risk reduction to ensure that the lowest possible residual risk or net risk is all that is retained. The decision to accept the risk should always be done in conjunction with a contingency plan to manage any consequences.

Neurological injury after cardiac surgery has multiple causes some of which are clearly defined while others are harder to identify. Whilst research has established that pre-operative screening may detect those at higher risk of this complication and certain surgical approaches such as off-pump techniques and epi-aortic scanning may reduce the likelihood of post-operative stroke, there will still be patients who unfortunately suffer some kind of neurological injury despite the implementation of best practice as far as it can be defined. The organization will have to retain the risk of neurological injury and ensure that appropriate contingencies are in place to manage the aftermath such as prompt access to a neurologist and rehabilitation programmes possibly using a neurological care pathway.

Innovation and development of new treatments and therapies is associated with new risks, some of which may not be defined until the new intervention has been introduced. To manage this type of risk, organizations need to develop systems for introduction of new interventional procedures (NIPS), which include:

♦ assessment of the research evidence used to support introduction of the NIP,

♦ ensuring all relevant staff have received relevant training,

♦ ensuring that detailed risk assessment of both patients and procedure have been undertaken,

♦ ensuring that during the consent process patients are aware that the procedure is novel and that some of the risks and long-term results may be unknown,

♦ ensuring that any safety incidents are reported and analysed,

♦ ensuring that the NIP is registered with NICE and any guidance they have issued is implemented, and

♦ ensuring a robust system of clinical audit to monitor progress.

If all the above are in place, then the organization may elect to tolerate the risks involved on the basis that the intended benefits outweigh the risks. Should any safety incidents occur these will prompt a review and changes to the programme initiated or it may even be halted if the risks cannot be adequately controlled, or unexpected risks appear.

Contingency plan

This is not strictly speaking a method of risk control but used as an adjunct to risk control measures in any risk treatment plan to deal with the consequences when a risk is realized. In healthcare organizations, it is important to appreciate that risks are present in all healthcare environments even when optimal controls are in place. As a result, patient safety may be compromised and harm can occur. In order to reduce the likelihood of significant harm occurring contingency planning is vital. Having a contingency plan to respond to complications when they arise is an essential part of successful risk management and has been demonstrated to be effective in many disciplines. The failed intubation drill is a contingency plan, which is implemented in the 'can't intubate, can't ventilate' scenario.

Evaluating risk control options

When evaluating potential risk control options, it is important to note their varying levels of effectiveness. The most effective measures are clearly risk avoidance and risk prevention but these are the most difficult to implement since healthcare involves human beings operating in a technologically advanced environment using complex equipment and drugs. Avoidance and prevention are often just not possible.

Least effective controls are risk retention and risk transfer since they are reliant on policies, procedures, and guidelines, which can be ignored or violated in various circumstances and hence the risk remains. In these situations, it is preferable to have a number of controls that work both in sequence and in parallel. For example, a number of patients who have an allergy to penicillin have died following prescription and administration of penicillin-like drugs. A sequence of controls can be put in place to reduce the risk of this happening:

+ Asking the patient on admission about allergies
+ Documenting allergies on the drug chart and how the allergy is manifest
+ Including the information on the identity wristband
+ Requiring nurses to double check intravenous antibiotics with another qualified practitioner and the patient before administration
+ In some hospitals, computerized prescribing has been shown to reduce prescribing errors by up to 70% since alerts can be put into the system to indicate that an inappropriate drug has been prescribed.

Selecting the appropriate control measures also requires an understanding of the risk culture or appetite within the organization. This can vary from risk averse to actively risk seeking. Healthcare organizations tend to be generally risk averse although individual organizations are likely to differ with regard the type and amount of risk tolerated in pursuit of their strategic goals. The expectation in risk-averse organizations that all risk will be avoided can be counterproductive and sometimes prevents implementation of appropriate risk control measures. Successful risk management:

+ recognizes that risks exist,
+ has a reliable method of assessing the level of risk,
+ uses appropriate control methods which take account of human factors,
+ checks the impact of controls on other parts of the system, and
+ regularly reviews the control methods employed.

The control measures selected should ultimately result in a balanced and proportionate response to identified risks. This helps to avoid overreacting to risks, thereby limiting development and initiative within the organization. The risk register, which is the central repository of risk information at organizational level, should include information on all controls and how they are monitored (see Chapter 6).

The risk treatment cycle

Risk control or risk treatment is generally the final step/part of any clinical risk management programme. Successful risk treatment is seldom restricted to implementing only one sort of risk control measure. Rather, it is a cyclical process that involves identifying all possible control options for the risks to be treated, evaluating and then selecting the appropriate control options, and ultimately preparing and putting into action a risk treatment plan. When combined with facilities for continuous monitoring and review, it allows for a successful risk management programme.

The risk control or treatment cycle involves seven steps:

1. identify all possible risk control options,

2. evaluate these risk control options,

3. select appropriate control option(s),

4. prepare a risk treatment plan,

5. implement risk treatment plan,

6. review residual risk,

7. monitor the risk treatment plan.

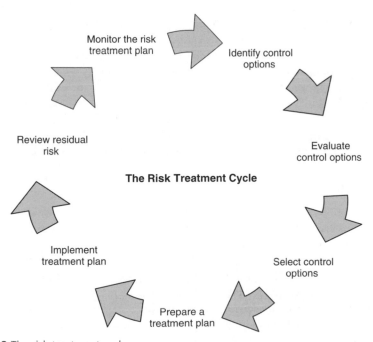

Fig. 5.2 The risk treatment cycle.

The risk treatment plan

The aims of any risk treatment plan are to:

◆ select suitable control options to effectively treat and manage risk, which must:
  • be implementable,
  • be subject to monitoring, and
  • not be associated with new or increased risk

◆ provide sustainable treatment options

◆ align with and meet organizational needs and risk management strategy

A risk treatment plan should include:

◆ details of the risks to be controlled,

◆ details of control options selected and how to implement them,

◆ details of resources needed for implementing controls – people, time, expenses,

◆ clarification of the lines of responsibility for implementation of control measures,

◆ a timetable for implementation, and

◆ review and monitoring details.

Before formulating a risk treatment plan, it is essential that there has been a thorough assessment and evaluation of the risks to be treated. This should also include the context and conditions in which the risk is likely to occur and any human factors elements, which are relevant such as hours of work, supervision of trainees, and communication issues such as handover. A careful assessment of existing risk control measures is also necessary to determine their adequacy and future validity. Consultation is a key feature in all aspects of risk management, especially when related to risk control and treatment. Engaging those who were involved in identifying and assessing risks as well as those who will implement risk control measures is essential. Where feasible those who are "end users" and affected by the risk, usually patients, should also be involved. For example, changes to out-patient services to solve throughput and flow problems must also be viewed from the patient perspective.

Summary

It is important that risk control is not applied in isolation but rather viewed as a part of an organization's global risk management strategy. Controlling risk in one area will invariably impact on risk in another area. Considering the potential interaction of risks and risk control measures is essential when developing a risk treatment plan. Controls entrenched within processes and activities are more likely to be successful than when applied as an added extra. It is vital to make risk control activities easy to comply with since this is the key to success. Making it easy to do the right thing and hard to do the wrong thing is fundamental in any risk control strategy. Any change must be closely monitored to ensure unforseen problems do not arise when changing the type or level of risk or transferring it elsewhere.

Further reading

Clinical Risk Management Guidelines for the Western Australian Health System. Information Series No. 8, http://www.health.wa.gov.au/safetyandquality.

JISC infoNet. Risk Management infoKit, http://www.jiscinfonet.ac.uk/InfoKits/risk-management.

Further reading

Chapter 6

Risk assurance

Elizabeth Haxby

Key points

- NHS Hospital Trusts are required to have in place systems of internal control which identify and control risks to an acceptable level.
- All identified risks: clinical, financial, and organizational should be assessed and recorded in a central repository called a risk register. Each division, directorate, or clinical area holds a local risk register which feeds into the main trust risk register.
- The risk register contains information on levels of risk, types of control, who is responsible, and time frames for action. New risks, which may be identified from a number of sources including internal issues, e.g. incidents and external reports, alerts, or requirements, must be entered onto the register in a systematic manner.
- The risk register informs the Board of the risk profile of the organization; the register should also inform decision making for business and financial planning so that investments in resources and services are directed at reducing risk and the Board can assure itself that risks are under control.

Risk management at organizational level

Trusts, through delegated responsibility from the chief executive, are required to have in place systems of internal control which identify and control risk to an acceptable level with a view to ensure the safety and well-being of staff, patients, and those affected by its operation. All National Health Service (NHS) staff members have a responsibility to ensure that, relevant to their seniority, all potential risks are identified and quantified through a process of risk assessment and systems, and processes developed to mitigate or control the risks. Implementation of control measures must be monitored and reviewed to ensure their continued effectiveness across the whole patient-pathway. Trusts monitor the effectiveness of internal control systems through the following range of indicators and assurances:

- An Assurance Framework and Risk Register provide a repository of all known risks and the effectiveness of their controls.
- Internal review to assess the robustness of the risk-management process is carried out by internal auditors as part of their annual audit plan.
- External review provides the Trust with assurance that its systems are working effectively, e.g. Care Quality Commission Inspections, National Health Service

Litigation Authority (NHSLA) risk-management standards, Audit Commission Auditors local evaluation.

Risk Management is an integral part of good general-management practice consisting of steps which when taken in sequence ensure sound decision-making and continual improvement in the quality of services provided. Every NHS Trust is required to have a Board approved strategy for managing risk which:

- clearly identifies the Trust objectives for managing risk,
- details the accountability arrangements, and
- details the main processes by which the objectives are to be achieved.

The strategy should also set out what is considered to be acceptable risk for the organization. Risk management is not about risk elimination, although risk reduction is clearly a key goal, but it is about encouraging appropriate risk taking, i.e. providing a framework within which risks are identified, assessed, controlled, and where appropriate accepted as tolerable. Only through appropriate risk taking will an organization be able to provide high-quality healthcare services and make progress towards the development of new and improved treatments and therapies. However inadequately managed risks have the potential:

- to prevent the Trust from achieving its objectives,
- to cause harm to those it cares for or employs,
- to incur losses relating to assets, finances, and
- to impact on good will, public confidence, and reputation.

Boards need to be confident through appropriate assurance processes that the systems, policies and people that they have put in place are operating in a way that is:

- effective,
- focused on key risks, and
- driving the delivery of objectives.

In order to achieve this the Board must regularly review the risk profile of the organization which is presented in the form of a risk register, and determine the level of assurance that should be available to it with regard to control of those risks. Since 2001/2002 all NHS Chief Executives have had to sign a Statement of Internal Control, which forms part of the statutory accounts and annual report. To provide this statement, Boards need to be able to demonstrate that they have been properly informed about the totality of their risks, not just financial, and have arrived at their conclusions with regards to the effective control of those risks based on all the evidence presented to them.

Risk management performance

A risk-management strategy is a fundamental part of a comprehensive assurance process which informs the Board; its efficacy can be measured through the following mechanisms:

- Statement of Internal Control,
- Assurance framework,

- Annual health check and healthcare standards,
- Auditors Local Evaluation,
- NHSLA Risk Management Standards,
- Performance reports to the Audit and Risk committee (subcommittee of the Board),
- Findings of external reviews and confidential enquiries,
- Monitoring patient-safety incidents, complaints, and claims,
- Monitoring non-clinical incidents and claims,
- Monitoring complaints and patient advice and liaison service (PALS) contacts,
- Monitoring the Risk register, and
- Health and Safety Executive workplace inspections.

Key indicators will be in place which are monitored and reported regularly for example numbers of serious untoward incidents, infection rates, mortality rates etc.

Statement of internal control

The chief executive must sign an annual statement of internal control which states whether an effective system of risk control is in place in the organization. To ensure such an effective system the Board is required to have in place:

- Clear objectives which provide the framework for all organizational activity,
- Risk-identification systems covering all risks,
- Robust controls in place for the management of risk, and
- Appropriate monitoring and review mechanisms which provide information (and assurance) to the board that the system of risk management is robust.

Integrated risk management links together clinical care (clinical governance), the environment of care, and financial resources and ensures the following:

- Risks are identified,
- Risks are assessed and quantified, and
- Controls are identified prioritized and implemented.

To be effective a committee structure is required, which can support the agenda and direct the development of risk management at all levels; this committee should be under the leadership of an executive director who will report to the Board. A culture of proactive risk ownership should be prevalent throughout the organization. An example of committee structure for large acute NHS Trust is shown in Fig. 6.2.

Assurance framework

The assurance framework provides a repository of all risks which threaten the attainment of the trust's aims and objectives and key controls to assure the board that risks are being managed appropriately. The framework will be regularly reviewed and consists of the following:

- The 'principal objectives' of the trust,
- The risks which threaten the achievement of the 'principal' objectives,

- The key controls applied to manage the risks,
- Assurances about the effectiveness of key controls, and
- Any assurance 'gaps'.

The assurance framework will include the most significant risks, i.e. high-level risks identified on the Trust risk register and together these will be regularly reviewed at Board level.

Risk registers

A risk register is a tool which enables a healthcare organization to understand its risk profile in relation to clinical, financial, operational, and reputational risks. According to the Risk Register Working Group at the Controls Assurance Support Unit (Keele University 2002) a risk register can be described as;

'A log of risks of all kinds that threaten an organisation's success in achieving its declared aims and objectives. It is a dynamic, living document which is populated through the organisation's risk assessment and evaluation process. This enables risk to be quantified and ranked. It provides a structure for collating information about risks that helps both in the analysis of risks and in decisions about whether or how those risks should be treated'.

A risk register comprises a number of components which are essential for tracking and monitoring how risks are being treated or controlled. The fundamental components of a risk register are shown in Table 6.1. These can be adapted to suit local practice and needs.

In the sample entry in the risk register shown in Table 6.2 (see end) the issue highlighted is blood sample mislabelling which is a ubiquitous problem in healthcare caused by human error resulting in a significant risk of delayed or even incorrect diagnosis. Each individual error on its own may only be a low-level error requiring repeat testing, but when aggregated the number of sampling and labelling errors may constitute a major risk for a healthcare organization affecting patients, operations (delays in treatment), and potentially the reputation of the Trust. To address this risk the Trust may decide to invest in electronically printed bar-coded wrist bands together with electronic requesting of samples to reduce risks. The initial investment may be in the order of several hundred thousand pounds to acquire all the relevant hardware, software, and staff training. This investment would have to be approved at the board level with a full review of the risk assessments including what new risks might be introduced by the system, e.g. how Information Technology (IT) failure would be managed and to what level the current risk rating would be reduced in the short and long term. The Board would also need to see detailed plans for implementation and how the progress would be monitored, as well as determining how it would be assured that the system was functioning as designed.

Sources of risk identification (see Chapter 3)

Risk identification must be both reactive and proactive and it should be a routine part of management activity across the organization, for example:

- Clinical risks can be identified from a variety of sources, e.g. incident reports, mortality reviews.

Table 6.1 Components of a risk register

Objectives	The link between strategic objectives and key risks for more major risks
Description of specific risk	This may be a simple phrase to describe the risk or a more detailed and complete description
Location	The department/place in the organization where this particular risk is an issue
Risk rating (likelihood × consequence)	Colour coding is used to group risks into general categories of risk and then within these categories risks may be ranked by number to allow more specific focus (see Chapter 4 Risk assessment) on significant risks
Lead individual/ department	Risk must be assigned to a lead individual or department who 'owns' the risk and is responsible for ensuring that the risk is monitored and mitigated or controlled
Existing controls	This describes what is currently in place to reduce the risk
Action/treatment plans	This describes what resources are required to mitigate the risk to an acceptable level. It may include a target risk-rating, achieving which is the overall aim. This risk level will be that which would be considered acceptable
Sources of assurance	How the organization will be assured that the controls/treatments in place are effective
Dates	The timeframes for implementation of any new controls and for review of the existing levels of risk
Cost-benefit analysis	To demonstrate that the controls are cost-effective. This may guide the approach taken if more than one solution is possible
Acceptance/Completion	Necessary to show which risks are still active or have been accepted at the current level or closed
Comments	For supplementary information such as relevant policies or dates of meetings at which a particular risk was discussed

- Financial risks may be identified through changes in funding or commissioning, or in relation to specific projects such as private finance initiatives or collaborations with other organizations or mergers.
- Operational risks may relate to staffing, provision of facilities, patient flows, or interruption / suspension of activities for refurbishment or building work.
- Reputational risks may relate to specific incidents or the publication of reviews by regulatory bodies such as the Care Quality Commission review.
- Risks to strategic objectives will also be included and these may relate to commissioning, development of new services, or specialist clinics.

Risk identification is both top-down, i.e. when the Board identifies risks to its strategic objectives, and bottom-up when the front-line staff identify key risks in relation to patient care, flows, and management. Trusts must have systems in place to ensure that risks are recognized, assessed and documented, and actively managed in a consistent way so that totally different risks can be compared in terms of severity.

Risk tolerability

The Trust, as part of its risk management strategy, will set out what levels of risk it is willing to accept relative to the perceived or potential benefit. The degree to which risks are considered acceptable may be specific relating to a particular issue, e.g. medication safety or generic considering the total level of risk an organization is prepared to tolerate at any one time. Each individual organization may decide what it considers to be an acceptable risk although this may vary depending on the type of risk. Most risk registers contain several hundred identified risks and clearly the Board cannot review all these risks on a regular basis. In general risks over a certain degree of severity, e.g. 15 or all those rated 'red' will be reviewed as a 'high level' in the risk register (forming part of the assurance framework) at every meeting until the Board is assured that reasonable levels of control, and risk reduction have been achieved. Low and very low-level risks (green and yellow) will be managed locally in divisions or directorates; however, if a high number of specific minor incidents is identified then the overall risk may be upgraded in terms of severity.

Managers are responsible for implementing and monitoring any identified control measures within their area of responsibility. In situations where risks are identified but local measures are inadequate managers must identify these risks through the committee structure. Regular reviews of identified risks are required to ensure compliance with control measures and to evaluate the degree of improvement. If significant financial investment or resources are required to manage the risk then these must be taken into account in deciding what is tolerable and what is reasonably practicable in terms of mitigating the risk. The Health and Safety Executive has proposed individual risk-criteria values specified as the risk of fatality per person per year and has said that an individual risk of death of 1 in 1,000,000 represents a very low level of risk and should

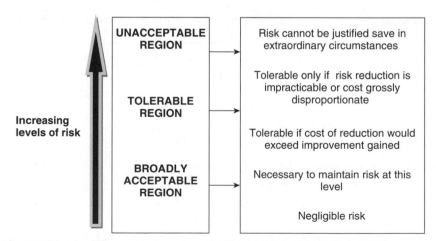

Fig. 6.1 Risk tolerability matrix (based on Health and Safety Tolerability of Risk Framework).

be used as a guidelines for the boundary between the broadly acceptable and tolerable regions (R2P2, HSE 2001).

Committee structure for managing risk within an NHS Trust

In order to ensure that risks are being monitored and controlled at an appropriate level each healthcare organization will have a series of committees and reporting structures in place. Ultimately the Board is kept informed of the risk profile of the organization and requires assurance that controls are effective, the Board will only review the more serious risks and may identify risks itself in relation to the overall organizational strategy. The names and functions of each committee will vary according to each organization but in general at the lowest level the committees are specific to a particular activity, e.g. blood transfusion, medicines management, clinical records etc. These groups will report regularly, although only annually in some cases, to committees with a broader remit for example a clinical effectiveness committee or risk committee which have responsibility for monitoring and directing activity across the organization and report up to subcommittees of the Board which are chaired by executives or non-executive directors such as the Audit and Risk Committee or Governance and Quality Committee. Ultimately the Board is provided with summary reports of the activities of the subcommittees and monthly performance reports of key indicators such as mortality, infection rates, compliance with national targets, e.g. 18-week wait etc. When working effectively this system should ensure that risks are dealt with at an appropriate level and the Board has assurance that risks are managed effectively. A sample committee structure is shown in the diagram.

The list of committees included is not exhaustive but illustrates the general idea of how risk-management systems and reporting might look in a secondary-care organization.

Summary

Effective risk management is fundamental to all healthcare organizations and systems and structures need to be in place to support a systematic approach to the control of all identified risks whether these are strategic, organizational, or at individual patient level. The Risk Register is the repository of all information about identified risks and the relevant controls and this should be reviewed regularly by an appropriate committee with the Board reviewing all high-rated risks and any others which threaten the organization's principal objectives. An assurance framework must be established to ensure that the Board can be confident that key risks have been identified and controlled to tolerable levels. Where risks are not adequately controlled the Board will be required to make decisions regarding allocation of resources to address the issue or acknowledge that the level of risk is acceptable at the current time.

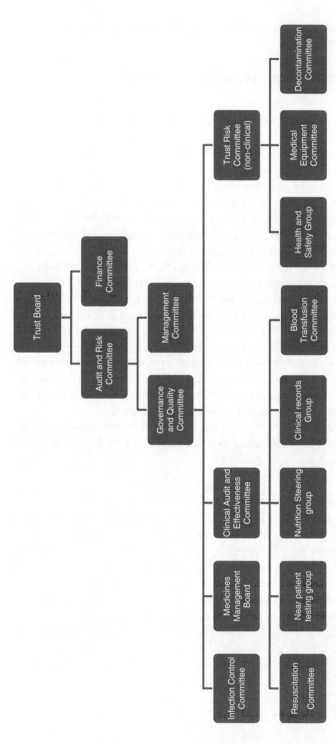

Fig. 6.2 Risk management committee structure.

Further reading

Tolley (2004). *Managing Risk in Healthcare: Law and Practice*, Vanessa L Mayatt (ed.), 2nd edition. LexisNexis, UK: Croydon.

Roberts, G. (2002). *Risk Management in Healthcare*, 2nd edition. Witherby & Co: London.

Table 6.2 Sample entry on a risk register

Objective	Specific risk	Location	Existing controls	Risk rating	Actions	Responsible individuals	Timescale	Costs	Target risk rating	Assurance
Improve patient safety	Sample mislabelling leading to diagnostic or treatment errors	Whole organization	Staff training Patient ID policy Phlebotomy service Incident reporting & review Laboratory sample checks	Amber 16	Highlight at induction Regular training updates Patient information Implement bar-coded wrist bands and electronic requesting	Director operations	On-going complete by October 2009	£750,000 for hardware, software, IT upgrades, £500 for patient leaflets, £10,000 for external trainers	Green 1	Monthly audits of rejected samples

Chapter 7

Complaints and claims

Ruth Symons

Key points

- Complaints and claims in the NHS are managed in accordance with national guidance and legislation.
- Analysis of complaints and claims data, together with patient-safety incidents, can provide a valuable source of learning and opportunity for risk identification particularly in relation to patient safety.
- From April 2009, if a complainant expresses the desire to make a claim as well, the complaints system will not automatically come to a halt as it has in the past. However, if a complaint is received after legal action has commenced, the NHS body is permitted to determine whether or not progressing with the complaint might prejudice the legal action.
- Complaints and claims management systems and processes should be audited to improve services.

The NHS complaints system

The basis of the current NHS complaints procedure was set out in April 1996 following the report of a review covering public sector bodies. It was set up as a three-stage system, which is:

- local resolution,
- independent review by the Healthcare Commission, and
- appeal to the Ombudsman.

In the White Paper *Our health, our care, our say* (Jan 2006) the Government had made a commitment to implement a single, comprehensive complaints process, across health and social care. This was launched on 1 April 2009 under the title *Making Experiences Count*, which supports the emphasis now being placed on learning from what has gone wrong. It is now a two-stage system in which complaints not resolved locally may be referred directly to the Health Service Ombudsman, so removing the intermediate independent review.

The new process includes:

- a greater emphasis on the prompt resolution of straightforward cases by managers and commissioners, with greater use of mediation to resolve complex cases locally,

- increased flexibility to allow complainants and NHS and social care organizations to agree on the timescale and approach to resolving a case,
- complainants can complain directly to the commissioner Primary Care Trust (PCT) or local authority (Adult Social Services) rather than to the provider of the service, and
- a complainant who is unhappy with the way their case has been handled can request the Health Service Ombudsman to review their case.

Around 140,000 complaints are made to the NHS annually. In 2007–08 approximately 9,000 complaints went to the Healthcare Commission for independent review, and more than 600 reports were issued by the Health Service Ombudsman related to the NHS in England, around half of which were fully or partly upheld. A complaint about any aspect of treatment or care can be brought by a patient or by someone else affected. A complaint must be submitted within 12 months of an incident happening or of becoming aware of the matter complained about. The patient advice and liaison service (PALS) will often be able to resolve patients' concerns on the spot in an informal way, or provide details of how to make a formal complaint.

Written complaints to an NHS body must be acknowledged within three working days, together with an offer to discuss the matter. A response should be made within six months. Agreement must be reached on how to get the most satisfactory outcome and this will depend on what the complainant is looking for. The new complaints procedure requires each body to have a 'responsible person' to ensure that a procedure is in place and that action is taken if necessary as a consequence of the complaint. This will usually be the Chief Executive, although the role can be delegated.

In addition, all organizations are to produce an Annual Report detailing the following:

- number of complaints received,
- the issues raised,
- how many were upheld, and
- where action has been or is to be taken.

The complaints manager within the organization will usually coordinate and administer the process and ensure that relevant information is fed into the clinical governance structure. The Care Quality Commission requires registered providers of services to prove that they investigate complaints effectively and learn from them.

Medical staff should understand the complaints process and know how it is managed wherever they work. All trusts will have a policy on complaints, setting out the system for complaints management including the responsibilities of staff to provide information and, in order to ensure that the issues raised by complainants are acted upon, many trusts will have a Complaints Working Group or similar committee as part of the Clinical Governance structure which will review the issues raised through the complaints systems and ensure that action plans are implemented and monitored.

Clinical negligence claims in the NHS

NHS Litigation Authority

In 1995 the NHS Litigation Authority (NHSLA) was established as a Special Health Authority to manage clinical negligence claims on behalf of NHS trusts in England. Its remit is to ensure that claims against the NHS are handled fairly and consistently, with due regard to the interests of the NHS and its patients. This centralized system means that expertise can be developed and lessons learned at a national level through compliance with the NHSLA's risk-management standards which provide a framework within which trusts can reduce the likelihood of further patient-safety incidents and consequential claims (see Chapter 8).

Clinical Negligence Scheme for Trusts (CNST)

The CNST, administered by the NHSLA, is a voluntary membership scheme which provides indemnity to member trusts and their employees in respect of clinical negligence claims arising from events which occurred on or after 1 April 1995. It is funded by member trusts on a 'pay-as-you-go' basis, through contributions calculated actuarially each year according to the risk profile and past claims history of the trust.

NHS employers are vicariously liable for negligent acts of their employees where these occur in the course of the NHS employment, so the Trust is the defendant and not an individual clinician. This also reflects the fact that many incidents are the result of systemic failure rather than the action of a single person. The medical defence organizations (MDOs) provide indemnity in respect of private practice and independent GP and dental practice.Currently all NHS trusts, Foundation trusts, and Primary Care Trusts in England belong to CNST and the DH is consulting on a proposal to expand the scheme to cover the liabilities of private companies providing clinical services to the NHS.

Negligence law

Negligence is a tort, i.e. a civil wrong, for which the remedy is compensation, and the standard of proof is a 'balance of probabilities'. This contrasts with criminal law which is intended to deal with offences against society; a person found guilty will be punished, and the standard of proof is 'beyond reasonable doubt'.

Criminal charges in healthcare are rare, and if brought will usually relate to a patient death. Once breach of duty has been established as causing the death, the jury must consider whether that breach should be characterized as gross negligence and therefore a crime. The test is 'whether, having regard to the risk of death involved, the conduct of the defendant was so bad in all the circumstances as to amount in their judgment to a criminal act or omission'. (*Adomako*). Less than 5% of negligence claims get to court, but those that do will begin in the County Court and criminal claims in the Magistrates' Court followed by the Crown Court, with either proceeding if applicable to the Court of Appeal and, ultimately, House of Lords.

Clinical negligence

The doctor – or other healthcare professional – has a duty of care towards the patient. However:

- That duty will be breached if the care or treatment provided by the doctor falls below the standard supported by a 'responsible body of clinical opinion' (the *Bolam* test) subject to logical analysis (*Bolitho*). Both sides may obtain reports from one or more experts, whose evidence will be based on medical literature and other indicators of what was accepted practice at the time of the event as well as relevant trust policies and protocols. Clinical records constitute the main source of evidence for what actually happened and the reasons for the action taken. Witness statements from those involved are certainly important, but if the claim relates to an event which occurred years before, it may be difficult to recall the details or even identify the people involved. It is for the claimant to show that an acceptable standard was not reached, with the court ultimately deciding whether the care provided was 'demonstrably reasonable' (*Bolitho*).

- The patient must have suffered injury which, on the balance of probabilities, was caused or materially contributed to by the breach of duty. This is often difficult to establish because the patient will usually have been suffering from some underlying illness. For example, substandard care may be shown to have resulted in a failure to diagnose a malignant tumour; however, if it can also be shown that any treatment would probably have been ineffective, and that the life of the patient was therefore not shortened as a consequence of this failure, then there will be no legal finding of liability. Again, expert reports and clinical records are fundamental to this stage of the process. A well-documented informed consent process can also be crucial; if it is evident that the patient was made aware, before undergoing surgery, that a loss of sensation is a recognized risk of the procedure, it will be more difficult to sustain an allegation of negligence if such an eventuality should occur.

Limitation period

A claim must normally be made within three years from the date of injury or the realization that an injury has been suffered which might have been related to treatment. The three-year period begins on the 18th birthday of someone injured as a child, and if the patient has a mental disorder within the meaning of the Mental Health Act 1983 there is effectively no limitation period until the patient ceases to be under a disability. A court may also decide to extend the limitation period.

Damages payments

The purpose of compensation in the law of negligence is to put the claimant – as far as is financially possible – into the position they would have been in had the injury not occurred. There are two elements to an award of damages:

- The first recognizes the 'pain, suffering and loss of amenity' caused by the injury, and varies from about £1,000–£2,000 for scarring following removal of a wart, through about £100,000 for infertility following unnecessary hysterectomy to about £250,000 for severe brain damage following anaesthetic error.

◆ The remainder of any award is wholly related to the financial losses and extra expenses caused by the injury, which is why figures cannot reliably be given for 'average' claims.

Currently fewer than 4% of the cases handled by the NHSLA go to court, and this figure includes those where the settlement involves a minor and thus requires court approval. About 1% of claims result in a contested trial. Most claims are settled by negotiation or mediation, and more than 40% of all clinical negligence claims brought over the past ten years were abandoned by the claimant. In 2007–08 the average time taken by the NHSLA to settle a CNST claim was 1.5 years from the date of notification.

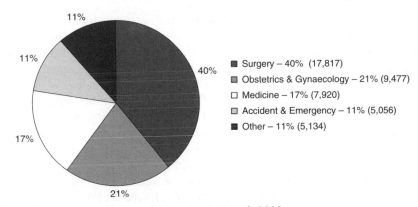

Fig 7.1 Total number of CNST claims as at 31 March 2008.
Reproduced from NHS Litigation Authority website (www.nhsla.com), with permission

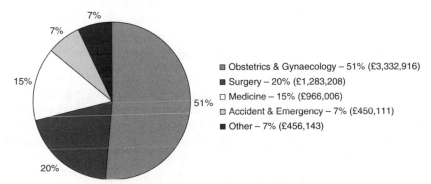

Fig 7.2 Total value of CNST claims as at 31 March 2008.
Reproduced from NHS Litigation Authority website (www.nhsla.com), with permission.

Damages and legal costs paid in respect of CNST claims closed in year

	No. of claims	Damages (£)	Defence costs (£)	Claimant costs (£)	Total costs (£)	Defence costs as % of damages	Claimant costs as % of damages
2003/04	6,259	140,222,642	29,296,621	40,876,343	70,172,964	20.89%	29.15%
2004/05	7,143	217,214,198	40,487,095	60,963,090	101,450,185	18.64%	28.07%
2005/06	6,261	245,844,124	39,391,251	69,757,289	109,148,540	16.02%	28.37%
2006/07	6,190	212,112,955	38,424,399	68,577,423	107,001,822	18.12%	32.33%
2007/08	6,212	264,943,382	43,309,237	90,729,857	134,039,094	16.35%	34.24%

Coroners' inquests

It is more likely that staff will be required to attend an inquest than a trial. An inquest is an investigation by the Coroner into a violent, unnatural or sudden death where the cause is unknown, to determine how, i.e. 'by what means', when and where the individual died. Although less formal than other legal proceedings, an inquest involves witness statements, cross-examination possibly by legal representatives of the interested parties, and on occasion a jury. The Coroner issues a verdict which, in cases involving medical care, is likely to be 'natural causes' or 'accident/misadventure', possibly qualified by 'neglect'. The Coroner must not make a decision as to civil or criminal liability, and if during the course of proceedings it appears that a criminal offence might have been committed, the inquest will be immediately adjourned.

A recent amendment to Rule 43 of the Coroners Rules 1984 (Amendment Rules 2008) increased the power of Coroners to ensure that lessons are learnt in light of evidence given at Inquests and that any such lessons are disseminated nationally. This places a statutory duty on healthcare organizations to respond to a report from a Coroner 'to prevent further deaths' and any such report will be put into the public arena. Prompt reporting and investigation at the time of an incident, together with evidence of any changes made or planned as a result, helps to show that the organization has taken steps to learn from what happened and seek to ensure that it does not recur.

Why patients make complaints and claims

People's expectations of healthcare have increased in recent years, so there is now greater likelihood than previously that these expectations will not be met, and a sense of unfairness or injustice may result. While many claims are undoubtedly brought for financial reasons, it has been accepted that a large number of complaints and claims arise from dissatisfaction at the way in which a patient-safety incident was handled, primarily:

- failure to acknowledge an error and say sorry where necessary;
- failure to provide an explanation; and
- desire to see that lessons have been learned and standards improved.

This is borne out by the fact that 'Complaints handling' was itself top of the list of issues raised in NHS complaints between Oct 2007 and Sept 2008 (*Healthcare Commission*). Two of the remaining top five: 'Treatment – delay, incorrect, unsuccessful'; and 'Diagnosis – delay, failure to diagnose, misdiagnosis' are also the two most common causes of clinical negligence claims (*NHSLA*). There is clearly a correlation between the causes of complaints and claims, and analysis at local level should consider the possibility that a claim has arisen because the original incident and/or complaint was dealt with poorly at the time. In addition to any damages and costs that arise from a legitimate claim, much time and money is spent on dealing with complaints and claims which could have been avoided.

To add emphasis to this, the NHS Constitution (2009) now sets out how patients:

◆ have a right to be treated with respect,
◆ have six specific rights related to complaints and claims.

The constitution includes three pledges that NHS staff must make:

◆ acknowledge mistakes when they happen,
◆ apologise, explain what went wrong, and
◆ put things right quickly and effectively.

What this means for the clinician

Apologise – If something goes wrong, staff should apologise, sympathize with the patient and relatives and express sorrow or regret at the outcome. This can be done without implying fault or blame. Staff prepare for such an eventuality by planning in advance what they might say should the situation arise.

Explain – An explanation of what went wrong should be provided. This should be factual and not an opinion and staff should take care how they provide this information. If what is said is later shown to be incorrect or misleading, this could cause difficulties in future litigation and will also prove upsetting and unhelpful to the patient.

Report – Any patient safety incident should be reported promptly. Early investigation will enable an appropriate explanation to be given to the patient and save time if a claim is subsequently brought.

Record – It is essential to keep thorough and accurate notes; the outcome of a claim (or Coroner's inquest) may well depend on the quality of the records. The following must always be included:

◆ signature, date and time (all legible),
◆ reasons for any decision to act or treat in one particular way especially if unusual or contrary to guidelines,
◆ review of a patient when no action is taken,
◆ matters relating to consent, and
◆ anything of particular concern to the staff or the patient.

Claims are often brought many years after an event, and it is very difficult to recall facts accurately. The patient will certainly remember the event, and should there be a disagreement as to the precise details the judge is likely to favour the patient in the absence of a written note. *'If it isn't written down, it didn't happen'!*

Ask – Being involved in a complaint or claim can be stressful, and despite strict time frames set out in national guidance, resolution can take a long time. Advice and support is available for all staff involved in a complaint or claim and appropriate use should be made of it.

All healthcare organizations will have policies on complaints and claims management as well as 'Being Open' (NPSA 2005) which set out the following:

- the processes for managing complaints and claims,
- advice on how to draft statements,
- who the key contacts are for advice and assistance, and
- how to approach a meeting with a patient or relatives who have raised concerns about their care management.

There should also be a policy on supporting staff involved in an incident, complaint, or claim. The Trust will regularly report on complaints and claims to the Board both in terms of numbers and outcomes as well as any 'high profile' cases which have the potential to cause reputational damage, and similar reports are also to be submitted annually to the Care Quality Commission and Monitor in the case of foundation Trusts.

Summary

It is important for doctors to understand the complaints system and the legal basis for clinical negligence claims even though for individual doctors personal involvement will be infrequent. Similarly attendance at a Coroner's inquest may only be required on a few occasions during a professional career . However it is very important that healthcare staff respond promptly when asked for information, engage fully in the process, and keep communication channels open with patients which facilitate the provision of open and honest explanation when things have not gone as planned. Hospital Trusts also have an obligation to provide support for staff who are the subject of complaints and claims to ensure they have access to appropriate advice and assistance.

Further reading

www.dh.gov.uk
www.ombudsman.org.uk
www.nhsla.com

Chapter 8

Risk management standards

Gaynor Pickavance

Key points

- The primary function of the NHS Litigation Authority (NHSLA) is the management of clinical negligence and non-clinical liability claims made against NHS organizations in England.
- Promotion of good risk management is integral to the remit of the NHSLA which sets standards, and assesses healthcare organizations against them.
- There is a set of NHSLA Risk Management Standards covering each type of healthcare organization: acute, mental health and learning disability, ambulance, primary care trusts, and independent sector providers of NHS care with separate standards for maternity services.
- Organizations demonstrating compliance with the NHSLA Risk Management Standards receive a discount from contributions (premiums) to the NHSLA Risk Pooling Schemes for Trusts (RPST).
- Results from NHSLA assessments are used by other bodies including the Care Quality Commission (CQC), Health and Safety Executive (HSE), Monitor, NICE, and the NHS Security Management Service (NHS SMS).

Introduction

The NHSLA is a Special Health Authority, established in 1995 to administer the Clinical Negligence Scheme for Trusts (CNST) and provide a means for NHS organizations to fund the cost of clinical negligence claims. It also covers clinical claims arising from incidents occurring before 1995, known as the Existing Liabilities Scheme (ELS). In 1999 the Liabilities to Third Parties Scheme (LTPS) and Property Expenses Scheme (PES), together known as the Risk Pooling Schemes for Trusts (RPST), were established to fund the cost of legal liabilities to third parties and property losses. Through the schemes the NHSLA seeks to support effective management of claims and the implementation of risk-management procedures and policies aimed at minimizing risk across the NHS and Independent Sector Providers of NHS Care.

On behalf of the NHS the NHSLA is also responsible for:

- monitoring human rights case-law through the Human Rights Act Information Service,

- resolving disputes between Primary Care Trusts (PCT) and independent contractors, and

- coordinating the management of equal pay claims.

Claims data

The average time taken to resolve a claim under CNST, from notification of the claim to the NHSLA to the date when damages are agreed (or the claim is discontinued), in 2007–08 was one-and-half years. At the end of 2007–08, the NHSLA estimated that its total liabilities (the theoretical cost of paying all outstanding claims immediately, including those relating to incidents which have occurred but have not yet been reported) was £11.95 billion, most of which related to clinical negligence claims. Most of the claims managed by the NHSLA are resolved out of court through 'alternative dispute resolution' (ADR): an analysis of the status of all clinical claims handled by the NHSLA over the ten years to the end of the 2007–08 financial year is shown in the chart below.

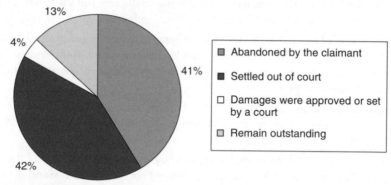

Fig. 8.1 Analysis of all clinical claims handled by the NHSLA over the past 10 years. Reproduced from NHS Litigation Authority website (www.nhsla.com), with permission.

NHSLA Risk Pooling Schemes

Membership of the schemes is voluntary and open to all NHS trusts, NHS foundation trusts, and PCTs in England. Funding is on a pay-as-you-go non-profit basis, and organizations receive a discount from their scheme contributions if they can demonstrate compliance with the relevant NHSLA Risk Management Standards. Actuaries appointed by the NHSLA analyse the available data and predict the total amount expected to be paid on behalf of members in respect of damages, costs, and other expenses in the ensuing financial year. This amount is then apportioned between the member organizations and the contributions reflect the risk-management status of the organization. Individual member contributions are based on a range of criteria including:

- Clinical activities,

- Type and total number of clinical staff,

- NHS income, and

- Property values.

Currently, legislation does not allow independent sector providers of NHS care to be members of the NHSLA schemes in their own right. However, where care is provided under specific Department of Health (DH) contracts, CNST cover is available via the membership of the referring PCT and contributions are collected from the PCT.

The standards and assessment process are designed to provide a structured framework within which to focus effective risk-management activities to deliver quality improvements in organizational governance, patient care, and the safety of patients, staff, contractors, volunteers, and visitors. The aim is to encourage and support organizations in proactive quality improvement and empower them to determine how to manage their own risks and thus reduce the number of patient-safety incidents and subsequent claims. Demonstrating compliance with the standards provides assurance to the organization, other inspecting bodies, and stakeholders, including patients and staff that effective clinical governance is in place.

The NHSLA consults widely on the development and ongoing maintenance of the risk management standards, a number of organizations, including Royal Colleges, professional bodies, national agencies, e.g. NICE, risk managers, and healthcare professionals have contributed to the current standards and assessment process.

The standards

Each set of standards contains five individual areas with ten equally weighted criteria, or risk areas, in each standard. Each risk area is addressed at the three progressive levels – policy, practice, performance – and organizations are only assessed against the requirements of the level being assessed. The structure of the standards is illustrated below in Table 8.1.

Each standard contains ten criteria which vary in some cases depending on the type of trust being assessed. As an example Standard 5 'Learning from Experience' contains the following criteria as shown in Table 8.2 which are assessed at each level (vide infra).

Table 8.1 Structure of standards

Standards (5 in each set of standards)				
Risk Areas– General Standards	Governance	Competent & capable workforce	Safe environment	Clinical care	Learning from experience
Risk Areas– Maternity Standards	Organization	Clinical care	High risk conditions	Communication	Postnatal and newborn care

Table 8.2 Criteria for standard of learning from experience

Criterion	Standard 5 (Learning from Experience)
1	Clinical audit
2	Incident reporting
3	Concerns and complaints
4	Claims
5	Investigations
6	Analysis
7	Improvement
8	Best practice (NICE)
9	Best practice (National Confidential Enquiries)
10	Being open

The full overview of risk areas covered by each criterion in all five standards can be accessed on the NHLSA website: www.nhsla.com.

Assessment process

◆ Discounts from CNST and RPST contributions are awarded on an increasing scale:
  • 10% for achieving Level 1,
  • 20% for achieving Level 2, and
  • 30% for achieving Level 3,
  (The same for maternity standard)
  A large acute trust can save more than £1 million on its contributions over two to three years by achieving Level 2 or Level 3.
◆ Organizations at Level 1 are assessed against the relevant standard(s) once every two years and those at Level 2 or Level 3 at least once in any three-year period. Organizations at Level 0 are assessed on an annual basis until they achieve Level 1. Organizations which fail an assessment and fall to a lower level are assessed at that lower level in the following financial year.

◆ Assessments are carried out on behalf of the NHSLA by a specialist team employed by an external contractor Det Norske Veritas (DNV) responsible for the administration of the risk-management programme. Annual informal visits provide support and guidance to organizations in relation to the standards and monitors progress against their assessment action plans.

The three levels are distinct, containing individual question sets and scored on a stand-alone basis. Lower level(s) are not reassessed as the organization progresses.

The progression of organizations through the three assessment levels follows the development, implementation, monitoring, and review of policies and procedures.

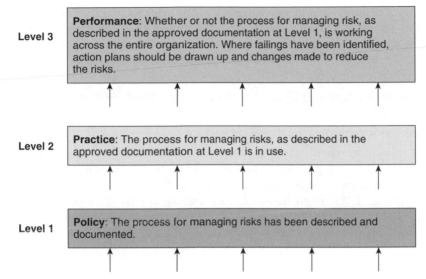

Fig. 8.2 Assessment Levels.

Level 1

A Level 1 assessment requires the organization to demonstrate the relevant documents, i.e. policies. This assessment is only concerned with the existence of the minimum requirements for each criterion within the documentation; the quality of the organization's documents will not be rigorously tested until the Level 2 assessment.

For example, in order to achieve compliance with Criterion 5.1 (Incident Reporting) the organization's approved document must contain all of the following requirements:

a. <u>duties,</u>

b. **process for reporting all incidents/near misses, involving staff, patients, and others,**

c. **process for reporting to external agencies,**

d. reference to the processes for staff to raise concerns, e.g. whistle blowing/open disclosure, and

e. process for <u>monitoring</u> compliance with all of the above.

The two minimum requirements in bold indicate those that are assessed in depth at the higher levels. The words underlined are hyperlinked to a clarification of terms section within the standards manual.

Level 2

A Level 2 assessment seeks to ensure that the organization's processes for managing risks, as described in the approved documentation, are in use and have been implemented. Organizations are required to provide evidence for a number of departments and/or staff groups and/or patient types, etc. The evidence may include risk assessments, records, e.g. training, incident reports, completed pro forma, evaluations, etc.

For example, to comply with the criterion on incident reporting at a Level 2 assessment, an organization would need to demonstrate implementation of the following minimum requirements:

b. process for reporting all incidents/near misses, involving staff, patients and others,

c. process for reporting to external agencies.

Most incident reporting policies state that staff will report all incidents which are graded and that appropriate action has been/will be taken. Statutory reporting to external agencies is also required in some instances, e.g. those involving medical devices to the MHRA and Reporting of Injuries, Diseases and Dangerous Occurrences Regulations (RIDDOR) to the HSE. At a Level 2 assessment the assessor would expect to see the reporting of incidents internally as well as the reporting to external agencies.

Level 3

A Level 3 assessment requires the organization to monitor whether or not its processes for managing risk, as described in the approved documentation, are working across the entire organization. Where deficiencies have been identified, action plans should have been drawn up and changes made to reduce the risks. Monitoring is normally proactive – designed to highlight issues before an incident occurs – and should consider both positive and negative aspects of a process.

To demonstrate compliance at Level 3 an organization would show the audit and the actions that have been taken (where necessary) to improve incident reporting, along with minutes of meetings where actions were discussed.

To achieve compliance with the standards at each level, organizations are required to pass at least 40 of the 50 criteria overall, and no fewer than seven in each standard.

Evidence templates

Each organization undergoing assessment must complete the appropriate evidence template(s) for the type of organization and level being assessed. In addition to being a basis for submitting evidence in a structured way, the evidence templates:

◆ Are designed to allow organizations to conduct a self-assessment,

◆ Are used by assessors to record their scores and findings, and

◆ Enable the organization to prepare an action plan.

Risk management handbook and template documents

There is a Risk Management Standards Handbook to support all the NHSLA Risk Management Standards (except maternity, where the information is contained within the standards manual), which provides both a general reference guide and contains references to all the documents which have been used as basis for the standards. In addition a number of template documents designed to assist organizations in developing their own local policies, procedures, etc. have been created.

Working with other organizations

The NHSLA collaborates with other organizations concerned with healthcare standards and the safety of patients and staff. It is a full signatory to the Concordat between bodies inspecting, regulating, and auditing healthcare, which aims to ensure effective regulation while reducing the burden of inspection on organizations. The NHSLA standards and assessments reflect the principles of the Concordat. The NHSLA is also a signatory to the Charter on Patient Safety which is a commitment to working with other organizations to improve the safety of patient care.

Assessment results and links with other organizations

Results and findings from NHSLA assessments are used in a variety of ways by other bodies which include:

- Care Quality Commission,
- Health and Safety Executive,
- Monitor,
- NICE,
- NHS Security Management Service.

Conversely, elements of the NHSLA assessment take assurance from work undertaken by the Audit Commission, and results of the Postgraduate Medical Education Training board (PMETB) national survey of trainee doctors.

Value of the NHSLA Risk Management Standards

A direct relationship between the NHSLA risk-management programme and improvements in patient and staff safety cannot be demonstrated since a very small number of safety incidents result in a claim. This would require the impact of NHSLA activities to be distinguished from those of others, including the healthcare providers themselves. However, anecdotal evidence, suggests that the standards provide a framework within which to manage risk and act as an indicator that effective risk management and clinical governance practices are in place. In addition, there is evidence to demonstrate an overall rise in the levels achieved by organizations in the standards since they were introduced, indicating an improvement in risk management and safety. The table below depicts the levels of standards of risk management achieved by maternity services in the CNST maternity standards from their introduction in August 2003 through to March 2008, and shows an increase in the number of services which have achieved higher levels.

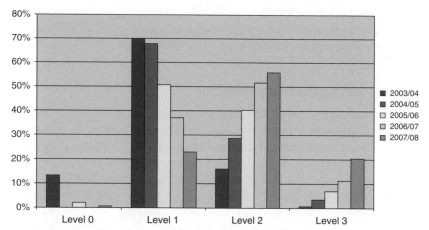

Fig. 8.3 Comparison of levels achieved in the CNST maternity standards.
Reproduced from NHS Litigation Authority website (www.nhsla.com), with permission.

Further reading

Further information about the NHSLA can be found at www.nhsla.com.

Section 2

Clinical effectiveness

Healthcare is increasingly complex and expensive. Clinicians can no longer treat patients in any way they see fit with the healthcare system picking up the bill. In this section, the drivers of effective healthcare are examined, from government and specialist society guidance on specific patients groups or conditions (*NICE and NSF's*) to how clinicians should evaluate scientific evidence presented to them as to the most effective treatments (*Evidence-based medicine*). Clinicians who wish to be at the cutting edge of medicine need guidance as to how a research project is run (*Research governance*) or how to introduce a novel procedure into practice (*New interventional procedures*). Finally, *Integrated care pathways* are a new patient-focused method of combining patient notes from all specialties, with guidance to carers as to how to manage a patient along the pathway, whilst flagging up deviations from the norm allowing appropriate and timely intervention if needed.

Chapter 9

Evidence-based medicine

Henry McQuay

Key points

- Published trials of efficacy relate to populations rather than individuals.
- Evidence-based medicine (EBM) involves applying population-based evidence appropriately to individual patients.
- Systematic reviews and large randomized controlled trials (RCTs) are the most reliable sources of evidence.
- Systematic reviews must include all relevant RCTs to be valid.
- Poorly randomized, or blinded, trials overestimate treatment effects.

Introduction

While testing the efficacy of medical interventions has happened for several thousand years, the high-quality trials, and the randomized and blinded controlled trials with which we are now familiar, date from the mid-twentieth century. The principle stimulus for the concerted effort to pull this evidence together was Archie Cochrane, who in 1972 wrote a book called 'Effectiveness and Efficiency', a collection of the best evidence available; it is his name which is used for the Cochrane Library. Subsequently, much of the development of the ideas and methods behind EBM came from McMaster University in the late 1980s and 1990s.

A definition of EBM is 'the conscientious, explicit and judicious use of current best evidence in making decisions about the care of individual patients'. The difficulty is ensuring that your patient does not differ from the population of patients that the evidence you are using is drawn from. That population may include people like your patient, or might be much healthier, or racially distinct, or different in other ways. The range of responses underlying that population estimate may be big, so an individual patient may not respond as well as the estimate implied, or indeed may respond better.

For example, codeine is the most commonly prescribed step 2 oral opioid, but 10% of people metabolize it poorly to morphine and so get little analgesia, and a smaller percentage of people are ultra-rapid metabolizers making proportionately more morphine. Clearly then, the population estimate of efficacy is incorrect for a significant percentage of individuals.

Systematic reviews and large randomized trials are generally considered to be the most reliable sources of evidence that we have; they are our best chance to determine what is true. Other study architectures, levels three to five in Table 9.1, are less robust as a basis for clinical decision-making.

Randomized controlled trials

A randomized controlled trial (RCT) is the most reliable way to estimate the effect of an intervention. The principle of randomization is simple. Patients in a randomized trial have the same probability of receiving any of the interventions being compared. Randomization abolishes selection bias because it prevents investigators influencing who has which intervention. Randomization also helps to ensure that other factors, such as age or sex distribution, are equivalent for the different treatment groups. Inadequate randomization, or inadequate concealment of randomization, lead to exaggeration of therapeutic effect.

Systematic reviews

A systematic review uses all the valid evidence available. To be systematic, qualitative, or quantitative, it needs to include all the relevant RCTs.

Problems in writing a systematic review include:

* Finding all relevant RCTs,

* Gaining access to original data,

* Assessing trial quality, and

* Assessing trial validity.

Table 9.1 Type and strength of efficacy evidence

Oxford CEBM levels of evidence (May 2001)	
Level	Therapy/Prevention, Aetiology/Harm
1a	SR (with homogeneity) of RCTs
1b	Individual RCT (with narrow CI)
1c	All or none
2a	SR (with homogeneity) of cohort studies
2b	Individual cohort study (including low quality RCT; e.g., <80% follow-up)
2c	"Outcomes" Research; Ecological studies
3a	SR (with homogeneity) of case-control studies
3b	Individual Case-Control Study
4	Case-series (and poor quality cohort and case-control studies)
5	Expert opinion without explicit critical appraisal, or based on physiology, bench research or "first principles"

Abbreviations: CEBM = centre for evidence-based medicine, SR = systematic review, RCT = randomized controlled trial, CI = confidence interval.

Commonly the number of eligible RCTs is unknown. The more comprehensive the searching, the more trials will be found, and subsequent conclusions will be stronger. The newer the intervention, the more sure reviewers can be of finding all relevant RCTs. Failure to find all relevant trials will lead to bias.

Retrieval bias can occur because trials are:

◆ still ongoing,

◆ completed but unpublished (= publication bias), and

◆ published but the search did not find them.

Registers of ongoing and completed trials can now be used to find data which has not yet been published.

Most systematic reviews use published trial results. Reviews where the individual patient data has been made available to the reviewer should produce more accurate efficacy estimates than those that only rely on the summary statistics from published papers.

Quality of trials

Having found all the reports of the trials relevant to the question posed, confirmation must be sought that they are of sufficient quality using a pre-agreed set scale. This is important as poor quality trials (non-randomized or non-blinded) overestimate treatment effects. Bias is the simplest explanation why poor quality reports give more positive conclusions than high quality reports (see Box 9.1). Thus, when faced with equal numbers of reports of trials for and against an intervention, the conclusion will be dependent upon the quality of the included trials.

A simple quality scale looks at measures of bias:

◆ Randomization (selection bias),

◆ Double blinding (rater bias), and

◆ Description of withdrawals.

The quality standards for inclusion in a review cannot be absolute because for some clinical questions no RCTs have been conducted. Thus, setting RCTs as a minimum absolute standard would be inappropriate for all reviews.

Validity of trials

A study may be both randomized and double-blinded, and describe withdrawals and dropouts in copious detail, so scoring well on this quality scale, and yet still be invalid. An example is a review published in the British Medical Journal in 2000, concluding that fewer patients would die after major surgery if they received regional plus general anaesthesia. The statistical significance which led the authors to this potentially important conclusion came from a number of small trials with 30% mortality rates, rates so high as to make one question the validity of the trials. A subsequent RCT published 2 years later in the Lancet rebutted the review's conclusion.

Judging validity is context dependent, but one simple thing to look for is whether there was enough of whatever it is that is being measured in the trial for any change to

Box 9.1 Some of the different kinds of bias

Selection bias:

Distortion of the evidence by the way the information is collected: e.g. the intervention only works in tall people. If you do not test it on short people then the evidence for the population as a whole (short and tall) is distorted.

Best defence = randomization.

Rater (or observer) bias:

Distortion of the evidence occurs by letting the person conducting the study know what treatment has been given.

Best defence = blinding.

Publication bias:

Distortion of the evidence occurs because studies with positive results are much more likely to be published than negative studies.

Best defence = difficult in an absolute sense – how do you know about unpublished studies? Also can one calculate how many negatives would need to be extant to overturn the positive evidence?

Duplication bias:

Distortion of the evidence occurs by publishing the same evidence multiple times (makes the evidence look better than it really is).

Best defence = review original data from papers to determine if same data used repeatedly.

Retrieval bias:

Distortion of the evidence takes place because your search did not find all the relevant trials (ongoing trial not yet published, published but missed by the search, and not published because of negative result [publication bias above]).

Best defence = searching of multiple databases, including trial registers and seeking advice from experts in field of study.

be measured reliably. An example from the pain world is trials where morphine was injected into the knee joint at arthroscopy, and the claim was made that the morphine produced analgesia. The problem is that we have no way of knowing whether or not the patients would have had any pain even if they had not been given the morphine. Thus, the trials are invalid because we do not know that the patients had enough pain before the morphine for any analgesic effect to be measurable.

Pooling of trials

It is often not possible, nor sensible, to combine (pool) data from different studies. A review which does not pool data is often called a qualitative, as opposed to a quantitative systematic review (in which data is pooled). Obstacles to pooling data include:

- Differing clinical outcomes, and
- Patients followed up for different lengths of time.

Where pooling is sensible, there are two 'does the therapy work' questions:

- How does the treatment compare with placebo?, and
- How does the treatment compare with other therapies?

What clinicians really need are the results of direct comparisons of the different interventions, i.e. 'head-to-head' comparisons. These are rarely available, as most comparisons are indirect comparisons about how well each of the interventions performs against placebo. This only tells us how fast each competitor runs against the clock, rather than who crosses the line first in a head-to-head challenge; making a judgment of one intervention against another more difficult.

Making decisions from systematic reviews

The four stages of examining a review are:

- L'Abbé plot,
- Statistical testing (odds ratio or relative risk),
- A clinical significance measure, such as number-needed-to-treat (NNT), and
- Safety evaluation, such as number-needed-to-harm (NNH).

When making decisions about whether or not a therapy works, a qualitative systematic review may look easy, count the successes and count the failures, but such simple vote counting may be misleading. This is because it ignores the sample size of the constituent studies, and the magnitude of the effect in the studies.

L'Abbé plot

A L'Abbé plot is a scatter plot of the data from trials included in the review, where the event rate in the experimental (intervention) group is plotted against the event rate in the control group, each point on the graph represents a single trial, the size of each point being proportional to the size of the trial. The plot is an aid to exploring the heterogeneity of effect estimates within the review.

Figure 9.1 contains data from a systematic review of single-dose paracetamol in acute pain.

Trials in which the experimental treatment (paracetamol) proves better than the control (placebo) (EER > CER) will be in the upper left of the plot, between the y-axis and the line of equality. Paracetamol was better than placebo in all the trials; although the plot does not say how much better. If paracetamol was no better than

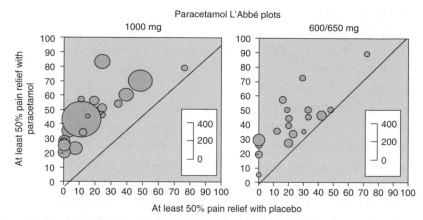

Fig. 9.1 L'Abbé plot.
The proportion of patients achieving at least 50% pain relief with paracetamol at two-dose levels (experimental event rate, [EER]) is plotted against the proportion of patients achieving at least 50% pain relief with placebo (control event rate, [CER]).

placebo then the point would fall on the line of equality (EER = CER), and if placebo was better than paracetamol then the point would be in the lower right of the plot, between the x-axis and the line of equality (EER < CER). Visual inspection gives a quick and easy indication of the level of agreement among trials as a check for heterogeneity, and gives a degree of confidence that apples are not being compared with oranges.

Statistical and clinical significance

When it is legitimate and feasible to combine data, accepted statistical tests to show that the intervention works significantly better than the comparator are:

♦ the odds ratio,

♦ relative risk (or benefit).

and, for how much better than the comparator:

♦ effect size, and

♦ number-needed-to-treat (NNT).

While odds ratios and relative risks can show that an intervention works compared with control, they are of limited help in telling clinicians how well the intervention works, i.e. the size of the effect or its clinical significance, for which we use effect size or number-needed-to-treat (NNT).

Effect size

An effect size is best explained using an example: if an alien being one day visited England, how many people would it need to see before realizing that, on average, men are taller than women? The answer relates to the effect size of the difference in average height between men and women. The larger the effect size, the easier it is to see that men are taller. If the height difference were small, then it would require knowing the heights of many men and women to notice that (on average) men are taller than women.

Effect size uses the standardized mean difference. The advantage of this is that it can be used to compare the efficacy of different interventions measured on continuous rather than dichotomous scales, and even using different outcome measures. The (major) disadvantage of effect size is that it is not intuitive for clinicians.

Number-needed-to-treat

The NNT is the number of people who have to be treated for one to achieve the specified level of benefit. NNT has the crucial advantage of applicability to clinical practice, and shows the effort required to achieve a particular therapeutic target.

Technically the NNT is the reciprocal of the absolute risk reduction, and is given by the equation:

$$NNT = \frac{1}{(IMP_{act} / TOT_{act}) - (IMP_{con} / TOT_{con})}$$

where:

IMP_{act} = number of patients given active treatment achieving the target.

TOT_{act} = total number of patients given the active treatment.

IMP_{con} = number of patients given a control treatment achieving the target.

TOT_{con} = total number of patients given the control treatment.

An NNT of 1 describes an event that occurs in every patient given the treatment but in no patient in a comparator group. This could be described as the 'perfect' result. However there are few circumstances in which a treatment is close to 100% effective and the control or placebo completely ineffective. Thus, NNTs of 2 or 3 often indicate an effective intervention. For some interventions an NNT of 1 is required, induction of anaesthesia being a good example. As much drug as is necessary is given to achieve the required result. It is important to remember that the NNT is always relative to the comparator, and applies to a particular clinical outcome. The duration of treatment necessary to achieve the target should also be specified.

For unwanted effects, NNT becomes the number-needed-to-harm (NNH) (see under Evaluating safety), which should be as large as possible.

The disadvantage of the NNT approach, apparent from the formula, is that it needs dichotomous data. In the induction of anaesthesia example, patients either went to sleep or they did not.

Figure 9.2 ranks the analgesics by their efficacy estimate; clinical choice might be to prescribe or take a safer although marginally less effective drug.

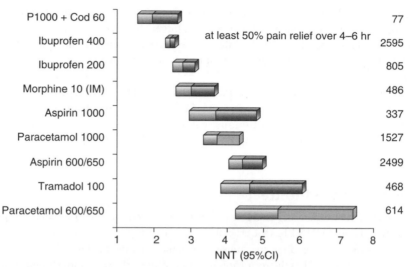

Fig. 9.2 Number Needed to Treat (NNT) for analgesics single dose postoperatively over 4 to 6 hours to achieve at least 50% of the maximum possible pain relief.
The point estimate for the NNT for each drug is the vertical line in the relevant rectangular box; the shaded areas to the left and right of those verticals are the 95% confidence intervals.
P1000 + Cod 60 = paracetamol 1000 mg plus codeine 60 mg. All dosing oral except 10 mg IM (intramuscular) morphine

Evaluating safety

Estimating the risk of harm is a critical part of clinical decision-making. Systematic reviews should report adverse events as well as efficacy, and consider the issue of rare but important adverse events. Large RCTs apart, most trials study limited patient numbers. New medicines may be launched after trials on as few as 1,500 patients, thereby missing rare but important adverse events. It is important to remember that mathematically if a particular serious event was not seen in 1,500 patients given the treatment, that only allows us to be 95% confident that the chance of it occurring is not greater than 3/1,500 = 1/500 (the rule of three).

Much the same rules apply to harm as to efficacy, but with some important differences, the rules of admissible evidence, and the NNH rather than the NNT. The absence of information on adverse effects in systematic reviews reduces their usefulness.

Rules of evidence

The gold standard of evidence for harm, as for efficacy, is the RCT. The problem is that in the relatively small number of patients studied in RCTs rare serious harm may not be spotted. Therefore, study architectures of lower intrinsic quality may be admissible for an adverse effect systematic review. An extreme example is that observer blinding is superfluous if the outcome is death. Such rare and serious harm cannot, and should not, be dismissed just because it is reported in a case report rather than in an RCT. The 'process rules' in this area have yet to be universally agreed.

Number-needed-to-harm (NNH)

For adverse effects reported in RCTs, NNH may be calculated in the same way as NNT. If the adverse effect occurs very rarely then an estimate of the NNH may be calculated but the confidence intervals may be huge (infinite).

Major harm may be defined as intervention-related study withdrawal in a set of RCTs, and may be calculated from those numbers. Precise estimates of major harm will require much wider literature searches to trawl for case reports or series. Minor harm may similarly be defined as reported adverse effects in a set of RCTs. The utility of these reports is limited because they are reported simply as present or absent, with no indication of severity or importance to the patient.

The safety of epidurals is a good example of where systematic reviews of harm can be useful. A recent national audit conducted on behalf of the Royal College of Anaesthetists provides safety estimates. However, three published systematic reviews of epidurals in different contexts reported greater numbers of harmful events. This demonstrates the potential advantage of systematic review over audit in estimating harm.

Using NNT and NNH to evaluate an intervention

In the ideal world a review would provide three numbers for each intervention:

◆ NNT for benefit,

◆ NNH for major harm, and

◆ NNH for minor harm.

These methods can be used to show the effectiveness, or otherwise, of a range of interventions, and if effective, to use the NNT as a benchmark of just how effective a particular intervention is. This then becomes the yardstick against which alternative interventions, each with its NNT for benefit, NNH for minor harm, and NNH for major harm should be judged, and when choosing clinically which (if any) intervention to use for an individual patient.

Conclusion

The methods described above can deliver high-quality efficacy estimates if there are randomized trials of adequate size and quality, but not if the trials are deficient in number, size, or quality. Safety estimates are more difficult, not least because the data from which they are derived commonly comes from study designs which are not randomized and hence more subject to bias. However, it must always be remembered that the practice of EBM means integrating individual clinical expertise with the best available external clinical evidence from systematic research. Thus, the 'cold numbers' provided by the reviewing process described above, must always be tempered by the judgement of the clinician to enable treatment to be appropriate for the individual patient.

Further reading

Cook, T.M., Counsell, D., Wildsmith, J.A., (2009). Major complications of central neuraxial block: report on the Third National Audit Project of the Royal College of Anaesthetists. *Br J Anaesth* Feb;**102**(2), 179–190.

Moore, A., McQuay, H., (2006). *Bandolier's Little Book of Making Sense of the Evidence.* Oxford: OUP.

Ruppen, W., Derry, S., McQuay, H.J., Moore, R.A., (2006). Incidence of Epidural Hematoma, Infection, and Neurologic Injury in Obstetric Patients with Epidural Analgesia/Anesthesia. *Anesthesiology* **105**, 394–399.

Sackett, D.L., Rosenberg, W.M.C., Muir Gray, J.A., Haynes, R.B., Richardson, W.S., (1996). Evidence-based medicine: what it is and what it isn't. *British Medical Journal* **312**, 71–72.

Chapter 10

National Institute for Health and Clinical Excellence (NICE), National Service Frameworks (NSF), and governance

Peter Littlejohns and Augustine J Pereira

Key points

◆ NICE and NSFs were introduced in 1999 as a means for standardization of healthcare and safety across the NHS.

◆ Health professionals are required to take NICE guidance into consideration in their practice.

◆ Primary Care Trusts: (PCTs) must make funding available within 3 months for an intervention supported by a positive NICE appraisal.

◆ NSFs address the 'whole system of care' and NICE guidance makes 'recommendations for practice (clinical and public health)'.

◆ NICE is now at the forefront of setting standards and has now taken over the responsibility for developing Quality of Outcome Framework (QOF) indicator standards.

The creation of NICE

The Department of Health 1998 white paper 'The New NHS: Modern Dependable' was set in the context of inequitable UK health service provision. Although many services demonstrated standards of excellence equal to the best in the world, others experienced serious problems. To address this issue the white paper announced the development of the National Service Framework (NSF) and the setting up of a new organization; the National Institute for Clinical Excellence (NICE). NICE was intended as a new body to give a strong leadership on clinical and cost-effectiveness by drawing up new guidelines from the latest scientific evidence.

Subsequently, NICE was established as a Special Health Authority in April 1999 with the aim of:

◆ Speeding uptake by the National Health Service (NHS) of interventions that are both clinically and cost-effective,

◆ Encouraging more equitable access to healthcare,

- Providing better and more rational use of available resources by focussing the provision of health care on the most cost-effective interventions, and
- Encouraging the creation of new and innovative technologies.

The Institute's stated vision is:

'to improve care for patients and the health of the country as a whole, by providing high quality advice and support to guide clinical and public health practice and by setting standards for the NHS'.

In 2005 NICE subsumed the public health functions of the Health Development Agency and became The National Institute for Health and Clinical Excellence (but the acronym remains the same).

NICE guidance

NICE only provides guidance to the NHS, and local authorities in England and Wales, on the effectiveness and cost-effectiveness of health care and public health interventions. In Scotland and Northern Ireland some guidance is applied, while others may be disseminated after local review. Nonetheless, NICE guidance is often referenced worldwide.

Despite the authoritative status NICE guidance has gained since its inception, it still remains an advisory body to health professionals. They need to take its guidance fully into account when making decisions on individual patient care, but ultimately it is their professional responsibility, in conjunction with the patient, to choose the final treatment. However, for PCTs the situation is different. If a NICE appraisal is supportive of an intervention, then the funding has to be made available within 3 months (unless waived by the Department of Health). This right is included in the UK's NHS constitution, first published in January 2009.

NICE has separate programmes (displayed in Table 10.1) for:

- appraising new and existing technologies,
- developing disease-specific clinical and public health guidelines,
- assessing new interventional procedures, and
- developing public health guidance.

In making its recommendations the institute takes into account:

- Clinical effectiveness
  The extent to which a specific treatment or intervention, when used under usual or everyday conditions, has a beneficial effect on the course or outcome of disease compared to no treatment or other routine care.
- Cost effectiveness
  Value for money; a specific health care treatment is said to be 'cost-effective' if it gives a greater health gain than could be achieved by using the resources in other ways.
- Efficacy
  The extent to which a specific treatment or intervention under ideally controlled conditions, has a beneficial effect on the course or outcome of disease compared with no treatment, or other routine care.

Table 10.1 NICE guidance programme: activity

NICE programme	Provides guidance on	What the guidance takes into account	Number of guidance published to April 2009
Technology appraisals	The use of health technologies, which include: ◆ pharmaceuticals ◆ devices ◆ diagnostics ◆ surgical and other procedures ◆ health promotion tools	Clinical effectiveness and cost-effectiveness	170
Clinical guidelines	The appropriate treatment and care of patients with specific diseases and conditions	Clinical effectiveness and cost-effectiveness	85
Interventional procedures	The safety of an 'interventional procedure' and how well it works. (An 'Interventional procedure' is any surgery, test, or treatment that involves entering the body through skin, muscle, vein or artery, or body cavity.)	Clinical efficacy and safety of the intervention. It does not take cost-effectiveness into account.	298
Public health guidance	Activities to promote a healthy lifestyle and prevent ill health (for example, giving advice to encourage exercise, or providing support to encourage mothers to breastfeed).	Effectiveness and cost-effectiveness of public health activities.	19

One of the key features that distinguishes NICE from all other guidance developers is the explicit expectation that cost-effectiveness (or value for money) is taken into account when assessing health and public health interventions. This has often led to controversial decisions, and since its inception NICE has rarely been out of the public or professional limelight.

Originally, NICE also had responsibility for the National Clinical Audit Programme and the four national confidential enquiries, but as part of a number of NHS reorganizations the former was transferred to the Commission for Health Improvement, and the latter to the National Patient Safety Agency.

NICE: Principles for decision making

Although NICE has a series of different processes to produce the different types of guidance they are all based on the same key principles:

◆ use of best available evidence,

◆ independence – all NICE advisory bodies consist of individuals drawn from the NHS, professional groups, patients, and the public and Industry,

- transparency of development – meetings are in public when possible, and all underlying evidence, as well as minutes of meetings, are available on the website, and
- regular updates.

Citizens council

NICE advisory bodies are expected to make scientific decisions, but as cost-effectiveness is part of the process value judgements must also be made. To help in this task NICE established a Citizens Council consisting of 30 members drawn from the general public. The members are drawn to reflect the age range, gender, socio-economic status, disability, geographical location, and ethnicity of adults in England and Wales. The council meets for 3 days twice a year to deliberate on the difficult societal issues that NICE has to face. Reports produced by the Council are presented at the NICE public board meeting.

The NICE social value principles

The Citizens Council's views, together with the experience of the advisory bodies, and advice from moral philosophers and ethicists, have been formulated in to a set of eight Social Values Principles that all NICE advisory bodies must take into account when developing recommendations.
Briefly, these eight principles are:

1. NICE should not recommend an intervention if there is no evidence, or not enough evidence, on which to make a clear decision.

2. Those developing clinical guidelines, technology appraisals, or public health guidance must take into account their 'cost effectiveness' when deciding whether or not to recommend them.

3. Decisions about whether to recommend interventions should not be based on evidence of their relative costs and benefits alone, but include the need to distribute health resources in the fairest way within the society as a whole.

4. If NICE decides not to recommend use of an intervention with a cost per quality adjusted life year (QALY) within, or below, the range of £20,000 to £30,000 per QALY gained, or decides it will recommend use of an intervention within or above this range, it must explain the reasons why.

5. NICE should not recommend interventions that are not effective and cost-effective enough to provide the best value to users of the NHS as a whole.

6. NICE should consider and respond to comments it receives about its draft guidance, and change it where appropriate.

7. NICE can recommend that use of an intervention is restricted to a particular group of people within the population (for example, people under or over a certain age, or for women only), but only where there is clear evidence about the increased effectiveness of the intervention in this subgroup, or other reasons relating to fairness for society as a whole, or a legal requirement to act in this way.

8. When choosing guidance topics, when developing guidance and when supporting people who are putting the guidance into practice, NICE should actively consider health inequalities, such as those associated with sex, age, race, disability, and socio-economic status.

NSFs and setting standards for quality

National Service Frameworks were established at the same time as NICE as a complementary process to establish national standards and guidelines. NSFs are long-term strategies for improving specific areas of care to help ensure consistent access to services and quality of care right across the UK.

National Service Frameworks:

◆ set national standards, identify key interventions, and put in place agreed timescales for implementation,

◆ set out where care is best provided, and the standard of care that patients should be offered in each setting, thereby reducing unacceptable variation,

◆ bring together the best evidence of clinical and cost-effectiveness,with the views of services, to determine the best ways of providing particular services, and

◆ are developed with the help of expert reference groups that engage a full range of views, bringing together health professionals, service users, carers, health-service managers, partner agencies, and other relevant groups.

In these respects, there are several parallels to NICE guidance development. The main points that are addressed in an NSF document are illustrated in Table 10.2.

The criteria which inform the selection of topics for National Service Frameworks include:

◆ a demonstrable relevance to the Government's agenda for health improvement and tackling health inequalities,

◆ an important health issue – in terms of mortality, morbidity, disability, or resource use,

◆ an area of public concern,

◆ evidence of a shortfall between actual and acceptable practice, with real opportunities for improvement,

◆ an area where care for a patient may be provided in more than one setting (for example hospital, GP surgery, or at home) and by more than one organization (for example, NHS and/or local authority/voluntary sector),

◆ an area where local services need to be reorganised or restructured to ensure service improvements,

◆ a problem which requires new, innovative approaches, and

◆ the Chief Medical Officer's Annual Report.

Table 10.2 Main Points addressed in a NSF document

Each National Service Framework will include:

- A definition of the scope of the Framework
- The evidence base
  - Needs assessment
  - Present performance
  - Evidence of clinical and cost-effectiveness
  - Significant gaps and pressures
- National standards, timescales for delivery
- Key interventions and associated costs
- Commissioned work to support implementation
  - Appropriate R&D, including through the NHS R&D programme (including Health Technology Assessments – HTA)
  - Appraisal
  - Benchmarks
  - Outcome indicators
- Supporting programmes
  - Workforce planning
  - Education and training
  - Personal and organizational development (OD)
  - Information development
- a performance management framework

The Department of Health requires NSFs be used in collaboration with NICE guidance, and that NSFs are updated by any new guidance or recommendations published by NICE.

The NSF programme was set up as a rolling programme with new topics introduced at regular intervals. There are, as of 2009, 12 NSFs in existence (Table 10.3).

Table 10.3 National Service Frameworks

Published National Service Frameworks (2009)

- Blood pressure	- Long-term conditions
- Cancer	- Long-term neurological conditions
- Children	- Mental health
- Chronic obstructive pulmonary disease (COPD)	- Older people
- Coronary heart disease	- Renal
- Diabetes	- Vascular

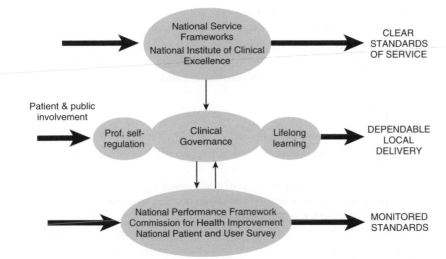

Fig. 10.1 Quality in the new NHS.

Reproduced from *Clinical governance: Quality in the new NHS*, Health Services Circular 1999/065, Department of Health, with permission

The governance and safety role of NICE and NSFs

When NICE and NSFs were established in 1999 their position in the broader quality assurance agenda (described in Table 10.2) reflected the fact that they were part of the government's approach to improving the quality of the care provided by the NHS. How NICE and NSF's fit into the government's plan of quality improvement in healthcare is illustrated in Figure 10.1.

This approach to improving care was initially presented as a 'quality improvement' model, with education and support being the key driving forces. However the various institutions involved in this initial quality initiative at that time, the Commission for Health Improvement (later became Healthcare Commission, and is now the Care Quality Commission), NICE, the National Clinical Governance Support Team, and the National Patient Safety Agency, indicated that their contribution was in supporting the NHS in addressing the daily challenges of delivering high-quality health care.

In this context, the Institute considered that one of its main roles was to provide guidance on controversial health issues where lack of clarity has resulted in regional variation in the care provided by the NHS. The guidance produced was expected to be incorporated into local clinical governance mechanisms via the use of local guidelines and protocols. Primary Care Trusts and NHS Trusts have all been required to set up governance mechanisms to ensure that NICE guidance and NSFs are fully implemented. These arrangements enable implementation of guidance within the required timeframes and also enable forward planning using horizon scanning tools provided by the Institute.

Lord Darzi's 'Next Stage Review' of the NHS, published to coincide with its 60-year anniversary in 2008, placed a new emphasis on 'quality' and places NICE unequivocally at the centre of standards in the NHS, with a brief to create a complete set of national clinical standards based on its guideline programme, as well as providing the underlying evidence for the Quality Outcome Framework for use in general practice. It has also been given the task of developing a new web-based portal called 'NHS Evidence', building on the work of the National Library for Health to help drive up quality of service within the health and social care sectors.

Conclusion

NICE is now part of the routine NHS world. It is consolidating on its first 10 years of producing guidance, and is now beginning to diversify into setting standards and providing a broader range of evidence. NSF's have provided a solid framework for standardizing care within the areas for which they have been published. Together they enable the Institutes' stated vision to be realized, leading to an improvement in the safety and quality of care for all NHS patients.

Further reading

Department of Health (1997). *The New NHS: Modern and Dependable.* HMSO: London.

Department of Health (1998). *A First Class Service: Quality in the New NHS.* HMSO: London.

Department of Health (2008). High quality care for all: NHS Next Stage Review final report. HMSO, http://www.dh.gov.uk/en/Publicationsandstatistics/Publications/PublicationsPolicyAndGuidance/DH_085825.

Chapter 11

Clinical guidelines

Gillian C Leng and Chris Connell

Key points

- Clinical guidelines are systematically developed statements to help clinicians and patients make decisions about appropriate health care for particular clinical conditions.
- Clinical guidelines help ensure that patients receive high-quality care.
- Clinical guidelines should be informed by the best available evidence.
- Clinical guidelines should support and inform, but not replace, the judgement of individual clinicians.
- Clinical guidelines are also relevant to health service managers and commissioners by helping inform the decisions that they make.

Introduction

A clinical guideline is a document designed to support decisions regarding the diagnosis, care, and treatment of a particular disease or condition. Historically, these may have been based on observation, received wisdom, convention, and or religious beliefs. Today, however, the most robust clinical guidelines are based on a systematic appraisal of the evidence.

Increasing emphasis on an evidence-based approach to healthcare is leading to a growing number of clinical guidelines being produced. Moreover, there is an expectation from professional bodies such as the Royal Colleges, healthcare regulators, healthcare providers, commissioners, and patients themselves that they should be implemented and followed.

Clinical guidelines, such as those produced by the National Institute for Health and Clinical Excellence (NICE), often cover broad areas of care, for example heart failure, depression, or head injury. As a result of the breadth of the topics covered, implementation of guidelines can sometimes be complex and time-consuming, involving a number of different professional and patient groups within a region.

The implementation of clinical guidelines can deliver clear and wide-ranging benefits for patients, clinicians, and healthcare organizations. Large numbers of guidelines are now published; in 2009 NHS Evidence listed around 1500 evidence-based guidelines for the United Kingdom alone. These have been produced by organizations such as the Medical Royal Colleges, patient and carer organizations, and health service bodies such as NICE and the Scottish Intercollegiate Guidelines Network (SIGN). NHS Evidence has now established a formal accreditation programme for guideline producers using internationally accepted criteria (http://www.agreecollaboration.org) to help users identify the best, most trusted sources of guidelines.

Developing NICE guidance

NICE is one of the best-known guideline-producing organizations in the world publishing around 20 clinical guidelines each year covering a broad range of topics from perioperative hypothermia to donor breast milk banks. The structured approach taken by NICE in developing clinical guidelines is described below.

Proposing and selecting topics for NICE clinical guidelines

Anyone can suggest a guideline topic for consideration by NICE. Suggestions are considered by NICE using a checklist based on Department of Health selection criteria. These criteria take into account

- 'the burden of disease' covered by the proposed guideline,
- the likely cost to the NHS and to other public sector organizations,
- the importance of the proposed guideline in relation to government policy,
- whether there is variation in clinical practice, and
- any other reason why the proposed clinical guideline is needed urgently.

Topic suggestions are reviewed by one of NICE's topic selection consideration panels, which are composed of experts in the topic area, other healthcare professionals, and patient and carers. The recommendations of the topic selection panels are passed to the Department of Health, and the Secretary of State for Health makes the final decision on which topics are referred to NICE for the development of clinical guidelines.

Producing the clinical guideline

Once the Department of Health has asked NICE to produce a clinical guideline, NICE commissions one of its National Collaborating Centres (NCCs) to co-ordinate the guideline's development. The fundamental basis of every clinical guideline is that it will be founded on an appraisal of the best evidence available, and that recommendations will take into account both clinical and cost effectiveness.

There are four NCCs (Table 11.1), all of which were established by NICE to develop clinical guidelines in particular fields. The NCCs bring together the expertise of the medical and nursing royal colleges, NHS trusts, professional organizations, and patient and carer organizations.

Table 11.1 The National Collaborating Centres

- National Collaborating Centre for Cancer
- National Collaborating Centre for Mental Health
- National Collaborating Centre for Women and Children's Health
- National Clinical guidelines Centre for Acute and Chronic Conditions

---

For each clinical guideline the NCC

- prepares a draft scope which defines what will and will not be included in the clinical guideline,
- establishes and works with the Guideline Development Group (GDG) (see below) to develop the clinical guideline,
- undertakes systematic reviews of the literature and health economic analyses,
- ensures that due process is followed,
- together with the GDG prepares a draft of the clinical guideline for consultation,
- together with the GDG makes appropriate changes to the clinical guideline in response to comments received during the consultation,
- publishes the full guideline, and
- advises NICE on the publication, implementation, and updating of the clinical guideline.

Guideline Development Groups (GDGs)

The NCC sets up an independent GDG for each clinical guideline to work with the NCC to develop the guideline recommendations. Specifically, during the development of the guideline the Guideline Development Group

- agrees the questions about treatment and management of the condition that will guide the search for evidence,
- considers the evidence and reaches conclusions based on the evidence,
- uses expert consensus to reach conclusions and make decisions where evidence is poor or lacking,
- formulates the guideline recommendations,
- considers comments made by stakeholders during consultation, and
- agrees the necessary changes to the guideline after consultation.

Membership of the GDG

Each GDG is made up of healthcare professionals, technical experts, and patients or carers and reflects the range of stakeholders and groups whose professional activities or care will be covered by the guideline. In addition, expert advisors may also be invited to attend meetings for specific discussions.

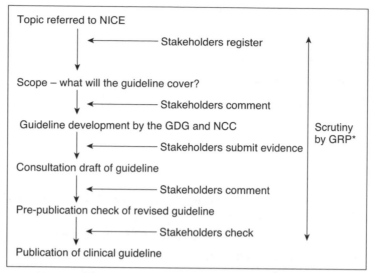

Fig. 11.1 The key stages of NICE clinical guideline development.
*Guideline Review Panel

Neither NICE nor the healthcare industry is represented on the GDG in order to ensure the group's independence and to prevent conflicts of interest.

Becoming a member of a GDG

All vacancies for GDGs are advertised on the NICE website. When appointing GDG members, the following factors are taken into account:

- The suitability of individual applicants, e.g. the relevance of their skills and experience to the clinical guideline under development.
- The requirement for the best combination of people to maximize the skills and experience of the GDG.

There will be at least two GDG members with experience or knowledge of patient and carer issues, and between six and eight members who are healthcare professionals and who either treat people directly with the condition or manage services. There will also be expert systematic reviewers who carry out analyses of statistical and health economic issues, and a health economist.

All members of the GDG have to have

- an interest and commitment to developing the clinical guideline,
- time to attend all meetings – usually 10–15 in total, held monthly,
- time to complete the background reading and help formulate the recommendations, and
- good communication and team working skills.

Table 11.2 Organizations that can register as stakeholder for NICE clinical guidelines

- National patient and carer organizations that represent the interests of people whose care will be covered by the guideline.
- National organizations that represent healthcare professionals who provide services described by the guideline.
- Companies that manufacture drugs or devices used in the treatment covered by the guideline.
- Providers and commissioners of health services in England and Wales.
- Statutory organizations, e.g. the Department of Health, Welsh Assembly Government, NHS Quality Improvement Scotland, Care Quality Commission.

Stakeholders

Stakeholders play a vital role in the development of clinical guidelines. Professional, patient and carer groups, healthcare organizations, and government bodies can all register with NICE as stakeholders for a clinical guideline (Table 11.2).

Stakeholder organizations can comment on the clinical guidelines at various stages in its development (see Figure 11.1).

Looking at the evidence

The GDG is required to make recommendations on the best available evidence of both clinical and cost effectiveness.

Assessing clinical effectiveness

The basis for assessing clinical effectiveness is a literature search of the areas covered by the guidelines scope. This will involve four key steps:

- Selecting relevant studies
- Assessing the quality of the studies
- Synthesizing the results
- Interpreting the results

Assessing cost effectiveness

Cost effectiveness is assessed in order to maximize health gain from available resources. The health economist on the GDG

- advises the GDG on economic issues,
- conducts economic evaluations and modelling, and
- prioritizes questions and issues for further economic analysis.

Cost effectiveness is assessed using a number of measures. If there is sufficient information, quality-adjusted life years (QALYs) are used to measure and compare the cost effectiveness of different interventions. QALYs are an internationally used measure of health outcome that attempt to weight the life expectancy of a patient with their quality of life on a 0 to 1 scale. A QALY score of 1 would indicate that a treatment would 'give' a patient 1 year of good quality of life.

Where there is insufficient data to estimate QALYs other measure of effectiveness may be considered such as the number of cases prevented, number of life years gained, or a more disease-specific outcome.

Guideline Review Panels (GRP)

NICE has established four independent Guideline Review Panels, each of which has four or five members. Each clinical guideline is allocated to one of the GRPs. The panel

* comments on the draft scope and the draft guideline,
* ensures that stakeholder comments have been considered appropriately by the GDG, and
* ensures that due process has been followed.

Publishing clinical guidelines

It usually takes NICE around 18–24 months from the time of referral to clinical guideline publication.

The timetable for the production and planned date of publication of each clinical guideline can be found on the NICE website (www.nice.org.uk). Guidelines are normally published on the fourth Wednesday of each month. Four versions of the clinical guideline are published:

* The *full guideline*, which contains all the recommendations, plus details of the methods used and the underpinning evidence.
* The *NICE guideline* presents the recommendations from the full version in a format suited to implementation by health professionals and NHS bodies.
* The *quick reference guide* presents recommendations in a summary form for health professionals.
* *Understanding NICE guidance* is written for people without specialist medical knowledge.

A range of tools are also published to help healthcare professionals and organizations implement the clinical guideline. These will include costing tools, audit data collection tools, slide sets, and increasingly tools that are specific to individual guidelines.

Benefits of clinical guidelines

Good, evidence-based clinical guidelines, properly implemented and evaluated, can deliver benefits to patients and their carers, clinicians, health service managers, and whole healthcare systems. By highlighting the best available evidence of clinical and cost effectiveness, clinical guidelines can

- improve quality of care,
- increase patient safety,
- help patients take decisions about their own care,
- help educate healthcare professionals,
- reduce inappropriate variations in standards of care,
- support healthcare managers,
- ensure resources are used wisely, and
- be used to set standards.

Improving quality of care

By translating the best available evidence on what works in every day practice, clinical guidelines can raise the quality of care received by patients and improve outcomes, although the picture with respect to uptake of clinical guidelines is arguably mixed.

For example, a review in 2008 by the Healthcare Commission on the NICE clinical guideline on schizophrenia found that 86% of mental health service users had received a baseline physical health assessment on admission, in line with NICE guidelines. Similarly, a NICE review of the clinical guideline on the management of hypertension in 2008 showed a sharp drop in the prescribing of betablockers, an increase in the number of prescriptions for angiotensin-converting enzyme (ACE) inhibitors, and increased use of calcium channel blockers, all in line with the recommendations of the NICE guideline. However, by contrast, the Healthcare Commissions review of the NICE clinical guideline on heart failure in 2007, which looked at 303 health communities against criteria in the guideline, assessed only 32% as providing good or excellent services.

Increasing patient safety

Adverse clinical incidents may be caused by ignorance, or inappropriate disregard, of clinical guidelines and healthcare standards, leading to the actions taken by clinicians not being supported by best evidence.

Clinical guidelines, therefore, have a valuable role in promoting patient safety by ensuring that healthcare professionals are aware of the best evidence-based approach to support their clinical judgement and expertise.

Helping patients and members of the public take decisions about their own health

Clinical guidelines can help patients and members of the public to look after their own health. Some clinical guidelines are written with the lay person in mind and offer advice on how they can treat or prevent ill health and promote good health.

For more specialist clinical guidelines, some organizations, such as NICE, write versions of their guidance specifically for patients, helping them to understand and make informed decisions about the treatment options that are available to them.

Education, training, and professional development

The number of high-quality, peer reviewed articles published each year is vast.

Clinical guidelines can also be useful teaching aids for those undertaking both initial and further training.

Reducing inappropriate variation in standards of care

A systematic approach to the implementation of clinical guidelines should ensure that patients being treated for the same condition receive the same high-quality care and have similar clinical outcomes. This helps remove the 'postcode lottery' whereby people receive different treatment, and experience different clinical outcomes, for no other reason than that they live in different parts of the country.

Clinical guidelines can also help overcome inappropriate variation due to other factors such as age, sex, and social circumstance by highlighting the needs of particular groups.

Supporting healthcare managers

The benefits of clinical guidelines can extend beyond clinicians and patients, and can be used by health service managers to help inform their decisions in the planning, commissioning, and running of services. For example, NICE has produced a clinical guideline on obesity, which is so comprehensive and broad in scope that it can be used to guide the provision of services in schools and local authorities, yet also inform decisions about the provision of bariatric surgery in specialist hospitals. Other NICE guidelines, such as those on the care of acutely ill patients in hospital, dementia, schizophrenia, and stroke can also be used to support managers' decisions.

Ensuring resources are used wisely

Some clinical guidelines, notably those published by NICE, make evidence-based recommendations about what is both cost-effective and clinically effective. By doing this, the guidelines aim to achieve improved outcomes for patients whilst also ensuring the most efficient use of health resources, such as money, staff time, expertise, and equipment, so that treatments are available to as many patients as possible. By implementing and following clinical guidelines, staff and patients can also be reassured that they will not be wasting time and resources on ineffective treatments.

Helping set standards

Clinical guidelines can be used to help set relevant, measurable standards to assess the clinical practice of healthcare professionals, and of the quality and safety of services provided by healthcare organizations as a whole.

In 2008 the Department of Health published the document 'High Quality Care for All', setting out a vision for establishing quality as a defining factor in the NHS in England. This report recommended that in future NICE should set Quality Standards for health and social care. The new standards will be evidence-based, and will act as markers of high-quality, cost-effective patient care within a specific clinical area, effectively a distillation of key aspects of a clinical guideline where change is required to improve the quality of care. They will be accompanied by quality indicators to enable progress to be measured. The NICE quality standards have the potential to enable local clinicians, commissioners, and service providers to use them to help address local priorities.

In addition, the Care Quality Commission and NHS Litigation Authority incorporate clinical guidelines in the standards that they use nationally to assess healthcare organizations. More locally, clinical governance groups and commissioners may also use clinical guidelines as the basis for local standard setting.

Next steps: NHS evidence

Actually finding the relevant clinical guideline, and being confident of the evidence on which it is based, is a significant challenge to many healthcare professionals given the large numbers of articles and guidelines that are published each year. One medical director likened it to 'looking for a snowman in a snowstorm'.

To help address this issue, NICE launched a new service in April 2009 called NHS Evidence (www.evidence.nhs.uk). It is a web-based service that provides access to a comprehensive evidence base for all those who work in health or social care and who make decisions about the treatments, care, or use of resources. NHS evidence will manage the synthesis and spread of knowledge through the NHS, and users will be assured about the quality and evidence base of the guidelines that they are using.

Summary

The NICE approach to developing clinical guidelines is rigorous, and this rigour is essential to ensure that guidance is consistent, high quality, and based on the best available evidence. Many other bodies produce clinical guidelines, however, a common feature of the highest quality clinical guidelines is a thorough appraisal of the best available evidence.

Rigorous implementation initiatives are also required, at national and local level, to ensure guidelines support a change in practice and drive improvements in care for patients.

Further reading

Greenhalgh, T., Robert, G., Bate, P., *et al.* (2005). *Diffusion of Innovations in Health Service Organisations: A Systematic Literature Review.* Blackwell BMJ Books: Oxford.

Fixsen, D.L., Naoom, S.F., Blasé, K.A., *et al.* (2005). Implementation Research: a synthesis of the literature. University of South Florida: Tampa, FL, Louis de la Parte Florida Mental Health Institute, The National Implementation Research Network (FMHI Publication # Available from: http://nirn.fmhi.usf.edu/resources/publications/monograph/.

Sutherland, K. and Leatherman, S. (2006). *Regulation and Quality Improvement. A Review of the Evidence*. The Health Foundation: London.

Wensing, M. and Grol, R. (2005). 'Educational interventions', in *Improving Patient Care: the Implementation of Change in Clinical Practice*, R. Grol, M. Wensing, and M. Eccles (eds.). Elsevier: Edinburgh.

NICE (2009). How NICE clinical guidelines are developed: an overview for stakeholders, the public and NHS, 4th ed.) ref 1233 # Available from http://www.nice.org.uk/aboutnice/howwework/.

Chapter 12

Clinical audit

David Hunter

Key points

◆ Clinical audit can be defined as a quality improvement process that seeks to improve patient care and outcomes through systematic review of care against explicit criteria and the implementation of change.

◆ Clinical audit is central to effective clinical governance as a measure of clinical effectiveness.

◆ Clinical audit is a cyclical process consisting of the following steps:

1. Identify problem or issue
2. Set criteria and standards
3. Observe practice/data collection
4. Compare performance against criteria and standards
5. Implement change to address deficits

◆ Clinical audits may address areas of structure, process, or outcome.

◆ The GMC publication 'Good Medical Practice' states that all doctors have a duty to 'take part in regular and systematic audit' and 'participate in regular reviews and audit of the standards and performance of the team, taking steps to remedy any deficiencies'.

Introduction

The most general definition of an audit is an evaluation of a person, organization, system process, project, or product. Most commonly, the word 'audit' has been associated with financial audit where the financial performance of a business is evaluated. However, audit is now part of most quality control systems and its application in medicine is no exception. There is, however, a rather fundamental difference between financial audits and clinical audit, in that the former are performed by external auditors who play no part in the system they are evaluating. By contrast, it is important in clinical audit that healthcare professionals have ownership of the audit, and design, participate, and act upon the results relating to their own team's performance.

History

One of the first clinical audits in modern times is attributed to Florence Nightingale, undertaken during the Crimean War (1853–1855) at the Barrack Hospital in Scutari on the Asian side of Constantinople. She kept meticulous records of the mortality rates among the wounded soldiers and demonstrated a fall in mortality rate from 40% to 2% by applying improved hygiene and sanitation standards. She returned to England in 1856, continuing her work in mortality rate analysis. In 1860 she became the first woman to be elected a Fellow of the Statistical Society for her contribution to Army statistics and comparative hospital statistics.

Ernest Amory Codman (1869–1940), a surgeon, conceived the 'End Result Idea', unpopular with colleagues at the time, according to which every hospital should follow up all patients, recording their final outcome to determine whether treatment was successful or not, and if not why not. He worked at the End Result Hospital in Boston with such luminaries as Charles Mayo and Harvey Cushing. Unfortunately the hospital closed after the First World War and Codman put his energies for the next 13 years into developing a sarcoma tumour registry.

The next step forward in evaluation of quality of healthcare was made by Avedis Donabedian (1919–1990) an Armenian by birth, who became Professor of Public Health at the University of Michigan in 1961. He stated that measurements of the quality of complex medical systems could focus on structure, process, or outcomes.

In the United Kingdom, the first large collaborative confidential audit between surgeons and anaesthetists looking at outcomes following surgery was in 1982. The Confidential Enquiry into Perioperative Deaths (CEPOD) looked at anaesthetic and surgical practice over 1 year in 3 regions in the UK. In 1988 the National Confidential Enquiry into Perioperative Deaths (NCEPOD) was established supported by government funding, and its first report on the deaths of children aged 10 years and under was published in 1990. Since then, NCEPOD has published over 20 reports. Samples for study have ranged from a percentage of all deaths within 30 days of surgery to those deaths within a specific age range or due to specific procedures. Two similar studies have also been undertaken (1995/96 and 2002) on the pattern of operating within hospitals regardless of outcome.

Although, rather surprisingly, there has been great historical resistance by doctors to measuring the quality of care delivered, it is now a General Medical Council (GMC) requirement of employment and registration in the UK to 'take part in confidential enquiries and adverse event recognition and reporting to help reduce risk to patients'.

Definitions of clinical audit

The definition of clinical audit has evolved over time. The 1989 white paper, Working for Patients, which required doctors' participation in medical audit, defined it as

> the systematic critical analysis of the quality of medical care including the procedures used for diagnosis and treatment, the use of resources and the resulting outcome and quality of life for the patient.

However, it became apparent that distinctions between

◆ medical audit (audit initiated by doctors),

◆ clinical audit (audits of clinical care by nursing and paramedical staff), and

◆ organizational audit (administrative audits).

were counterproductive, and that the totality of patient care should be studied, with all members of a team delivering a particular service being involved in auditing their work. This multidisciplinary approach was given the name 'clinical audit'. In 1994 the NHS Executive defined clinical audit as:

> the systematic analysis of the quality of healthcare, including the procedures used for diagnosis, treatment and care, the use of resources and the resulting outcome and quality of life for the patient.

In 2002 the then National Institute for Clinical Excellence (NICE) published the paper *Principles for Best Practice in Clinical Audit*, which defines clinical audit as

> a quality improvement process that seeks to improve patient care and outcomes through systematic review of care against explicit criteria and the implementation of change. Aspects of the structure, processes, and outcomes of care are selected and systematically evaluated against explicit criteria. Where indicated, changes are implemented at an individual, team, or service level and further monitoring is used to confirm improvement in healthcare delivery.

This definition demonstrates the modern concepts of the multidisciplinary, patient-centred, continuous nature of auditing against previously identified explicit criteria. Above all, clinical audit is a process that is instigated, conducted, and discussed by teams of healthcare professionals examining their own practice. It should not be a study designed by external auditors. Indeed, the GMC states in *Good Medical Practice* (2006) that doctors have a duty to participate in regular and systematic audit, taking steps to remedy any deficiencies.

Components of clinical audit

The component parts of a clinical audit are:

1. Standard setting

2. Measuring current practice

3. Comparison of results with stated standards

4. Implementing appropriate changes

5. Re-auditing to ensure practice has improved.

This is a constant, reiterative process, and is known as the audit cycle (Figure 12.1).

What is the difference between audit and research?

This is not such an easy question to answer as might appear. One of the frequent reasons for posing such a question is that all research requires Research Ethics Committee (REC) approval, and audits usually do not. It is possible that an audit

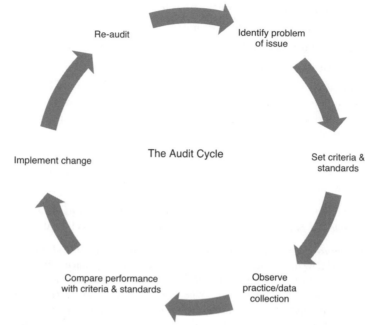

Fig. 12.1 The audit cycle.

project might require ethical approval and it is best, if in any doubt whatsoever, to ask the advice of the local REC chairman. Ethics aside, there are differences between most audits and research, which can be summed up as 'research is concerned with discovering the right thing to do; audit with ensuring it is done right' (Smith R BMJ 1992). Thus research is about defining best practice and audit determines whether we are following best practice or not.

Some of the major differences between the two are summed up in Table 12.1.

As audit compares clinical practice against agreed standards, and research is often needed to identify the appropriate standards, then research is sometimes seen as 'pre-audit', or put another way, audit is the completion of a research cycle. Certainly, audit may identify areas that require further research, and research may identify areas for audit.

How to do an audit project

1. Choose a topic

Audit projects can look at the following:

Structure

Audit of structure looks at the things that need to be in place to enable a high standard of care or treatment – staff, environment, equipment. For example, acceptability of premises to patients, clinic waiting times, staffing levels, availability of equipment/test results, appropriate qualification, and training of staff.

Table 12.1 Differences between Audit and Research

Audit	Research
Aim to monitor and improve local clinical practice	Aims to increase body of scientific knowledge
Is a systematic and critical analysis of patient care	Is a systematic scientific enquiry
Tests care against knowledge from research	Creates new knowledge
Measures against standards	Tests hypothesis
Should never involve anything beyond normal clinical management (but see patient surveys note)	May involve experiments on patients and/or volunteers
Abides by an ethical framework but doesn't usually require ethical approval	Requires submission to a Research Ethics Committee (REC) for ethical approval
Never involves random allocation or placebo treatment	May involve random allocation to different treatment groups, including placebo
Different methodology from research, usually smaller sample sizes	Rigorous methodology and statistical analysis
Results only applicable locally. May be publishable for interest particularly in audit process	Results should be publishable and applicable elsewhere

Process

Audits of process look at the clinical care given to the patients. How well do we apply our own guidelines? If treatment X has been shown to have the best outcomes, are we giving our patients X, or are we giving inferior Y? If we aim to give all patients X, Y, and Z, how often do they get all three.

Outcome

Audits of outcome look at the results of interventions. The most obvious would be mortality and morbidity rates. Another example could be patient satisfaction surveys.

Patient surveys These are a popular audit tool as many 'outcome' measures can include questions that only the patients can answer. However, there are problems with audits involving patient surveys. Firstly, a patient survey clearly involves doing something to patients beyond normal clinical management, and so is not strictly audit. Secondly, it can be very difficult to design a patient survey that is not offensive, is ethically correct, and also delivers the answers required. An oft-cited example is of a survey into adequacy of patient information provision. However, the suggested questionnaire to be applied to random in-patients included the question:

1. When your doctor told you that you had cancer did you....

    (a) feel he explained it well

    (b) have enough time to ask questions

    (c) receive adequate written information

It is easy to see the problems with such a survey, but others may have more subtle problems.

In all patient surveys, the patients' rights, dignity, and time must be considered.

In general, most successful audits focus upon process. This is because when closing the audit 'loop', it is difficult for staff to change structure as this usually requires budgetary changes. Similarly, audits of outcome are frequently complex and it is difficult to alter outcomes without changing process. Most audits are therefore audits of process ensuring that we are following the practice that has been shown by research to have the best outcome. Ideally though, we would aim to audit both process and outcome, to ensure that the published best practice truly leads to best outcome in our population.

Prioritizing audit projects

There is a limit to how many audit projects can be run simultaneously, or indeed sequentially, to avoid staff experiencing 'audit burnout', with low interest and compliance. Thus, audits need to be prioritized. Sometimes audit topics are imposed; e.g. National or regional projects the Trust has agreed to participate in, audits of NICE guidance required by the Care Quality Commission or purchasers, or re-audits to ensure closure of the audit loop. Other topics chosen should be important to participants. Examples might include:

- An identified problem (e.g. from complaints or patient safety incidents)
- High risk, or high volume of lower risk, or high cost areas of practice
- Published evidence about clinically effective treatment
- Availability of clinical guidelines from national bodies (e.g. NICE, Royal Colleges)

Audits should not be undertaken simply because 'it might be interesting to know whether...'.

2. **Form an audit team**

It is vital that audits be supported by colleagues who have the authority and commitment to implement changes shown to be necessary by the audit. It is a waste of time, to demonstrate that something needs to be done without having the ability to effect necessary change.

Audits may be unidisciplinary (i.e. only involving doctors or nurses) or multidisciplinary, involving team members from different staff groups. It is unusual that process audits will only involve one healthcare group. Consider inviting patient group representatives to be part of the audit team, or at the least have some input into the audit design.

3. **Set objectives and standards**

The audit objective should be identified at the start and written down. This may take the form of a question that needs to be answered, or of a standard to be achieved. The standard of care aspired to should be appropriate and based on recent best evidence. If there are no published local or national evidence-based standards in existence, then some should be set based on current published research. Ensure that the audit has not recently been undertaken, or that the topic does not overlap with another audit.

4. **Select the audit sample**

Use a patient population with similar characteristics, or undergoing the same procedure (e.g. patients receiving epidural analgesia, or patients attending a specific clinic), and ideally capture all patients on a rolling basis. In practice, this may be difficult to achieve and it is common to use a 'snapshot' sample, ensuring it is large enough to be representative of the whole population.

5. **Plan and carry out data collection**

Decide whether the audit will be retrospective or prospective. It is easier to ensure data capture prospectively, and much easier to collect data personally. Ensure that the questions posed on any questionnaire will supply the data required to achieve the audit's aims. Decide whether this data be collected on a computer or on paper. It may be possible to use IT-based data collection, or analyse data already collected routinely. In any event, the 'form' needs to be designed so that it is easy to fill in and collate. A pilot audit is a useful step to ensure that the correct sample is collected without missing patients, or bring to light problems with the data collection form. Prior to starting the audit, ensure that all members of the team are aware of the audit start and finish dates, and which patients (if it is patients) are included. The sudden appearance of a form with exhortations to fill it in when no one has any idea of its purpose, or how long the extra work is to go on for leads to poor data capture. All audits may suffer from the 'Hawthorne' effect (subjects changing their behaviour as a result of being observed), but this usually abates as the study progresses.

6. **Analyse the data**

Data should be collated in a timely fashion, and compared with the explicit standards set at the start of the audit. Complicated statistics are not required for audits, the simpler the better. Usually, percentage compliance with the standard is the most effective statistic. Nonetheless, in some cases, it may be advisable to discuss the audit design in advance with a statistician to ensure an adequate and representative sample is that is truly reflective of the practice being audited.

7. **Present the data**

Present the data at a meeting where all interested parties are present allowing plenty of time for discussion. Ensure minutes are recorded. Large numbers of changes in practice should not be recommended by the presenter, any changes should be decided by the group. It should be remembered that audit presentations are disclosable information, and Care Quality Commission inspectors have been known to ask why recommendations in presentations have not been acted upon.

8. **Write a report**

Finally, a written report of the audit data and results and the recommendations of the audit group and stakeholders at the presentation discussion should be made. All Trusts keep a register of audits and reports of results and recommendations, and any audit should be registered via the Trust audit department.

Acknowledgement

I would like to acknowledge the large amount of input to this chapter provided by Chris Swonnell, Clinical Governance Manager and Eleanor Bird, Assistant Clinical Audit Manager of the University of Bristol Hospital NHS Trust.

Further reading

http://www.uhbristol.nhs.uk/healthcare-professionals/clinical-audit.html (last accessed 20th April 2010).

Principles for Best Practice in Clinical Audit. Radcliffe Medical Press Ltd. ISBN: 1-85775-976-1.

Making Use of Clinical Audit: A Guide to Practice in the Health Professions. Open University Press. ISBN-13: 978-0335195428.

The Clinical Audit Handbook. Bailliere Tindal. ISBN-13: 978-0702024184.

Implementing Change in Clinical Audit. Wiley Blackwell. ISBN-13: 978-0471982579.

Chapter 13

Research governance

Paul Farquhar-Smith

Key points

- Research governance is a system to ensure the delivery of high-quality research.
- The UK Government's Research Governance Framework provides a structured means to achieve high standards for all research.
- The core standards include: ethics, science, health and safety, information and financial and intellectual property.
- Good clinical practice (GCP) is pivotal to the implementation of the research governance framework, and therefore high-quality research.
- Trial monitoring and surveillance are paramount in the management of high-quality research.

Introduction

In 2005 the UK government published a revised Research Governance Framework, which outlines principles of good governance that apply to all research within the remit of the Secretary of State for Health. This document sets out the principles, standards, regulations, and requirements that together provide the framework for good practice in research, and the mechanisms needed to improve practice and ensure high quality.

Research governance is one of the core standards for healthcare organizations and applies to all aspects of healthcare research, including any research that involves humans, their tissue, or their data, and also includes everyone involved in research from the chief investigator to support staff. Research governance is designed to protect not only participants in research but also the researchers, and also applies to those responsible for any aspect of research including those who are in

- planning and design,
- management,
- funding bodies, and
- organizations hosting/sponsoring research.

Having a defined framework is beneficial as it gives clear boundaries for researchers to operate within. This framework is intended to promote ethical and scientific quality and to enhance safeguards for those involved. Analogous to clinical governance, risk management and reduction of risk are pivotal to the principles of research governance (Fig. 13.1).

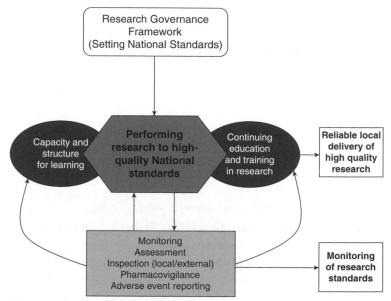

Fig. 13.1. What the research governance framework means for participants.

Core standards

Health and social care research is not the province of a single discipline, profession, or organization, and no single document adequately captures the full range of legislation, standards, and good practice guidelines that apply to this wide-ranging body of work. It is useful to consider the standards in five main domains:

1. Ethics
   Ensuring the dignity, rights, safety, and well-being of research participants.

2. Science
   To assure the validity and quality of research proposals.

3. Health, safety, and employment
   Priority given to the health and safety of the participants and the researchers.

4. Information
   Maintaining confidentiality, adherence to the Data Protection Act, free and unhindered access to information about the conduct and results of the trial.

5. Financial and intellectual property
   The importance of financial probity and compliance with the law including mechanisms for compensation for negligence.

These domains work within a quality research culture that defines the responsibilities and accountability of those involved in research.

1. Ethics

The National Research Ethics Service (NRES) is a directorate of the National Patient Safety Agency (NPSA) and has a dual mission:

- To protect the rights, safety, dignity, and well-being of research participants
- To facilitate and promote ethical research that is of potential benefit to participants, science, and society

The NRES comprises of:

- All NHS Research Ethics Committees (RECs) in England (111 in 2009)
- The volunteer members and chairs that sit on those RECs
- REC coordinators and local managers
- The NRES NPSA division.

All clinical trials conducted in the United Kingdom must be subjected to approval by an ethical review body independent of institutional, political, or other influences. No research study within the NHS involving individuals, their organs, tissue, or data can begin until it has a favourable opinion from a Research Ethics Committee (REC).

Research Ethics Committees

Each local REC consists of a minimum of 7, and a maximum of 18 volunteer members comprising:

- Lay members
  People whose primary personal or professional interest is not in a research area. At least one-third of committee members must be lay.
- Expert members
  A broad range of specialists including doctors, other healthcare professionals, and academics.

Research Ethics Committees must

- be independent and impartial,
- primarily assess the interests of the potential participants,
- weigh benefits against burden (to the person or society), and
- consider the needs and safety of the researchers.

The role of the REC should be to promote good research ensuring timely return of decisions rather than being an obstacle. Each year, NHS RECs consider approximately 7000 applications, and usually give an opinion after 35 days, well within the 60-day maximum allowance.

RECs must be recognized as fit for purpose and also have a detailed governance framework. In specialized studies, the REC can ask for independent expert opinion. Although all research studies have to be approved by REC, the named principal investigator is still responsible for the ethical conduct of the trial.

The process of informed consent is regarded as key part of a study's ethical assessment and involves detailed consideration of:

+ how consent is taken,

+ what and how information is supplied,

+ time given to subjects to consider participation, and

+ provisions made for those unable to give consent themselves (the Mental Capacity Act 2007 adds safeguards to this population).

All members of the research team taking consent should be specifically trained and able to address questions. The researcher should give sufficient time for subjects to make their decisions, and make efforts to assess if the subject understands the implications and potential burdens and risks of taking part. It must also be made clear that subjects can withdraw at any time without reason and without prejudice.

Some trials, e.g. phase I (first trials in humans) cancer therapy trials, may expose a subject to a high probability of risk. Clearly, these risks must be minimized, weighed against the potential benefit, and clearly stated in the information given to subjects in order to obtain a fully informed consent. For example, the potential harm from novel, or a novel combination of cancer therapies in phase 1 trials is only considered in patients with cancer refractory to existing treatments. However, the design and conduct of the trial must still aim to minimize any potential suffering and maintain scrupulous pharmacovigilance. Since the events following the first in man trials of the anti-CD28 antibody (TGN1412) in London in March 2006, which led to multiple organ failure in six volunteers, RECs must now confirm that there is provision for sufficient compensation in the case of non-negligent harm to the subjects. This incident also led to the requirement for establishments carrying out phase I trials to be specifically accredited for this purpose.

2. Science

All existing sources of evidence, especially systematic reviews, must be considered carefully before undertaking research. Research, which duplicates other work, or which is not of sufficient quality to contribute something useful to existing knowledge, is unethical.

Every proposal for health and social care research must be subjected to review by experts in the relevant fields able to offer independent advice on its quality.

Arrangements for peer review should be in proportion to the scale of the research, and the risks involved. For example, in some circumstances, an external panel of independent experts may be invited to review a programme, or a controversial or costly proposal. For student research projects, the university supervisor is normally able to provide adequate review.

There must also be evidence of robust data retention systems that permit detailed examination for surveillance and monitoring, and allow free access (with consent) for others to undertake further analysis.

Since implementation of the Medicines for Human Use (Clinical Trials) Regulations 2004, any trials that involve an investigational medicinal product (IMP), even if already licensed, require authorization by the Medicines and Healthcare Products Regulatory

Agency (MHRA). This approval is known as the Clinical Trials Authorisation (CTA). Explanation and guidance documents are available on the MHRA website.

The online Integrated Research Application System (IRAS) allows single data entry to be used to request appropriate permissions and approvals from most of the necessary regulatory bodies. The IRAS automatically identifies and generates the application for those studies that require authorization and also generates the REC form. The IRAS system is streamed so that only the necessary parts are accessed and only the appropriate permissions obtained.

However, prior to applying for CTA, the investigator is required to gain a European Union Drug Regulating Authorities Clinical Trials (EudraCT) number so that the trial information is added to the European Clinical Trials (ECT) database.

3. Health and safety

Certain aspects of research may be potentially hazardous to both participants and researchers. The potential and actual risks of using equipment, medicine, and organisms must be assessed and minimized. The Health and Safety at Work Act (1974) dictates that adherence to health and safety guidelines is a legal requirement.

4. Information

The research governance framework highlights the requirement for transparency and freedom of information, not only for the conduct of research (such as the ECT database), but also allowing public access to the final results of the research. It is therefore important that the following occur:

- Write up and submission of completed studies for peer review.
- Publication, independent of outcomes (i.e. even if negative).
- Free access to the trial results for trial subjects.
- Access to the study findings for patients for whom the conclusions are pertinent.

The provision of such open public access may be compromised by charges made by publishers for papers, but nonetheless the onus is on the authors to promulgate important results and to promote ways of using these for clinical benefit. This reflects the desire to ensure potentially beneficial results impact on patient care. Indeed, many grant review bodies require evidence that a research project has the capability of translating findings into a meaningful clinical advance, such as the development and introduction of novel medicines.

5. Finance

Financial probity, especially when public funds are being used for research, is vital. Organizations employing researchers must be in a position to compensate anyone harmed by their negligence. The financial management of intellectual property rights must also be considered.

Good clinical practice

The principles and standards that comprise Good Clinical Practice (GCP) form the basis of the implementation of the research governance framework.

Box 13.1 What is good clinical practice?

"Good clinical practice is a set of internationally recognised ethical and scientific quality requirements which must be observed for designing, conducting, recording and reporting clinical trials that involve the participation of human subjects."

Definition from EU Directive 2001/20/EC, article 1, clause 2

All those involved in research concerning patients are required to undergo regular training in GCP and to comply with its tenets. GCP defines the responsibilities and roles of the investigators, and of the sponsoring establishment.

Standard operating procedures (SOPs) are tools used to facilitate the implementation of GCP, and are usually drawn up by the sponsoring establishment to reflect local practice. Normally a research project would include SOPs for

+ serious breaches of GCP,

+ approvals of trial amendments,

+ obtaining and documenting informed consent for research, and

+ reporting adverse events (part of pharmacovigilance).

Monitoring and surveillance

Pharmacovigilance concerns the monitoring and evaluation of adverse events in patients taking part in drug trials. Investigators are responsible for recording adverse events and notifying sponsors, who in turn must report to regulatory authorities (including RECs), and generate regular safety reports. Quality control must be shown in data collection and documentation, evaluation, and reporting adverse events. The events recorded will depend on the drug used (i.e. new or established), aims of the trial and the trial patients, but should be agreed prior to commencement of the trial and contained in a SOP. Events are assessed for seriousness, causality and expectedness (Table 13.1). If possible, event reporting should maintain blinding but patient safety is paramount and takes precedence.

Local systems should be in place to ensure audit and monitoring of trial conduct. Data monitoring committees are one part of the ongoing surveillance. Regular, formally minuted research meetings act as a focal point for monitoring trial management and pharmacovigilance. All necessary documentation to allow surveillance must be kept impeccably in the Trial Master File.

A Trial Master File is required for any trial involving a drug and contains 'essential documents', which must enable both the conduct of the trial, and the quality of the data to be assessed. Essential documents would include:

+ Protocol (with inclusion and exclusion criteria)

+ Investigators' Brochure containing
  • Drug documentation (if not licensed for sale), pharmacology and efficacy, toxicity and safety, including risks and possible adverse reactions. Phase 1 trial drug information must also include preclinical data.

- Summary of Product Characteristics (SmPC) for licensed products refers to similar information including the conditions of use.
- Patient Information
- Signed Consent Form
- Financial Agreements
- Insurance Statement
- Signed Amendments (if any)
- Subject recruitment advertisement (if applicable)

Any drug trial can be externally assessed at any time by the Medicines and Healthcare Regulatory Agency's Good Clinical Practice (GCP) inspectorate, which is part of the Inspections & Standards Division of the MHRA. This inspectorate assesses the compliance of organizations conducting clinical trials using investigational medicinal products with UK and EU legislation.

The MHRA has five medicines inspectorates. The other four being

- Pharmacovigilance (GPvP) Inspectorate,
- Good Distribution Practice (GDP) Medicine Inspectorate,
- Good Laboratory Practice (GLP) Monitoring Authority, and
- Good Manufacturing Practice (GMP) Medicine Inspectorate.

After any MHRA review, a report is generated identifying any deficiencies and dictating any remedial actions required. Sanctions for breech of GCP (or any other the other areas of the inspectorates) include termination of clinical trial authorization, and could even incur criminal investigation.

Table 13.1. Definitions of various adverse events encountered in trials

Adverse event (AE)	Any untoward medical occurrence in a patient or clinical trial subject administered a medicinal product and which does not necessarily have a causal relationship with treatment (includes those in untreated control group).
Adverse reaction (AR)	Any untoward and unintended response to an investigational medicinal product related to any dose administered ('related' defined after assessment as 'reasonable causal relationship').
Unexpected adverse reaction (UAR)	An adverse reaction, the nature and severity of which is not consistent with the applicable product information. Available in the 'Investigator's Brochure', which contains clinical and non-clinical data about the investigational medical product (IMP).
Serious adverse event (SAE), serious adverse reaction (SAR), serious unexplained adverse reaction (SUSAR)	Any AE, AR, UAR that at any dose results in • death, • is life-threatening, • requires hospitalization or prolonging of existing hospitalization, • results in significant or persistent disability or incapacity, and • consists of a congenital anomaly or birth defect.

Summary

Research governance aims to facilitate the conduct of high quality, ethical scientifically valid research, while protecting both subjects and investigators. Good research governance mandates meticulous record keeping and trial surveillance, and drives a quality research culture. The Research Governance Framework explicitly sets out national standards supported by legislation for research conducted within the NHS in the United Kingdom. This document defines the roles and responsibilities of all those involved in research, and the implementation of the framework using GCP principles and SOPs. It also highlights the importance of meticulous documentation and monitoring (local and external) during any trial. These mechanisms ensure continual assessment of the quality of conduct of research and allow continuing trial development and improvement.

Further reading

Messer, J. (2006). Pharmacovigilance in clinical trials of investigational medicinal products. *Clinical Discovery* **4**, 12–13.

Jefford, M., Moore, R. (2008). Improvement of informed consent and the quality of consent documents. *Lancet Oncol* **9**(5), 485–493.

Research governance framework for health and social care: Second edition. Department of Health Publication DH_4108962. http://www.dh.gov.uk/en/Publicationsandstatistics/Publications/PublicationsPolicyAndGuidance/DH_4108962 (accessed May 6, 2009).

Implementation of the Clinical Trials Directive in the UK. MHRA http://www.mhra.gov.uk/Howweregulate/Medicines/Licensingofmedicines/Clinicaltrials/ImplementationoftheClinicalTrialsDirectiveintheUK/index.htm (accessed May 6, 2009).

Chapter 14

New interventional procedures

Carole M Longson and Mirella Marlow

Key points

- An interventional procedure (IP) is one used for diagnosis or treatment that involves incision, puncture, entry into a body cavity, or electromagnetic or acoustic energy.
- An IP should be considered *new* if a doctor no longer in a training post is using it for the first time in his or her NHS clinical practice.
- NICE IP guidance covers the safety and efficacy of the procedure, and whether special arrangements are needed for patient consent and audit.
- Randomized controlled trials are often not appropriate for evaluation of new IPs and attention must be paid to case reports and adverse events reported.
- Trusts must have clinical governance systems in place to ensure that new IPs can be introduced safely.

Introduction

Historically, unlike new pharmaceutical products which undergo rigorous routine safety and efficacy testing in the course of their development, new interventional procedures (IPs) were introduced into the National Healthcare System (NHS) without systematic testing or guidance on their use.

The balance of possible disadvantages and unproven advantages can make it difficult for both patients and clinicians to judge the risks and benefits of undergoing, or using, a new treatment.

The decision to carry out a new IP does not just lie with the clinician and patient. Healthcare trusts need to be able to decide what new procedures can safely and sensibly be offered, bearing in mind local clinical skills and facilities. This needs to be matched by the willingness of commissioners to pay for them. When considering whether to pay for novel procedures as a priority, commissioners will be interested in the potential for the intervention to improve the health of their population. Commissioners will want to be reassured that such procedures are being introduced in a managed way, with the correct infrastructure, and that they are affordable.

New IPs can lead to resource-releasing changes such as shorter lengths of hospital stay, or a lowering of the intensity of the setting in which the procedure is carried out, which may benefit both the trust and the commissioners who may want to take advantage of innovation to carry out service reconfigurations.

Table 14.1 Advantages and disadvantages of new interventional procedures

New interventional procedures	
Advantages	**Disadvantages**
Often less surgically invasive	Small evidence base
Shorter patient recovery times	Operator learning curve
Reduction in intensive care requirement	Novel devices at early development stage

As well as leading to procedures being carried out in less resource-intensive settings, it is sometimes clear that a new intervention makes use of scarce skills or resources, or needs the input of a multi-disciplinary team in order to be carried out safely, such that it should only be carried out in settings where these are available.

New IPs and techniques can therefore have a significant impact both on individual patients and on the organization of health services.

Characteristics of new interventional procedures

The Department of Health definition of a new IP is as follows:

- An IP is one used for diagnosis or treatment that involves incision, puncture, entry into a body cavity, or electromagnetic or acoustic energy.

- An interventional procedure should be considered *new* if a doctor no longer in a training post is using it for the first time in his or her NHS clinical practice.

New IPs are assessed by the National Institute for Health and Clinical Excellence (NICE) using the above definition, and usually fall into one of the following categories:

1. Minimally invasive procedures
   Techniques or instruments used to carry out procedures that were previously done via open incision. For example, laparoscopic techniques for cystectomy and pros-tatectomy, or use of endovascular stents for abdominal aortic aneurysm repair.

2. New energy sources
   Use of either a completely new energy source or more usually use of an established energy source for a new indication. Examples are photodynamic therapy techniques for skin cancer, the "gamma knife" for treatment of brain tumours, or Grenz rays for inflammatory skin conditions.

3. New devices
   Use of a new device that has been designed specifically to
   - make an existing procedure easier to perform, or potentially more effective, perhaps because access is difficult with conventional instruments or approaches,
   - allow treatment of a condition for which there was previously no comparable surgical intervention, e.g. intraocular lens insertion to correct refractive error, and
   - target more closely a specific part of the body, e.g. stereotactic radiosurgery for trigeminal neuralgia using the gamma knife.

4. New to the United Kingdom

Sometimes, a procedure is 'new' under NICE's definition just because it has not been performed in this country before. This type of innovation classically takes the form of diffusion from large, specialized centres to other hospitals, or other countries, often as a by-product of being publicized at international conferences or training sessions.

5. Newly described procedure

Sometimes clinicians simply "invent" procedures, which may bear their name.

Common to all of the above is the concept that new procedures are likely to have a different efficacy and safety profile from the comparator procedure.

The following are generally *not* considered to be new IPs:

◆ A minor modification of an established surgical technique, e.g. a minor variation in size or site of an incision.

◆ Development of a device similar to an established one (or a "me-too" device).

NICE's interventional procedures programme

The IP Programme is part of NICE's Centre for Health Technology Evaluation, and was set up in 2002 with the aim of promoting the safe introduction of efficacious, innovative procedures into the NHS. In line with its remit from the Department of Health, the programme assesses these procedures' efficacy and safety at the point at which they are about to be used for the first time outside clinical research, and issues guidance to the NHS.

This function is carried out by a NICE independent advisory body, The Interventional Procedures Advisory Committee (IPAC).

The Interventional Procedures Advisory Committee (IPAC)

The Committee is made up of 25 members, all independent of NICE and with a range of expertise. It includes

◆ clinicians who carry out interventional procedures,

◆ people who are familiar with the issues affecting patients, carers, and trusts,

◆ experts in regulation and in the evaluation of healthcare, and

◆ a representative from the medical technologies industry.

IPAC considers the evidence base for the new IP, using advice from amongst others:

◆ Specialist Advisors, who are clinicians involved in the use of the identified interventional procedure and are nominated or approved by their professional bodies such as Royal Colleges, specialist societies, and other professional associations.

◆ Patient commentators who have undergone the procedure, are the carer of someone who has done so, or have been offered the procedure and declined it.

The Committee then makes recommendations in one of four categories:

1. Use with normal arrangements for clinical governance, consent, and audit

2. Use with special arrangements for clinical governance, consent, and audit or research

3. Use only in research

4. Do not use

These recommendations bear on how the procedure should be used in relation to clinical governance, consent, and audit:

1 Where the evidence indicates the procedure is efficacious and safe, clinicians should make 'normal' arrangements for consent, audit, and clinical governance, i.e., the same arrangements they would have in place for any established procedure.

2 Where there is less evidence that the procedure is efficacious and/or safe, clinicians should notify their clinical governance leads or Medical Director and ensure when consenting the patient that they understand both general and specific uncertainties there might be about the procedure's efficacy or safety. Clinical outcomes should be audited and reviewed. NICE's guidance describes these as 'special arrangements'.

3 Sometimes a procedure's evidence base is so lacking in quantity or quality that the guidance recommends it should only be available to patients under a research protocol.

4 Occasionally there is no evidence of efficacy and/or safety – or occasionally, evidence of *lack of* efficacy or safety – and in these cases NICE's guidance prohibits use of the procedure in the NHS.

The evidence base for new interventional procedures

Randomized controlled trials (RCTs) do not provide the most relevant evidence on the efficacy and safety of a new procedure for the following reasons:

- The procedure is frequently too new for an RCT to have been conducted.
- It may be difficult to blind the technique in a meaningful way, or to develop a sham version of the procedure that would allow an RCT to be conducted ethically.
- It may be necessary to make technical modifications to procedures or the devices as experience of carrying out the IP accumulates. Modifications if carried out in the course of an RCT may fatally undermine its validity.
- RCTs are often not the best design for the identification of significant safety outcomes, which may only be available in the form of published case reports or unpublished conference abstracts.

The efficacy and safety of a new procedure can also be significantly affected by other conditions surrounding the operation, particularly the training and expertise of the surgical team, the number of procedures they have carried out, and the equipment available to them. None of this is true for conventional pharmaceutical products or the trials they undergo where RCTs offer the best evidence of efficacy. Any assessment of new procedures, such as those carried out by the NICE Interventional Procedures Programme, must therefore be capable of evaluating observational data, and of taking into account clinical advice on use of the procedure in clinical settings.

New implants or devices

Where new procedures involve an implant or device, the duration of follow-up in studies will be of great importance in the assessment of their efficacy and safety.

However, if they are being used for the first time in the NHS, follow-up is likely to be generally relatively short. The potential for deterioration or failure of an implant is of primary interest in considering the risks and benefits of a procedure. Patients need to understand whether such implants or devices are permanent, and whether 'failure' will be harmful to them and/or lead to the need for a re-operation at some point in the future. Any uncertainties about the efficacy or safety of new procedures in the short or longer term should always be discussed with patients when obtaining consent, and should reflect the current state of knowledge about the procedure and its evidence base.

Surveillance and development of the evidence base

NICE's recommendations on new procedures closely correlate with the maturity and size of the evidence base. Clinicians' audit data, registers, and other data collection exercises are of vital importance in maintaining the currency of the evidence base on new procedures as they are introduced into the NHS. Although such data collection systems are sometimes facilitated by clinicians' professional bodies or device manufacturers, there remain many new procedures for which there is no structured research study or evidence-gathering in place. National databases with well-established infrastructure, such as the UK Central Cardiac Audit Database (CCAD), are capable of providing long-term surveillance data on new interventional procedures and, in combination with other sources such as Hospital Episode Statistics (HES) data, can support NICE's reassessment of procedures in the future, with a view to making changes to recommendations if the evidence indicates this. However, even where such data collection does exist, failure to publish the results of analysis of the data means that decision-making bodies such as NICE will have difficulty reviewing follow-up data in the future.

Reports of adverse events for new interventional procedures should not simply be dismissed as anticipated side-effects: particularly for procedures with a small evidence base, adverse event reporting can add substantially to the knowledge base on safety. Operators must be aware of the arrangements for adverse event reporting locally and should ensure reported adverse events occurring during new IPs are reported to the National Reporting and Learning System (NRLS) run by the National Patient Safety Agency (NPSA). Adverse events involving equipment, or implants, should be reported to the Medicines and Healthcare Products Regulatory Agency (MHRA). The adverse event report should include the reference number of the NICE IP guidance along with the OPCS procedure code to ensure patterns of adverse events can be picked up across all centres carrying out the procedure.

If the NPSA or MHRA receives reports that give rise to serious concerns about the safety of a procedure or the device(s) used in carrying it out, they may notify the procedure to NICE, which will prompt NICE to consider assessment of it; this applies whether or not the procedure has already been the subject of guidance.

Corporate governance and new interventional procedures

An effective clinical governance structure in healthcare trusts is paramount to ensure that new interventional procedures are introduced safely. Healthcare systems have a duty to introduce innovative procedures that have been demonstrated to be of benefit to patients, and Strategic Health Authorities now have an important role in the promotion of innovation. The NICE Interventional Procedures Programme is a major element of the support necessary to introduce innovation safely, and Trusts can make use of the Programme's guidance as a focus for bringing the various elements of clinical governance together, with the aim of offering safe and efficacious treatment to patients.

The provision of innovative procedures places demands on all levels of the organization (Fig. 14.1).

Trust Boards should consider the implications of the risks and benefits of new procedures for clinical governance, risk management, medicolegal protection, and inspection. Failure to follow NICE's interventional procedures guidance is increasingly regarded as a risk for the organization.

Medical Directors need to consider the impact of innovative procedures on the requirements for advanced specialist training and revalidation, and on service design and delivery. The Medical Director and Trust Clinical Governance lead should be aware of any new procedure that is being carried out by their clinicians in their Trust.

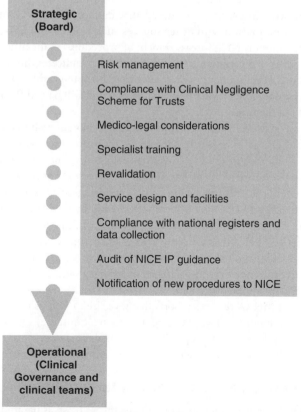

Fig. 14.1 Responsibilities of trusts offering new interventional procedures.

The safest way of ensuring this is to stipulate that clinicians about to embark on new procedures must explicitly gain the permission of their Trust to carry them out, as well as being encouraged to notify them to NICE for assessment. NICE's guidance often also makes recommendations on other conditions that are important to the safety or efficacy of the procedure, e.g. that special training is required in order to carry it out safely, or that patients being selected for the procedure should be assessed by a multi-disciplinary team.

Medical directors via the Trust's clinical governance department should

- establish a reliable means for disseminating NICE's guidance on new interventional procedures among their clinicians,
- require that clinicians inform them if they are carrying out a procedure for the first time,
- use NICE's audit support for those procedures where they are recommended,
- insist clinicians comply with national data collection exercises – particularly where this is a condition of carrying out a procedure in NICE's guidance, and
- encourage clinicians to report adverse events relating to new interventional procedures, ensuring onward reporting to the NRLS.

Auditing outcomes for new interventional procedures

Where a procedure is judged to require 'normal arrangements', outcomes should be audited locally in a standard fashion.

Where 'special arrangements' are required, NICE provides an audit tool for the purpose.

When the data on the efficacy and/or safety of a procedure are inadequate in quantity or quality, IPAC may recommend that data be collected on all patients who undergo the procedure in order to

- accrue data for future review of the guidance,
- monitor the use and dissemination of the procedure, and
- encourage audit of outcomes.

A recommendation for data collection may stipulate submission to

- an established register specific to the procedure,
- an established register which includes a number of related procedures, and
- a new register, created as a result of the IP guidance.

Before an established register is recommended, the IP Programme team confirms that

- its dataset is adequate to inform future review of guidance,
- all data required for future review will be made available to NICE,
- the register has independent clinical supervision (i.e. it is independent of commercial concerns, and is clinically supervised by a body that has the recognition and support of its clinical community), and
- data submission is likely to be practical for all clinicians involved.

No matter how the IP is categorized, all results should be audited and disseminated.

How to introduce a new interventional procedure

A clinician intending to perform a novel procedure should first check to see if NICE has already issued guidance on the procedure. If there is no guidance, they should tell their trust Medical Director or clinical governance lead about their intention. They should also notify the procedure to NICE so that it can be considered for assessment. Notifications should be made via NICE's website, which asks for basic facts about the procedure, including how it is carried out, its indications and comparators, and current evidence.

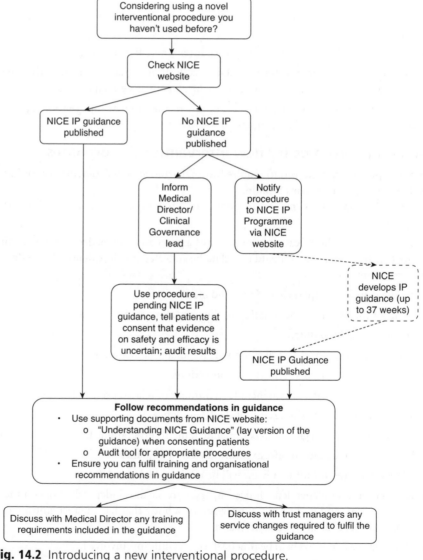

Fig. 14.2 Introducing a new interventional procedure.

Most importantly, pending the development of guidance by NICE, clinicians should only use the procedure with the 'special arrangements' set out above. The flow diagram above shows the process clinicians should follow when including a novel procedure in their own practice. They should also take account of any local arrangements for introducing new interventional procedures in their trust (Fig. 14.2).

Summary

The NICE IP Programme is intended to introduce new procedures safely into the NHS. The basic requirements for achieving this remain the same as they were when it was formally established by the Department of Health in 2003: where there are uncertainties about the evidence on a new interventional procedure, clinicians should take special care to inform their trust clinical governance lead that they are planning to undertake it, tell the patient about those uncertainties, audit and publicize their results.

Further reading

Health Service Circular 2003/011. The Interventional Procedures Programme: Working with the National Institute for Clinical Excellence to promote safe clinical innovation.

NICE Interventional Procedures Programme Process and Methods Guides (www.nice.org.uk).

Department of Health (2001). Good practice in consent implementation guide: consent to examination or treatment.

Chapter 15

Integrated care pathways

Helen Goodman

Key points

- An integrated care pathway (ICP) determines multidisciplinary locally agreed practice for a specific patient group.
- ICPs assist communication and team working by ensuring all documentation is in one place in a standardized format.
- ICPs increase the adherence to guidelines and assist effective clinical practice.
- ICPs may allow less experienced staff to care for patients whilst maintaining standards of care.
- ICPs can assist with audit of process and measurement of outcomes against agreed targets (protocols or guidelines prescribe care but do not demonstrate whether it has been achieved).

Introduction

An integrated care pathway (ICP) is an outline of the care required for a specific procedure or disease providing structured integrated documentation and consistent records.

ICPs were introduced in the United States in the 1980s driven by insurance companies demanding competitive rates for their clientele and attempts to reduce litigation costs. ICPs offered a way to both improve and maintain quality of care at lower cost through standardization, and also ensure that there is always a plan of care which can be used to track and monitor reasons for delays or complications.

ICPs are patient-centred following the patient through the healthcare episode, as opposed to profession-centred traditional clinical records, which have separate records for each discipline. Previously, as the patient came into contact with each new discipline, they were asked the same questions repeatedly; the patient may be asked their past medical history by a doctor, nurse, and physiotherapist in the course of one admission. ICPs, by integrating records, allow all staff to see the same information and so questions need only be asked and recorded once; duplication of paper and time is avoided.

ICPs are written by the multidisciplinary team (MDT) to reflect

- current best practice,
- the evidence base, and
- current guidelines.

ICPs also contain parameters and timeframes so that all members of staff know what care should take place and when, the expected outcome of care, and whether this has been achieved. ICPs, therefore, also act as educational tools and can demonstrate adherence to evidence-based guidelines.

ICPs require signatures at each stage to ensure that the care is either recorded as delivered or reported as a variance. This assists communication so that staff can see what care has been completed and what is still to be done. Moreover, planned care can be compared with actual care by analysis of variances from the ICP, and this allows for evaluation of care given and subsequent quality improvement to take place.

Advantages of ICPs include the following:

- Staff know what should be done, when, and in what order.
- Outcomes that necessitate further action are highlighted.
- Standardization of documentation layout aids finding of relevant information.
- Incorporation of approved guidelines protocols and algorithms allows less experienced staff to be able to care for the patient safely.
- Embedded alerts enable staff to know when intervention is needed.

ICPs still allow care to be individualized by deviating from the pathway as long as the clinical justification for doing so is recorded.

Integrated care pathways and safety

Healthcare systems commonly fail due to poor communication, often due to illegible notes. This can result in poor outcomes from good clinical work or technical procedures because the rest of the patients' care is not coordinated. ICPs seek to reduce communication errors by standardizing care and integrating the notes of the multidisciplinary team.

All ICPs should consider the specific risks relevant to the patient's condition, and where appropriate, the ICP should be developed in such a way so as to reduce these risks.

ICP layouts are standardized so that information can be found easily; checklists and protocols are embedded enabling each patient to receive safe care regardless of the experience of the member of staff caring for them. Each element of care is signed off, demonstrating compliance, and identifying the team member who delivered that care element.

Finally, ICPs can be used to help to continuously monitor and improve clinical quality by

- including explicit clinical standards,
- providing a standardized system for clinical record keeping,
- incorporating evidence-based guidelines for everyday practice, and
- identifying and managing risk.

Designing an ICP

The writing of the pathway, especially when a process map is drawn first, allows care to be streamlined and synchronized and ensures roles and responsibilities are clarified.

1. Select topic/area to be reviewed

Topics for ICPs are chosen generally because they are either

- high volume: the condition or procedure is one which is used frequently and with little variation in the care needed for each patient,
- high cost: there is a need to justify each element of care,
- high risk: there is a need to ensure that each member of staff involved knows their role, protocols are in place, and a clear audit trail available, or
- new guidelines or standards have been issued.

National guidance from professional bodies or organizations, such as the National Institute for Clinical Excellence (NICE), often contain evidence-based guidance for ensuring safe and effective care, and this should be included in local care pathways.

2. Set up a multidisciplinary steering group

It is vital to hold meetings with representatives of each of the multi-disciplinary teams involved in the care of the specific patient group. This allows the scope and objectives of the pathway to be agreed by all teams and prevents unnecessary duplication. The exact composition of the steering group will vary depending on the topic and targets for the ICP. Often it is useful to include someone from finance or clinical audit, and if there is the possibility of the pathway having an electronic format, an information technology team member should be involved from the start to understand the users' requirements. Due to the technical nature of most ICPs, it may not be appropriate to have a patient on the steering group, nonetheless, where there are appropriate patient and public involvement groups or forums they should be asked if they would like to be involved.

3. Agree project lead

The project lead, or leads, must be clinically credible and influential, frequently a consultant or nurse, but may be another member of the MDT depending on the pathway (e.g. a physiotherapist for pulmonary rehabilitation, or radiographer for radiofrequency ablations). The leads must commit to promoting the pathway to colleagues, and to being involved in the implementation process.

4. Process map the topic/procedure

Before the pathway is written, it is important to review the current service. Mapping the process helps the MDT review where potential risks, duplication of work, bottlenecks, or time wasting occur. The care pathway can then be clarified, or redesigned, as part of the pathway writing process. Process maps allow people to see what their job is and how their work fits in with the work of others in the system. Fig. 15.1 is an example of part of a process map for cardiac surgery. It includes the process, actions, and the decisions needed.

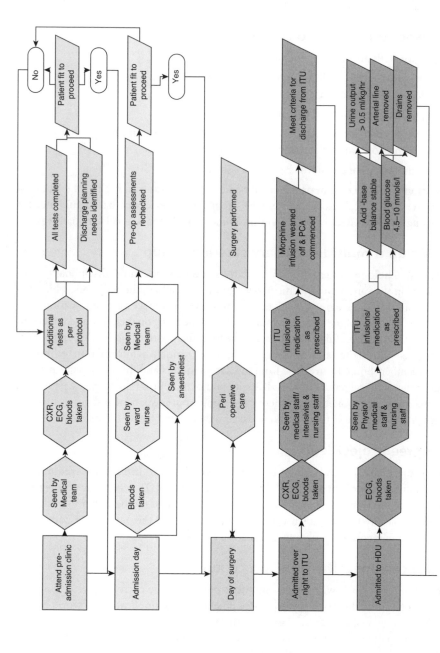

Fig. 15.1 An example of a process map for cardiac surgery.

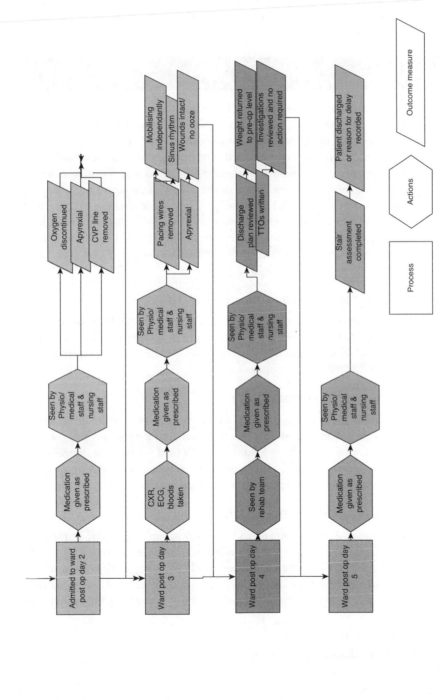

Fig. 15.1 Cont'd

5. Define objectives and indicators for specific topic

Specific measurable objectives with targets for achievement should be identified that will show the value of the pathway in improving care. A baseline audit of these indicators or outcomes should be carried out so that the effectiveness of the ICP can subsequently be measured.

Box 15.1

Example: A team set out to write a pathway for chronic heart failure patient admissions. NICE guidance states that these patients should be prescribed a beta blocker, loop diuretic, and ACE inhibitor. Baseline audit showed that this information was not recorded routinely in the medical record. The team designed the new pathway to record if the patient was prescribed these medications and if not, why not. Re-audit occurred following introduction of the ICP. This demonstrated that all 3 medications were now prescribed in 85% of patients, or had a reason recorded as to why it was not appropriate (9%). The remaining 6% of patients did not have the medication prescribed, nor a reason why not recorded. This was fed back to the ward staff to seek further improvement.

---

6. Gather and review available information

Establish what paperwork, polices, and data are available locally, and in other centres, so as to reduce duplication and 're-inventing the wheel'. It is important to review what national standards, NICE and specialist society guidelines, and relevant research data need to be included in the ICP.

7. Produce a draft care pathway

The care pathway should be clear, precise, and guide the user easily through each step of the patient journey. The focus should be on the needs of the patients and users of the service rather than those of the individual disciplines. Realistic goals, timeframes, and measurable outcomes should be included, and made explicit, to ensure variance or deviance from the pathway is captured at each stage.

8. Write a supporting action plan

The multi-disciplinary steering group needs to identify actions required to implement and review the care pathway together with relevant timescales and inception dates. Some actions may be as basic as deciding where the ICP is going to be kept, or where it will be filed. Frequently staff are used to keeping separate notes, and so it is essential that the pathway is easily accessible and that all staff know its location. Other things to consider are:

◆ Training in the use of the ICP
◆ Education about changes to care as a result of the ICP

- Writing new patient information leaflets
- Writing new patient group directives
- Running initial pilots
- Review and evaluation strategy

9. Consult with stakeholders, practitioners, and users

Circulate the draft pathway as widely as possible to inform people of its content, but also to ensure it has been looked at from as many perspectives as possible, and that no groups have been overlooked. Aim to include patient involvement in this process if they are not represented on the steering group. ICPs also support other departments such as clinical coding, and audit, and it is therefore important to ask them to check the documents to ensure that information will be collected in a meaningful way.

10. Implementation

Once the planned training, education, and publicity has been carried out in accordance with the action plan the implementation can commence. Ensure that the start date is widely advertised.

11. Evaluation and review

Review compliance and gain user feedback, both formally and informally, soon after the introduction of the ICP, as it is often not until the document is in use that problems become apparent.

Also review the ICP in relation to

- process,
- content,
- previously agreed targets and outcomes, and
- variance.

The results of all audits and feedback sessions should be reported to the steering committee and appropriate changes made. The steering committee should regularly review any newly published evidence, guidelines, or standards, and the pathway revised appropriately.

12. Maintenance and dissemination

After the initial pilot, pathways would be expected to run for a year prior to review unless there are major changes affecting care in the interval.

Variance analysis and measurement of outcomes

The pathway is more than a record of clinical care. The information obtained through variance analysis can be used to review and improve standards of care.

Variance

- ◆ Is any variation from an entry set out in an Integrated Care Pathway document?
- ◆ Can be positive or negative? A positive variance might be a length of stay shorter than expected.
- ◆ Can be used to evaluate and improve care?
- ◆ Is one element unique and essential to all ICP documents; by contrast, protocols or guidelines prescribe care but do not demonstrate that it has been delivered?

When care has taken place as planned the pathway is signed, but if there is a variance a 'V' for variance is placed in the signature box and the variance coded. The code for the action can then be used to write a variance report. An example of the recording of variance can be found in Fig. 15.2. All ICPs should have a mechanism to undertake regular analysis of variations.

Variance analysis

- ◆ Is a mechanism for determining the impact of variation in care.
- ◆ Allows the ICP to be used as a tool to support clinical governance and audit.
- ◆ Allows changes to the ICP to be evaluated.

The ICP will also have specific targets or outcome measures set within it. Not all variances need to be included in each review of the ICP, but it is important that attainment of targets or outcomes should be reported, so that staff can assess how well they have achieved the planned care.

No:	Name:	Stage 2 of Assisted Discharge Pathway	AM	-PM	code
TESTS	Weight checked		*HG*	*HG*	2.0
RESP.	Sputum clear		V	V	3.0
	Respiratory rate and SAO_2 within normal limits		*HG*	V	3.1
	Breathing pattern acceptable to the patient		*HG*	*HG*	3.2

Code	Variance record	Sign
3.0 3.1	Sputum thick and green, sample sent to lab for analysis Oxygen saturations dropped from 96% to 92%, doctor informed and deep breathing exercises encouraged. To be re-assessed in 2 hours	*HG*

Fig. 15.2 An example of ICP record completed with signatures and variances.

Box 15.2

Variance analysis of an ICP for cardiac surgery demonstrated variances in 6 out 25 patients having post-operative day 5 mobility assessments. This led to delayed hospital discharge of these patients. The reason given was that these assessments were due at the weekend when no physiotherapists were available on the ward. Following discussion with the physiotherapy team, physiotherapists based in the intensive care unit at the weekend were made available to carry out these ward assessments to allow the patients to be discharged.

Common concerns encountered

◆ 'Pathways stop the staff from thinking from themselves.'
There are some pathways produced that do nothing to improve patient care. The challenge is to write pathways that provide guidance, whilst also giving a template for the care that most patients with that condition, or procedure, are expected to have.

◆ 'ICPs replace clinical judgement'
All ICPs include a statement that this is not the intention. ICPs are intended as a guide to providing care for patients and their families. Professionals are encouraged to exercise their own judgement, but any deviation, or removal from the ICP, must be recorded as a variance and justified.

◆ 'An ICP wouldn't work here: all the patients are different.'
Start initially with a process map and see if there are areas which can be standardized, such as the admission documentation. It is a good idea to start with either a high-volume patient procedure or one where the most errors occur.

◆ 'Are care pathways legal documents?'

ICPs meet all legal requirements for record keeping as long as they are completed according to standard record keeping guidelines, i.e. the patient's name, and the date of entry, appear on all pages. It is good practice to include an accountability log (a record of names and signatures/initials) at the beginning of each pathway so that individuals providing the care can be easily identified from their signatures or initials.

Summary

In order to achieve successful ICP implementation, vision and organizational commitment from both senior managers and staff in all departments and disciplines is essential. Good clinical leadership for individual pathways, as well as a feeling of ownership by the staff using the pathways, is the key to success. Each pathway must have a team dedicated to its development and facilitation and there must be continual education and information dissemination, usually using workshops and training programmes, to keep up with constantly changing staff. Successfully designed and implemented ICPs improve the quality and safety of patient care.

Further reading

Integrated care pathways, http://www.medicine.ox.ac.uk/bandolier/painres/download/whatis/What_is_an_ICP.pdf.

Layton, A., Morgan, G., Mchardy, G., Allision, L. (2002). *How to Successfully Implement Clinical Pathways: A Step by Step Guide*. Kingsham: London.

Middleton, S., Roberts, A. (2000). *Integrated Care Pathways: A Practical Approach to Implementation*. Butterworth Heinemann: London.

Nicola Davis (ed.). *Integrated Care Pathways: A Guide to Good Practice*, http://www.wales.nhs.uk/sites3/Documents/245/ICPGGP.pdf.

de Luc, K. (2001). *Developing Care Pathways: the Handbook*. Radcliffe Medical Press: Oxford.

Section 3

Strategic effectiveness

The safety of patients within a Trust is the responsibility of its leaders (*Trust Board*), who set the agenda for the organization (*Strategy and strategic planning*) and are accountable for its safe operation. The Board needs to understand and buy into the fact that enhancing patient safety is a strategic and financial imperative in the post-Darzi era (*Capacity, efficiency, and targets*). Effective clinical governance and thus high-quality patient care, within a Trust will depend upon clinical engagement at all levels (*Service provision*) and a framework to support the delivery of safe, effective healthcare (*Policies and procedures*). A structured approach to quality improvement can bring significant benefits to both the process and outcome of care and current techniques have been adapted from other industries with success (*Quality improvement*). To ensure this all occurs, Performance Management systems will need to be in place.

Chapter 16

The Trust Board

Paul Williams OBE

Key points

- The Board ensures that the organization is fit for purpose to deliver its key objectives and overall vision
- Boards comprise a Chair, non-executive directors, and executive directors, who must all operate as a cohesive unit
- The culture of the organization is set by the Board
- Trust Boards must be able to demonstrate the seven key standards of public life: selflessness, integrity, objectivity, accountability, openness, honesty, and leadership
- Board functions can be divided into five key areas: strategy, risk, performance management, information, and relationships

Board structure and roles

First, and foremost, NHS Trusts are legally constituted, publicly funded bodies, responsible for providing safe and sustainable services within the resources made available to them. These responsibilities are discharged through the Board, consisting of executive and non-executive directors.

	Non-executive directors	Executive directors
Appointed by	Ministers of State	Non-executive directors
Duration of term	Fixed term	Variable
Contract	Part-time	Full-time
Required to	Provide checks and balances	Run organization
Example	Chair	Chief executive (CEO)

Although Board members have different levels of responsibility and skills, there is no legal distinction between the Board duties of executive and non-executive directors.

Sub-committees

It is usual for Boards to set up a number of sub-committees to handle the key areas of business of the organization. These committees go into a level of detail of Board business that cannot possibly be considered within the time available at a full Board

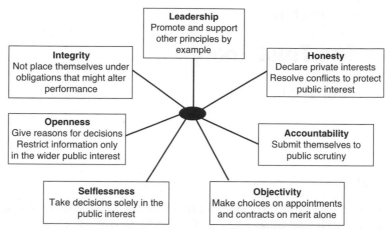

Fig. 16.1 The seven general principles of conduct in public life.

meeting. An important committee required of all Boards is the audit committee. This provides an overarching view of the organization's financial health, ensuring that there is sound financial stewardship and effective planning. In many Trusts, audit committees have now taken on the broader role of controls assurance, i.e. they are the primary Board committee overseeing risk management and general governance. For any health organization, clinical risks will be a significant area of concern, and the arrangements by which Boards receive assurance on this critical area can vary. Some Boards have a sub-committee responsible for clinical (increasingly termed as healthcare) governance.

Boards, as public bodies, are expected to behave in an exemplary fashion. The Nolan Committee on *Standards in Public Life* (1995) defined the seven general principles of conduct which should underpin public life (Fig. 16.1).

Roles

Executive and non-executive directors have specific roles, but it is vital that they work together as a cohesive team.

The Chair is responsible for the performance and development of the Board, probity and holding the Chief Executive to account. He/she also has an ambassadorial role. *The Non-Executive Directors* (NEDs), working with the Chair, will take particular responsibility for:

- Accountability
- Governance
- Performance
- Learning and development

The accountability for the organization's performance ultimately rests with the *chief executive* who acts as the *Accountable Officer* and is responsible for setting:

- The direction of the organization
- Service delivery
- Governance

- Performance management
- Communications
- Connecting with the whole organization
- Advising the Board

Executive Directors have defined responsibilities for leading specific aspects of the business of the Trust. These will vary between Trusts, but will include: medical and nursing directors, and directors of operation, finance, communication and governance.

The chief executive will rely on executive director colleagues to carry significant responsibility on the delivery of performance in their particular areas. It is therefore important that the executive directors operate as a team.

The relationship between the chair and the chief executive is of paramount importance, and it is critical that the difference between the non-executive role of the Chair and the executive role of the CEO is understood.

Board functions

The functions of the Board can be divided into five key areas:

- Strategy
- Risk
- Performance management
- Information
- Relationships

Strategy

A plan or course of action leading to the allocation of an organization's scarce resources over time, to reach identified goals.

Setting the direction of the organization requires the development of well thought out strategies and service plans. These must make best use of the organization's resources: financial, workforce, capital, information and intellectual properties. Once these plans are developed into a coherent strategy, the focus of direction for the organization should be set. Clearly this is easier said than done, and first and foremost there must be clarity on the purpose and vision for the organization. This, together with a careful analysis of the key issues confronting the organization, will lead the Board to set objectives for the organization and to produce plans and actions in order to deliver them. These plans and strategies cannot be developed in isolation, and the Board will be responsible for ensuring key staff (especially clinical staff) and partner organizations are engaged fully in this process.

Effective Boards will develop a corporate culture where there is a shared vision within the organization of:

- What needs to be done
- How it will be done

- When it will be done
- Who will do it

It is important to remember that strategy cannot be divorced from the day to day operational efficiency of an organization and service quality; this is how care is measured and provided to patients. A high level of efficiency must be regarded as the norm. Well-run organizations have effective strategies to ensure the delivery of the overall objectives of the organization. They provide sufficient resources to allow empowered clinical teams to provide consistently high standards of care, improve services, and drive innovation.

Michael Gerber says of organizations: 'If everybody is working *in* the organisation who is working *on* the organisation'. To be successful the Board must ensure the organization is fit for purpose, and able to deliver its key objectives and overall vision.

Strategies, therefore, must take into account the environment in which hospital Trusts operate, and in particular their interface with primary care Trusts, key partners, (including commissioners, social services and the voluntary sector) and the community they serve.

Risk: from both internal and external factors

Every action has a consequence and Trusts face a wide range of risks:

- Strategic
- Operational
- Financial

These may prevent them from achieving their objectives. Successful organizations will have an effective risk strategy, identifying all the risks that may confront them. This does not require a catalogue of every possible thing that could go wrong, nor should it cause decisions to be avoided. It is about ensuring that:

- Key risks are identified and managed (so service to patients continues improving)
- When things do go wrong, the risk is minimized and lessons are learned to avoid recurrence

In order to do this, Boards set in place mechanisms to ensure risk management is embedded in the organization through appropriate processes and structures. Risks may be clinical in nature, or relate to finance, systems, information, staff, buildings etc. When things go wrong, this may result in litigation. In 2006 an NHS Trust was prosecuted and convicted of corporate manslaughter, 3 years after 2 doctors were convicted of negligence. This resulted from the decision that the Trust had failed to manage and supervise the doctors. The precedent that Board members can be identified as 'the controlling mind' responsible for the negligence was thus laid. In addition to legal ramifications, incidents can (and do) affect the way in which the organization is viewed within the wider community. A Trust, which has a poor reputation, is hardly likely to engender confidence in its patients, its staff or indeed its partners.

Performance management

The Board needs to satisfy itself that the organization is delivering its key objectives. Such targets may be set by:

+ Government
+ Commissioners
+ The Board itself

These objectives will cover a wide range of areas including performance on waiting times, infection control rates, financial performance, and workforce matters. There are a variety of key performance indicators and critical success factors which need to be mapped to do this.

Clearly the Board has the potential to be overburdened with data that does not add value. To avoid this, Boards will agree what data needs to be considered routinely and what should be considered on an exceptional reporting basis. Some organizations, recognizing the importance of integrating fields of data, use a balanced scorecard approach to measure performance across a range of indicators. The balanced scorecard recognizes that strong performance in one area is unlikely to be sustained if there are poor performances across other key areas of a Trust's operation. Adopting this approach ensures improvement across a whole range of areas and does lead to sustained improvement.

Information

Information is the life blood of any organization. For the Board to discharge its responsibilities effectively, the information that it receives must be accurate and timely. The Board must also be satisfied it has:

+ The right information – to set the strategic direction and ensure plans are being achieved
+ Good quality information – providing evidence to support options for action

This significantly reduces the risk of taking decisions that either fail to meet the objectives of the organization or that will have unintended consequences.

Due to the nature of the service provided by Trusts, the importance of the Board receiving sound professional advice is critical. It is for this reason that Boards are required by law to have executive directors qualified in medicine, nursing, and finance. The Board will look to the executive directors to provide them with key information, required to demonstrate it is discharging its responsibilities. The Board will normally establish a set of key indicators allowing it to monitor both qualitative and quantitative aspects of the services for which it is ultimately responsible. Information technology systems have not had a good reputation for delivering what was claimed of them, and have often led to costly over-runs and disappointment at outcomes. In view of the importance of timely information and robust information technology systems, the Board will wish to satisfy itself that it has effective plans and regular reports on this important area of its function.

Relationships: internal and external

Effective communication, supported by an effective communication strategy, will be key to establishing a dialogue with clinicians, staff, managers, professional organizations, and advisory committees. The best form of communication is face to face. It is therefore essential that the chairman, chief executive, executive directors, and non-executive directors are visible and approachable within the organization. The importance of effective communication strategies cannot be overestimated.

As Boards are public bodies, it is important they make decisions in an open and transparent way. They are required to meet in public and anyone is entitled to attend. This is done routinely, through an annual general meeting (AGM). It is good practice, as part of induction and development, for clinicians to attend the Board and get to know the executive and non-executive directors. In many organizations, non-executive directors spend time getting around the organization, meeting clinical staff within their own departments as part of their function of being the eyes and ears of the chairman.

The Board is ultimately responsible for setting the culture of the organization and how it is seen by others. It therefore needs to manage its external relationships with key partners including:

- Commissioners, including Health authorities and GPs
- Neighbouring Trusts
- Local authorities
- Voluntary organizations
- Local and national politicians
- The media: ensuring that stories are covered fairly and accurately and that the Trust uses the media in a positive way, rather than reacting when negative stories appear

Underpinning this is the need for the Board to establish a dialogue with the people it serves, and to whom it has a direct accountability. To make this real, Boards will set in place mechanisms that welcome both positive and negative feedback on its services (e.g. thanks and complaints), and arrangements to consult with service users and the public on the services it provides and any plans to change these.

Summary

The Board determines the strategic direction for an organization, and is responsible for the day to day performance and culture of the organization. Boards which fail in this, not only fail their organization but also the people they are there to serve. It is therefore imperative that clinicians, who form a critical component of the organization, know what is going on at Board level and form an integral part of its working.

Trust Boards then can make a significant difference to the way healthcare is provided in setting a clear direction, making sure the staff and other resources are available to meet the objectives of the organization, and ensuring value for money and risks are managed. This is a hugely challenging role that is made easier when there is clinical leadership and involvement.

Further reading

Gerber, M.E. (2003). *The E-Myth Physician: Why Most Medical Practices Don't Work and What To Do about It*. HarperCollins. ISBN 0-06-621469-6.

Kaplan, R.S., Norton, D.P. (2001). *The Strategy-Focused Organization: How Balanced Scorecard Companies Thrive In The New Business Environment*. Harvard Business School Press. ISBN 1-57851-250-6.

The Committee on Standards in Public Life Homepage. http://www.public-standards.gov.uk/ (last accessed May 2010).

Chapter 17

Strategy and strategic planning: Setting the direction at a Trust level

Gareth Goodier

Key points

- Strategic planning should reduce risk and increase benefits to patients.
- The Trust Board is responsible for setting the strategic direction.
- Divisions, directorates, and departments should align their plans to the Trust plan, focusing on how to achieve the Trust's vision and mission.
- Clinicians and stakeholder engagement is essential for successful strategic planning.
- Strategic planning helps assist in the prioritization of investments for new services, equipment, and buildings.

Introduction

Whether robbing banks, walking to the centre of Antarctica, or winning an Olympic gold medal, it helps to underpin ambition with some key objectives and an understanding of the strategies required to achieve these. Better still if it is written down as a plan. And so it is with a health service. The larger the organization and more complex the service, the more difficult to ensure cohesive team behaviour and prioritize the next investment; the greater the need for a strategic plan.

The strategic plan will identify the ambition or vision of the organization over a period of 2–10 years, detailing how that ambition might be achieved. It sets the direction of travel for the organization. Each department or service should develop their own strategic plan, but these must be informed and guided by the overall Trust strategic plan. In a similar way, the Trust plan must reflect the NHS plan and government policy. This represents a hierarchy of governance, with each service aligning its future to the NHS plan.

Establishing a strategy and a strategic plan is one of the key responsibilities of the Board. Enterprise governance is 'the set of responsibilities and practices exercised by the Board and management with the goal of providing strategic direction, ensuring that objectives are achieved, ascertaining that risks are managed appropriately and verifying that the organisations resources are used responsibly'.

Supporting enterprise governance are a number of processes and structures shown in the figure below:

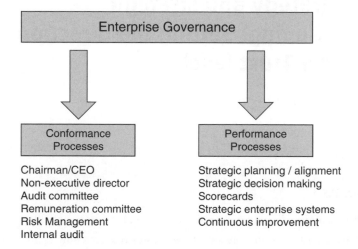

Because the physical life span of a hospital building is usually at least 25 years, the planning process is often required to anticipate the future of clinical services for a period of 10–20 years. Obviously, the more distant the prediction, the less accurate it is.

Poor strategic planning can be very wasteful. In recent years the NHS has wasted millions of pounds by not fully anticipating the move towards:

♦ Ambulatory care and day surgery

♦ Day of surgery admissions

♦ The reduction in the length of stay (LOS)

As a consequence, the number of beds built in some areas has been excessive; average LOS remains long and clinical teams do not have the appropriate fabric to care for patients in the most efficient and effective way.

Each pound spent on healthcare has an opportunity cost. A pound wasted is a pound that could otherwise have been spent on patient care. All staff must understand the importance of good strategic planning. Ultimately, the strategic direction of clinical services can only be determined by clinicians.

Unfortunately, all too many strategic plans remain dormant upon an executive's bookshelf. The aim of the strategic planning process is to have an active plan; one that informs and guides many of the decisions of a health service. In a good organization, every:

♦ Job description would place each staff position within the context of the overall vision and purpose of the service

♦ Investment decision would fit within the priorities of the strategic plan

The generic language and vocabulary of strategic planning is that of a management tool; a tool that has been used in many industries for several decades. Experience shows that clinical staff often prefer to adopt a lexicon reflecting a health environment and culture. It is important that the language used in planning documents is owned by clinical staff and reflects their culture.

The elements of a strategic plan

Typically the strategic planning process will identify and define the Trust's:

Vision: The desired future state the Trust is trying to achieve; its ambition. It should stretch the service to achieve its very best (e.g. be the best academic health science centre in Europe).
The vision statement should be ambitious but realistic. It should inspire and motivate staff to want to achieve difficult objectives, even if the early steps are painful or require a relative redistribution of resources.

Mission: The purpose or primary function of the Trust (e.g. Cambridge University Hospital's: 'innovation and excellence in health and care'). The mission statement must represent the views of a large section of the organization.

Strategic objectives: These are the overarching, intended outcomes, or the goals of the Trust (e.g. to be recognized as a top 5 NHS hospital within 5 years). Typically there are 4–10 strategic objectives, and they should be:

◆ General and broad
◆ Related to a single topic
◆ Specific and measurable within a time frame
◆ Challenging but achievable

Strategies: The actions describing what the Trust has to do to achieve a strategic objective. For each strategic objective, there might be 4–10 strategies.

The strategies are usually accompanied by a set of *metrics* to measure progress. Possible examples are shown in the table below.

Values: The core behaviours and beliefs that staff should uphold (e.g. Cambridge University Hospital's 'kind, safe and excellent').

Objectives	Strategies	Potential metrics
Become a top 5 NHS hospital	Clinical outcomes	Standardized mortality ratio < 80 MRSA < 10 cases/year
	Patient experience	Score > 8.8 on National survey
	Value for money	Average length of stay better than upper quartile
Achieve upper quartile in-patient lengths of stay	Ensure no significant delays in diagnostic processes	All CT scan in-patient requests performed in < 6 h

The importance of culture, behaviours and values in driving performance

The best-performing organizations have a positive culture; one in which staff feel supported, engaged, and valued. An organization's culture reflects the 'way things are done here' and is based upon behaviours and values. Staff should feel that:

◆ Their suggestions and feedback are taken seriously: they control their own destiny

◆ They are empowered to perform at their best within a strong culture of team working

◆ Decisions are based upon objective problem solving: facts and logic, rather than politics and hierarchy

Most strategic plans reflect a values statement the Trust aspires to uphold. It would be easy for a leadership team to list their perceived values for the organization in a matter of minutes, but that misses the point. All staff must have the opportunity to affect the values statement. The process of gathering and understanding the values driving an organization, and distilling them into one short statement is time-consuming (often taking a year). It is typically done as a separate, parallel piece of work by a team representing a cross-section of staff. It is both a reflection of what currently happens, but also what needs to be strengthened within the culture of the Trust. Once the values have been determined it is useful to establish a set of desired behaviours.

The benefits of a successful strategic plan

A successful strategic plan will focus and formalize thinking about the future, and engage as many staff and stakeholders as possible. This will:

◆ Enable better teamwork, communication, and ownership of future developments, be they services or buildings

◆ Assist in the prioritization of investment in new services and equipment

◆ Foster a culture of cooperation and collaboration, rather than political intrigue and unhealthy competition

◆ Help individual staff members understand their role in the big picture

The very process of trying to anticipate the future and develop the direction of travel brings disparate departments together, building a cohesive, collaborative team culture with a common view of the future.

The role of stakeholders in developing a strategic plan

The process must engage with a variety of stakeholders. For example, a teaching hospital may well include the following stakeholders (by no means an exhaustive list) in the planning process:

◆ Strategic health authority (SHA)

◆ Specialist commissioners (e.g. national or regional commissioners purchasing complex patient care, such as heart transplants)

◆ Leading primary care trusts (PCTs)

- Other organizations providing care in the community (e.g. non-governmental and charitable agencies delivering hospice care)
- Local district general hospitals (DGHS)
- Local clinical networks (e.g. cancer networks)
- Universities and other organizations training, educating, or developing staff
- Ambulance services
- County or borough councils
- Patient representative groups
- Regional economic growth and development organizations
- Local business representatives

The engagement process should be positive and seen as an opportunity to build stronger relationships and a wider understanding of the broader community.

The difference between strategic thinking and strategic planning

Mintzberg's work (1994) exposed one of the major weaknesses of strategic planning: planners simply extrapolate dots on a graph, extending the trend line. Strategic planning also demands lateral and innovative strategic thinking:

- *Strategic planning* is about analysis: breaking objectives down into steps, formalizing those steps and articulating the expected consequences
- *Strategic thinking* is about synthesis: involving intuition and creativity

Clinical examples of new 'disruptive' treatments or technologies having an impact upon health service development have occurred and are likely to continue to do so:

- Significant changes in treatments occurred during the last few decades with the introduction of thrombolysis and then interventional cardiology. This has resulted in a reduction in coronary artery bypass graft surgery
- Looking forward, if an intervention to prevent premature labour were discovered, the need for neonatal intensive care cots (and support services of neonatologists and nurses) would reduce more than 30% almost overnight

All changes of this nature are best anticipated and reflected by clinicians within the strategic planning process.

The elements of a strategic plan and how to develop them

Developing a strategic plan requires central control and facilitation, whilst capturing the creative input from a diverse number of staff and stakeholders. Often large organizations have an executive with specific responsibility for strategic planning.

The process cannot be rushed if a meaningful outcome is to be achieved, but the timeline is important. Typically the process (shown in Fig 17.1) will take 9–12 months to complete. The process should be run as a project with:

- Set objectives
- A detailed timeline for outcomes

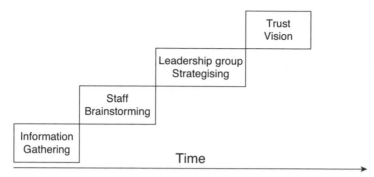

Fig. 17.1 The strategic planning process.

Information gathering

This involves gathering current data including demographics, clinical service changes, costs, trends, research articles on breaking technologies, government policies, clinical frameworks, service standards, clinical network documents, and regional and national plans.

Staff brainstorms

Gather together a large number of staff (especially clinical) and stakeholders to review the current environment and to brainstorm the future, an Environmental Scan (ES). This group can consist of volunteers or they can be handpicked, but must reflect a diverse cross-section of the Trust.

Some organizations choose to run several focus groups; others enjoy one large session of environmental scanning. If time permits, one large group should establish the key issues for discussion and then use focus groups to examine issues in more detail.

Some organizations develop specific scenarios of the future to help with the creative side of innovative strategic thinking. For example, examining the worst-case, best-possible, and most-likely scenarios.

Each clinical service/department must develop a clinical strategic plan that gives the broader strategic planning group some insight into the developments on the horizon for that service. It is essential that clinicians take a leadership role.

The usual problem is that each service will develop a plan requiring a significant increase in investment. When all clinical departmental plans are collated, the clinical leadership must prioritize the proposed developments into a single clinical strategic plan for the Trust. This process determines the clinical priorities for the Trust.

It is useful for staff and patients to give feedback via the focus groups on subjects such as:

◆ What is working well
◆ What is not working well
◆ What are the opportunities for improvement

Typically, all groups should consider the ES under a set of systematic headings such as:

+ Social/demographic/lifestyle/values/markets
+ Technology/information systems
+ Scientific
+ Economic
+ Political, including government policies
+ Health services

There are various possible methodologies to follow in an ES. It is, in essence, used to scan the global, national, regional, and local environments in a systematic way. The expectation is that the process will:

+ Identify new and emerging trends
+ Give an early warning of impending problems or difficulties
+ Maximize opportunities by identifying developments earlier than competitors
+ Enable the team driving the strategic planning process to understand current and potential changes taking place within their Trust and the external environment
+ Promote a future orientation in the thinking of both the leadership team and staff

The most famous methodology is the SWOT analysis. This is an exercise evaluating both the internal strengths and weaknesses of the organization as well as the opportunities and threats imposed by the external environment. Examples are shown in the table below.

Internal	
S	*Strengths*: Good brand/reputation, e.g. best outcomes for transplant patients Superior technology, e.g. imaging, Da Vinci robotics Close links to other units, e.g. 5* medical research, strong university
W	*Weaknesses*: Poor information systems Excessive political in-fighting, poor leadership Expensive area to live, with associated recruitment difficulties
External	
O	*Opportunities*: Strong brand with opportunities to increase private practice Laboratory innovations with potential commercial spin-offs PCT provider interested in joint polyclinic venture
T	*Threats*: PCT encouraging private sector to take over day-case work Too many local hospitals/beds

The issues that arise are fed back into the next stage of the process.

Leaders strategize

The Board of Directors is responsible for the outcomes of the whole process. Leadership of the strategic planning group is important but it is also important to have a diversity of opinion to achieve the best outcome. The frisson between differing opinions can help the creativity and innovation required.

It is worth pausing to consider the characteristics of innovative thinkers. They are more often:

- Younger rather than older
- Not necessarily found on the Board of Directors nor at the head of a department
- Rather challenging and difficult personalities

The key issue is to know who they are and where they exist within the health service.

Trust vision and mission

Having considered the ES, the strategic planning group develops the vision, mission, objectives, strategies, and values. At each stage, the outcomes of the deliberations are communicated to the larger group (if possible, all staff) asking for comments and feedback. Experience shows that staff will not implement a strategic plan they:

- Do not understand
- Are not committed to

The language of these statements is important. It must be clear to all, i.e. simple. The length of statements is also important. It is desirable that all staff can remember statements and understand where their job fits into the Trust's vision and mission.

An example from an leading site is Cincinnati Children's hospital:

Vision: To be the leader in improving child health

Mission: Cincinnati Children's will improve child health and transform the delivery of care through fully integrated, globally recognized research, education and innovation.

For patients from our community, the nation and the world, the care we provide will achieve the best:

- Medical care and quality of life outcomes
- Patient and family experience
- Value

Today and in the future

It is often difficult in health services to keep these statements short because of the tripartite mission of patient services, education, and research. Cincinnati has achieved this by focusing upon outcomes, experience, and value for all aspects of the mission they are referring to.

The leadership group of the strategic plan then identifies and develops objectives and strategies. The whole plan must then be presented to all staff and processes developed to ensure that as many staff as possible understand the key components of the plan.

When to do a strategic plan and how often to refresh

A Trust must complete a strategic planning process at the commencement of a new organization or when there is a new major initiative, e.g. a significant new building or service. It is normal to completely review a strategic plan at least every 3 years and refresh it every 1–2 years.

The difficulties and limitations of strategic planning

Many of the difficulties and limitations in formulating a strategic plan have been covered. Others not yet mentioned include:

- Gaining the support and engagement of the clinical staff, determining which clinical specialties are the priority for development and investment during the next 5–10 years
- Significant changes in government policy
- Limited access to major capital expenditure
- Political interventions overriding due process

Summary

The Board sets the strategic direction for the Trust, taking into account information and views from all stakeholders. Staff and patients are crucial in this, but information must also be sought from external sources.

Further reading

Williamson, S., Stevens, R.E., Loudon, D.L., Migliore, R.H. (1997). *Fundamentals of Strategic Planning for Healthcare Organizations*. The Haworth Press. ISBN 0-7890-0060-1.

Davis, J.A., Savage, G., Stewart, R.T. (2003). Organizational downsizing: a review of literature for planning and research. *J Healthcare Manage* **48**(3), 181–199.

Schreter, R.K. (1998). Reorganizing the departments of psychiatry, hospitals, and medical centers for the 21st century. *Psychiatr Serv* **49**(11), 1429–1433.

Chapter 18

Putting the business into the NHS

Heather Shearer

Key points

- The NHS needs to be responsible with taxpayers' money.
- Contracts signed between commissioners and providers contain both quality and quantity targets.
- Understanding and managing variation in patient flows has a significant impact upon the efficiency of a service.
- Services need to find cost efficiencies every year.
- Focusing on high-quality, safe services can reduce costs and increase efficiency.

Balancing financial considerations and healthcare needs

In tax-funded systems such as the NHS, it is important that money is used wisely: tax payers can be viewed as customers. NHS services are accountable to the public for the judicious use of funds. Government and government-bodies (e.g. Audit Commission, Quality Care Commission), and wider democratic processes of local and general elections provide the mechanisms for this accountability.

Successive recent governments have emphasized the position of the patient as 'customer', and used market levers as a method to improve the quality of healthcare services. It is arguable whether these levers are the only, or most effective, approach to achieve this end. Policies including patient choice and a national tariff (payment by activity) to facilitate that choice are designed to give healthcare providers an incentive to make their services as attractive and efficient as possible. Moreover, contracts with private providers and experiments with primary care provision have created competition between providers.

Some key 'market' policy areas

The more recent introduction of 'Quality Accounts' and 'Commissioning for Quality and Innovation' are an attempt to add strong quality levers into the market policies. These levers include the cost of non-payment for episodes of care where a patient experiences certain adverse safety events.

Patient Choice – emphasizing the role of the customer. Patient chooses:

- Provider they receive their care from (NHS/private/UK/overseas)
- Appointment times

Payment by Results – better described (thus far) as 'payment by activity'

- Essentially the agreement of a national pricelist for patient care episodes
- Designed to prevent hospitals competing for patients on the basis of price, and encourage efficient use of resources

Competition – increased opportunity for private firms to provide services

- Private healthcare may be provided by for-profit or not-for-profit organizations
- Private care is subject to the same regulatory framework and national pricelist
- Debate exists around levels of government subsidy to encourage providers into the field

Foundation Trusts (FTs) – independent trusts under the regulation of Monitor

- FTs have greater freedom than non-FTs to generate and retain financial surplus
- Considerable constraints are applied upon how the surplus can be generated and what it can be used for

How money flows round the NHS system (see Fig. 18.1)

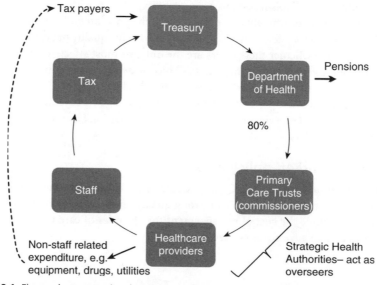

Fig. 18.1 Figure demonstrating how money flows round the NHS.

The Department of Health negotiates with the Treasury to agree budgetary settlements for the NHS, typically for a period of three years. Over 80% of this money is allocated to Primary Care Trusts (PCTs), which are responsible for purchasing the healthcare provision for their population; most of the rest goes towards NHS Pensions. There are approximately 150 PCTs in the UK and the Department of Health (DH) has a resource allocation method to determine the amount of money each PCT receives. This method includes an assessment of the relative health needs of the population served.

PCT functions include:

- Provision of primary care services
- Commissioning and agreeing of contracts with providers to ensure their catchment population has access to the necessary healthcare. Most contracts are agreed with NHS providers:
  - Primary care providers (e.g. GP practices)
  - Acute services
  - Community services
  - Mental health services
  - Specialist Trusts
  - Foundation Trusts

However, under the DH competition policies, PCTs can also contract with non-NHS providers who demonstrate that they meet the same clinical standards and price as NHS providers.

The providers spend the money on service delivery. The majority of this supports staff salaries, of which some feeds back into the general taxation pot and the circle starts again.

There are 10 Strategic Health Authorities (SHAs) across England alone, with responsibility to oversee the process of healthcare purchase and provision in their area. This responsibility is leveraged through a combination of legislation, government policy, and political influence.

Within the context of three-year settlements for the DH and typically three-year plans between PCTs and providers, there is a cycle of annual planning, agreement, and monitoring of the contracts. Thus, broadly speaking, there is a predictable annual cycle to the contractual agreements (see Fig. 18.2).

1. Contracts are signed between commissioner and provider in April (the start of the financial year). They are then monitored for the remainder of that financial year.

2. In the autumn (the month varies between October and December, and even exceptionally January) the DH issues priorities for the following year. These inform the decisions commissioners make about the services they will purchase. Negotiations take place between commissioners and providers about the types and volume of the service to be provided.

3. In December (although on occasion there is a delay), the DH will issue the national tariff. This 'price list' is then added to the volume agreements and the total value of the contract agreed.

4. January to March is when final negotiations take place and contracts are agreed.

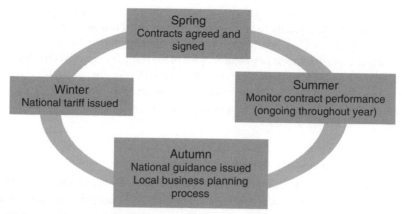

Fig. 18.2 Annual cycle of contractual agreements within the NHS.

Yearly savings requirement

A local obligation to ensure savings may be:

Nationally driven: The price list issued by the DH is adjusted annually and contains an inherent assumption of savings as the price is increased by less than the inflation rate. This forces the provider to find savings year on year.

Locally driven: If the local organization wishes to invest in new services or buildings, or has a financial deficit, greater savings may be sought. These savings need to be found through both greater efficiency and cutting costs.

Each organization therefore needs its own process of business planning to respond to the external environment and to plan how to deliver services to patients.

One might think that the need to find savings could be reduced by increasing patient volumes to increase income. Sometimes this is possible, but there are two major, and related, reasons why this needs to be considered carefully:

- As the total sum of money for the NHS is finite, the savings requirement placed on NHS trusts must include 'real' savings not just additional income
- Contracts with purchasers often contain an upper level of activity, above which payment is reduced or withheld

Organizational planning

The internal planning process relates to the commissioning cycle. Although the specifics will vary between organizations, the typical arrangement is as follows. In the autumn, service managers and clinical directors undertake business planning and:

- Review their existing budget
- Prepare bids for service developments
- Identify cost savings for the following year

These internal plans are then related to the agreements being made externally (e.g. how much of which service is to be bought) and negotiated to match internal and external demands as closely as possible.

Staff involved in organizational planning

Internal management structures do vary between providers. However, developing and delivering budgets for the service are the generally the responsibility of:

+ Managers – service, directorate or general
+ Clinical directors

They are also required to find yearly savings. Constructive approaches to service development requests, that recognize the balanced budget they are trying to achieve, will always be well received.

There will be some administrative staff with responsibility for agreeing contracts with commissioners. Job titles for these staff will vary and they may be part of the finance department, or a separate team that focuses upon service or business developments. These people are useful to clinicians looking to develop or start a new service.

The business planning process can be incredibly complex because:

+ Hospitals often have a turnover of several hundred million pounds a year
+ Most hospitals offer a vast range of services which all develop over time
+ The detail of each service varies:
  • Services may be largely outpatient, daycare, or inpatient
  • Patients may require theatre time or a significant medical management time
  • Admissions may be emergency or planned
  • Services place varying demands on support services (e.g. imaging)

However, there are some concepts that can be applied consistently across these variables to help measure the effective use of resources in that service.

Capacity: provides a measure of volume of a service
Efficiency: relates inputs to, and outputs from, a service
Targets: are created to assess whether plans are being achieved at service and Trust level (e.g. 18-week wait)

In economics, *capacity* is the point of production where costs per unit begin to rise, because some fixed factor needs a step change (e.g. new factory, new storage area, new machine). By contrast, in healthcare, it is often used to measure the volume of a service (e.g. the space in an outpatient clinic, the number of ward beds or theatre slots available). Changing capacity in one part of the health system will impact on other parts (e.g. increasing capacity in A&E to meet the 4-hour wait target moves the bottleneck to the transfer to other wards). Without reviewing systems as a whole, problems are simply shifted to another area.

Planning is made even more difficult since there is substantial unavoidable variation in healthcare systems (e.g. the number of admissions per day/week/month). Perhaps most surprising is that planned (elective) admissions typically vary more than unplanned (emergency) admissions over the course of a week, since patients are

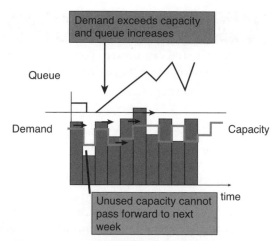

Fig. 18.3 Queues form if matching of demand and capacity is undertaken on the basis of averages.
Adapted from Silvester, K., Lendon, R., Bevan, H. et al. Reducing waiting times in the NHS: is lack of capacity the problem? *Clinician in Management* 2004;12(3):105–14. Used with permission of Radcliffe Publishing.

rarely admitted electively on Friday or Saturday. Such variation tends to increase queues and blocks in the system (see Fig. 18.3).

Capacity typically varies across a week or a month. This can be for planned reasons (e.g. annual leave, clinical education days, bank holidays, reluctance to have clinics on Friday afternoons), or unplanned reasons (e.g. no beds available, equipment failure, staff sickness). The crucial point to understand is that while average capacity may be sufficient for demand, it is not possible to 'pass forward' unused capacity (i.e. if you have four wards you can't create a fifth for one week because one of your four was closed the previous week). Therefore if you match average demand with average capacity a queue will form. Smoothing demand variation over time (for example, admitting electively at the weekend) will help mitigate the queue.

By regulating the flow of admissions, it is possible to reduce bottlenecks and increase patient flow through the system. There are statistical models for understanding variation in flow that are being applied across the NHS to reduce this fluctuation. It is also possible to apply techniques from manufacturing (e.g. lean, six sigma) that help design out activities that do not directly add value to the process (i.e. waste) (see Chapter 21).

Efficiency refers to the relationship between inputs and outputs. If no more output can be extracted from a system for the same input, then it would be considered efficient. It is rare to find a healthcare system in which this is true. In the case of the NHS:

- Input is tax payers' money
- Output is some measure of activity (e.g. number of patients seen, number of operations undertaken)

Using the principles of reducing variation outlined above, it should be possible to make a health system more efficient. Increasing output *per se* is not synonymous with improving outcome. A highly efficient system might still produce poor health outcomes (e.g. operations that fail to improve patient well-being or resolve a physical problem). However, there is a strong argument that delivering reliable, high-quality, safe care saves money.

Targets are created in order to assess whether the plan for activity is being met. These can be helpful, but managing to a target can have unintended consequences (e.g. transferring the bottleneck from A&E to the wards in the earlier example). All services will have variation; the key is to minimize and control it as much as possible. Statistical process control techniques may be helpful here.

When comparing two unequal numbers, one will always be larger than the other. This is a deceptively simple statement but it is surprising how many times people overreact to a single number comparison.

'We've seen fewer patients than last week, PANIC'

'We're seeing more patients than last month, we must have more staff NOW'

This can result in a lot of wasted energy, which would be better spent in other ways. In a sophisticated environment where the patient flows are well understood, it should be possible to predict the range within which the service would stay (bar exceptional circumstances). This is currently very uncommon in NHS services.

Finance and quality of patient care

Adverse clinical events are a major problem in hospitals. One in ten patients admitted to hospital in developed countries will unintentionally be the victim of an error. Around 50% of these events could be avoided if lessons from previous incidents were learned effectively and solutions implemented. A recent UK study concluded that 15% of adverse events led to impairment or disability lasting >6 months, and that 10% contributed to patient death.

Adverse clinical events also have an unfavourable financial impact. They are associated with longer length of stay, for which there is no additional income despite increased costs. For example hospital-acquired infections increase length of stay (and therefore cost) for affected patients.

Studies demonstrate that reducing adverse events can release cash and resources. A study of costs of healthcare-acquired infections in a district general hospital estimated that a conservative 10% reduction in the observed incidence of healthcare acquired infections would release resources valued in excess of £500,000. In the short term, a small proportion of these benefits are likely to be in the form of cash savings; however, over a longer period of time fixed costs may be also avoided. For example, for a 10% reduction in hospital-acquired infection, the number of bed days released for alternative use was estimated at 1413.

Summary

Focusing and investing in patient safety may reduce overall costs. This offers the potential for better quality of service to a wider number of patients, as well as increased income and reduced costs for hospitals.

Further reading

Department of Health (2006). Safety First – a report for patients, clinicians and healthcare managers.

Sari, A.B., Sheldon, T.A., and Cracknell, A. (2007). Extent, nature and consequences of adverse events: results of a retrospective case note review in a large NHS hospital. *Quality and Safety in Healthcare* **16**, 434–439.

Plowman, R. *et al.* (2001). The rate and cost of hospital-acquired infections occurring in patients admitted to selected specialties of a district general hospital in England and the national burden imposed. *The Journal of Hospital Infection* **47**(3), 198–209.

International Forum on Quality and Safety in Healthcare (last accessed December 2009). http://internationalforum.bmj.com/.

Institute for Healthcare Improvement webpage (last accessed December 2009). http://www.ihi.org/ihi.

Department of Health Website (last accessed December 2009). www.dh.gov.uk (look here for more information on Commissioning for Quality and Innovation, and Quality Accounts).

Chapter 19

Clinical governance at service level

David James

Key points

- Healthcare staff are responsible for improving the quality of care and are accountable for ensuring safe and reliable delivery at service level.
- The relationship between managers and clinicians is pivotal to efficient and effective provision of safe, high-quality healthcare.
- Effective clinical governance fosters multi-disciplinary activity, within and between services.
- Services must develop quality and safety agendas to align with organizational values and strategy.
- Data and information should be reported to the Trust Board, other services, and all relevant staff.

Introduction

There is currently no universal model of clinical governance at service delivery level. An individual service should devise a model that best fits its own circumstances, but which sits firmly within the overall Trust values and objectives. Delivering a clinical governance (CG) agenda requires staff participation, but the problem facing the frontline staff is how to apply broad CG concepts in the workplace.

The clinical governance cycle

A simple approach allows the concepts of CG to be tailored to various clinical settings (Fig. 19.1). The cycle is designed to ensure clinical services provide care to an acceptable quality. It seeks to compare current practices to reference standards, emphasizing that CG activities are undertaken iteratively, with considerable overlap of each component of the cycle, which may be entered at any point.

Quality standards: defining 'the right outcome'

Defined quality standards should ensure that service delivery or clinical care is acceptable in terms of safety, effectiveness, appropriateness, patient-focus, accessibility,

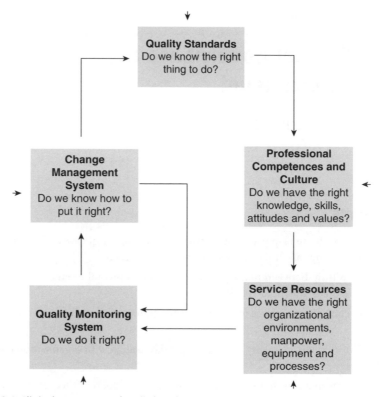

Fig. 19.1 Clinical governance (quality) cycle.

and efficiency. Standards development should be proactive and supportive, not reactive and policing. Locally developed standards have to stand up to external scrutiny.

Standards originate from a number of external sources, often assessed as part of an external accreditation scheme, including:

◆ Clinical standards defined by:
  • Department of Health (DH), e.g. in Standards for Better Health
  • NHS bodies, e.g. National Institute for Health and Clinical Excellence (NICE), Care Quality Commission (CQC), and National Service Frameworks (NSFs)
  • Professional organizations such as the Medical Royal Colleges or specialty associations

◆ Legal standards defined in UK law, e.g. Health and Safety legislation, conduct of bio-medical research such as The Medicines for Human Use Regulations 2004.

◆ Procedural standards, e.g. those defined by National Health Service Litigation Authority (NHSLA) through its Clinical Negligence Scheme for Trusts (CNST)

◆ Regulatory Standards, e.g. From the General Medical Council (GMC)

◆ Professional standards, e.g. defined by Medical Royal Colleges

- Training standards (and how they will be delivered) defined for example, by the Medical Royal Colleges, PMETB or the GMC

Standards may also originate internally:

- Organizational standards (defined at Board or service level): e.g. service level agreements (SLAs) with commissioners and suppliers, or defined aspects of the clinical service
- Local standards may be developed to help define service needs (see Chapter 21).

Professional standards: ensuring the right knowledge, skills, and behaviours are in place

Professional standards are covered in sections on resource effectiveness, learning effectiveness, and fundamental principles. However, individuals need to understand that whilst they are governed by national bodies, local standards will also be applied, e.g. mandatory training in the use of locally used equipment.

Service resources: checking if the organization has 'the right' resources available

The rational delivery of a service can be considered as a cycle (Fig. 19.2). This cycle starts with a plan (communicated as the Annual Business Plan) that defines the resources necessary to meet the stated objectives of the service. These objectives can be broadly defined in terms of finances, activity, and quality. The achievement of these objectives should be assessed regularly and defines the performance of the service (communicated as the Annual Performance Report).

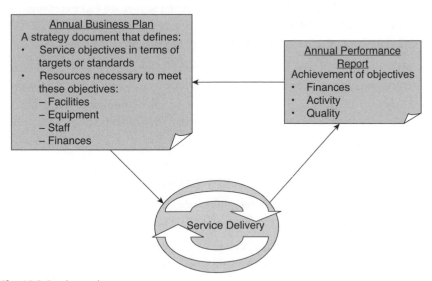

Fig. 19.2 Service cycle.

Service objectives are influenced by key stakeholders, notably patients, policy makers, purchasers, and professional groups. Clinicians and managers must work together to ensure that, for example, quality is not compromised by the need to cut costs or increase service activity.

Quality monitoring system: discerning if 'the right things' are done

An effective structure must be in place to allow appropriate processes to be implemented.

Structure

Clinicians must play a vital part in Trust and service clinical governance teams, the structure of which might be somewhat like that shown in Fig. 19.3.

Service Clinical Governance Teams are pivotal in monitoring quality.

Membership: A multidisciplinary grouping of doctors, nurses, professions allied to medicine (PAMs), a risk manager, a health and safety advisor (ideally), a service general manager and a clinical lead (e.g. clinical director), along with the service lead for CG.

Role: To act as a steering committee for service CG activities, ensuring quality issues are part of service performance monitoring and business planning.

Objectives: To meet regularly (e.g. monthly) and identify problems and trends, suggesting remedial actions to services. This will incorporate:

◆ Ensuring the service meets the requirements of NHSLA risk management standards

◆ Review of clinical incidents, complaints, and claims to identify areas of risk

◆ Planning audit priorities around identified safety issues

◆ Coordinating clinical risk assessment, identifying new risks, and monitoring the control of established ones

◆ Organization and review of patient surveys and feedback (see Chapters 36 and 37)

◆ Communication of risks to appropriate clinical areas, by means of alerts etc

◆ Development of standards/guidelines/integrated care pathways (see Chapters 12 and 15)

◆ Monitoring the implementation of any suggested changes in practice

This may require that they advise management on:

◆ Clinical information needs of the service

◆ Appropriate training needs of staff to ensure change of practice can be implemented

◆ Monitoring the appraisal and development of staff

◆ Business planning; ensuring CG is included at all levels

Leadership: The nominated service CG lead may be the clinical lead or delegated colleague, the latter does not necessarily need to be a clinician. They should have the authority and responsibility to negotiate with other services, and probably require

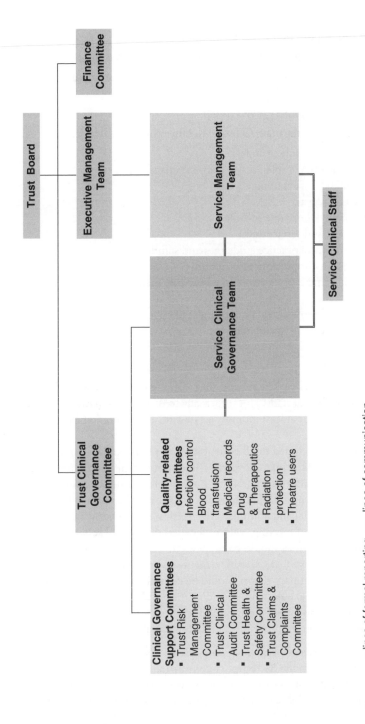

Fig. 19.3 Typical Trust CG structure.

an allocation of at least 1 session/week, along with appropriate training in clinical governance.

The CG lead's role and responsibilities include:

- Developing the service's CG processes in line with service, division, and Trust strategy
- Communicating relevant information up, down, and across the organization as indicated in Fig. 19.3
- Promoting wide multidisciplinary involvement
- Delegating and supervising the main CG roles to other colleagues, e.g. leads for:
  - Risk management, whose role includes:
    - Patient safety incident, complaint, and claims management
    - Statutory and mandatory training
    - Managing the risk register
  - Quality management, whose role includes:
    - Organizing clinical and service audit
    - Development of clinical practice guidelines and standards
    - Establishing a quality improvement program
  - Performance management of individuals, whose role includes:
    - Appraisal
    - Ensuring continued professional development of colleagues
    - Ensuring effective team performance

Communications: verbal and written.

If the CG programme is to succeed, it is vital that the team communicates regularly with service staff. This requires sufficient protected working time be included in normal service activities for clinical staff to meet formally to discuss CG matters and fuel the CG cycle (this should occur at least monthly). These meetings should be facilitated by the service CG team.

CG activities should be included in all consultant job plans, understanding that attendance is not optional. Meetings allow front-line staff to truly participate in all elements of CG cycle, whilst affording a training opportunity for juniors. Attendance can be varied according to the agenda, but these meetings should be multi-disciplinary and include service, managerial and administrative/clerical staff. The agenda may on occasion be best served by joint meetings with other specialty clinical services.

Regular reports of CG activities should be made to the Trust CG committee. This requires good record keeping so that CG achievements are transparent and visible for review. An annual service summary report should be compiled. It should commence with a clear statement of annual objectives, including measurable outcomes of change, along with minutes and attendance of meetings. All reports should be kept for a period of time (e.g. 10 years) with agreed procedures for confidentiality.

Clinical governance support committees and quality-related committees.

Many Trusts have established CG 'support committees' whose main functions are to inform, advise, and monitor the activities of the service clinical governance teams in the various CG domains, e.g. risk management and clinical audit (Fig. 19.3).

There are also often a variety of other Trust 'quality-related' committees who serve similar functions, but in defined clinical areas, such as infection control and blood transfusion.

Processes

Reflective of the need for accountability, for practical purposes four main components of management must be addressed:

- Risk
- Quality
- Information
- Performance

Each shares many of the individual CG activities (e.g. incident reporting can be considered a component of all parts). Further information on these areas is found in the relevant chapters, but reviewed briefly below.

Risk management With the objective of practicing safely, and always seeking to reduce the clinical and non-clinical risks associated with healthcare, each service should have a:

- Risk register
- Incident management system
- Complaints and claims management system
- Training and development system
- Policies and standards development system

Quality management The highest quality care requires the service to continuously improve its standards by having integrated systems of:

- Clinical risk management and audit
- Evidence-based practices
- Continuing practice and professional development

Data management and information Monitoring the quality of clinical services requires accurate, reliable, and relevant information (see Chapter 33). Trend analysis may help identify recurring problems warranting further investigation and remedial action. Data may be qualitative or quantitative, and relate either to individual patients or sample data of aggregated population. It may be acquired from several sources, including:

- CG tools
  - Clinical and service audit, e.g. an audit of the quality of post-operative pain management (outcome of care) or an audit of outpatient waiting times (process of care).
  - Complaints, incidents, and claims monitoring, e.g. individual case reviews of all recent complaints, or a risk cause analysis of a serious patient safety incident.

- Risk assessments, e.g. an electronic incident reporting system or health and safety environmental hazard assessment.
- Patient surveys, e.g. patient service experiences survey or patient-reported outcome measures (PROMs).

◆ Other sources
  - Service agreement performance monitoring
  - National indicators
  - Peer review of accepted standards of care
  - Reports from internal and external bodies including:
    - Health Ombudsman
    - Caldicott Guardian
    - Royal College visits
    - Care Quality Commission

Regular, high-quality data should be collected and related to specific clinical areas, teams, services, or directorates. The information should be fed back quickly so as to remain relevant. Examples might include:

◆ Patient deaths and cause

◆ Emergency re-admission within 5 days

◆ Unscheduled returns to theatre

◆ Patient safety incidents

◆ Unscheduled ICU admission

◆ Complaints and/or legal claims

◆ Data on finished consultant episodes for top ten OPCS4/ICD10 codes

◆ Performance against defined clinical indicators, e.g. meeting standards for the time between the diagnosis of a myocardial infarction and the administration of thrombolytic therapy

◆ Performance against national standards, e.g. set by NSF, NICE

Currently, data *routinely* collected by most services is of limited use in measuring quality of care. Most quality data is project-based (e.g. clinical audits, patient surveys) with labour-intensive data processing and analysis. The aim should be for routine capture of robust clinical data about the processes and outcomes of clinical care. Good quality data must be complete, accurate, and timely. This requires robust procedures and staff education so they can use the data systems and understand their roles and responsibilities.

The clinical dashboards programme is a national pilot programme developed after recommendations from both Lord Darzi's Next Stage Review (NSR) and the Health Informatics Review. Dashboards aim to give clinicians easy access to data being captured locally in a visual and usable format. Currently, the data available in the average acute hospital includes:

◆ Patient Administration System (PAS) – a relatively complex dataset designed around national standards and definitions that manages a patient pathway from GP referral to follow up (ICD-10 and OPCS-4 codes are included).

- A host of bespoke, isolated administrative, and clinical databases for theatres, pathology, pharmacy etc. These are often not based on national standards and definitions, so data comparison is problematic.
- Incident, complaints, and claims management systems – data from incidents are collected centrally as part of the NPSA National Reporting and Learning System, which allows data comparison between organizations.

Performance management Management of good and less good performance at service, team, and individual levels requires information. Performance has to be understood and assessed as a systemic phenomenon. Data may be derived from many sources, e.g. incidents, audits, external reviews.

At a service level, developing a range of 'quality indicators' will provide data on service performance and a guide to improvement, e.g. rates of defined complications, defined clinical outcomes, patient satisfaction.

Change management: ensuring problems can be addressed

The CG cycle should detect when either professional practice, service delivery, or both are below defined, acceptable standards. This may identify a need for change in a service, or rarely, raise serious concerns about the management of a service or an individual's performance. Clearly defined lines of procedure are necessary to address these outcomes. They may involve senior Trust management in addition to CG leads.

Service

Identified deficiencies in service provision, notably when they occur frequently, require an explicit remedial action plan. This plan should be focused, where possible, on positive actions to improve the system of care, rather than on negative actions to blame and discipline. Remedial action requires identification of an individual responsible for the implementation of changes, including the timescale. The service leadership remains accountable for completion of remedial action and monitoring of outcomes. Actions, which may be required for improvements in service, include:

- Operational policy rewrites
- Education and training programmes
- Manpower expansion
- Environmental, e.g. building works
- Equipment purchase
- Long-term funding alterations

The effectiveness of any action plan should be measured by improvement in the monitored data which identified the problem. Clinical services should have access to senior managers at Trust level to resolve quality issues which cannot be dealt with locally.

Individuals

Services need to assure themselves that individual performance management occurs, starting with recruiting talented motivated staff and adopting modern human resource practices to help establish a 'psychological contract' with them. This will include:

- Organizational orientation and training of new staff
- Annual performance appraisal with problem identification and resolution in a blame-free manner, along with development of meaningful professional development plans around aspirations/goals
- Clear graded disciplinary procedures with counselling and personnel development
- Managing under performance
- Staff sickness and turnover monitoring
- Exit interviews for all staff, to assess reasons for leaving and perceptions of the service
- Annual staff satisfaction surveys
- Team training programmes

Summary

It is over 10 years since clinical governance was introduced as the NHS approach to quality improvement; but frontline staff are yet to fully engage with it. The organization needs to be seen to value clinical governance from Board to ward and promote quality and safety at every level. It is the responsibility of service level leads to encourage this in all staff.

Further reading

The Kennedy Report. http://www.bristol-inquiry.org.uk/.

Scally, G. and Donaldson, L.J. (1998). Clinical governance and the drive for quality Improvement in the new NHS in England. *BMJ* **137**, 61–65.

Department of Health (1997). *The New NHS: Modern*, Dependable. DH: London.

Department of Health (1998). *Quality in the New NHS*. DH: London.

NHS Executive (1998). *Health Service Circular* 1999/065. *Clinical Governance: Quality in the New NHS*. DH: London.

Chapter 20

Processes and policies: Directorate level

Catriona Ferguson

Key points

- Clinical directorates are service delivery units led by a general manager, senior nurse manager, and a clinical director.
- When directorates function well, they improve quality and safety of outcome for patients.
- Policy can be made at national, regional, or local levels.
- Clinical involvement is vital for successful introduction of new processes and procedures.
- Good management skills and understanding the doctor/manager relationship will increase successful development of process.

Definitions

A *Directorate* is a service delivery unit. The clinical services within a Trust are split up into directorates usually putting allied specialties together, e.g. a critical care directorate might include, anaesthetics, intensive care, theatres etc.

A *Policy* is a deliberate plan of action to guide decisions, and achieve rational outcomes.

A *Process* is a series of actions, changes, or functions bringing about results or changes in outcomes.

Directorates

Directorates are responsible for:

- Delivery of safe effective care to patients
- Putting processes in place to implement policy decided on at a higher level (e.g. Trust, professional, national)
- Auditing and appropriate reporting of performance
- Budget management
- Developing services to meet the needs of users, in line with Trust strategy

Position of directorates within the NHS

See Fig. 20.1.

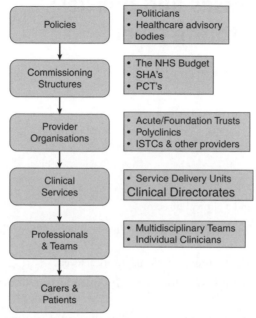

Fig. 20.1 Position of directorates within the NHS.

The position of directorates within a trust

There are many different organizational configurations of trusts; one example is shown in Fig. 20.2.

The structure of a Directorate

Directorates can be made up in different ways. Most directorates have a triad of leaders, a manager, a clinical director, and a nursing manager; each with their own teams and responsibilities (see Table 20.1).

Table 20.1

	Manager	**Clinician**	**Nurse**
Responsible for	Delivering service Improving quality and safety Managing the budget	Service delivery Improving quality and safety Managing the budget	Nursing hierarchy Managing allied specialities Managing support services (e.g. portering)
Answer to	Trust Board Chief executive	Trust Board Medical director	Trust Board Director of nursing
Lead team of	Service managers	Clinical leads for all specialities in directorate (these manage front-line doctors)	Matrons and senior sisters

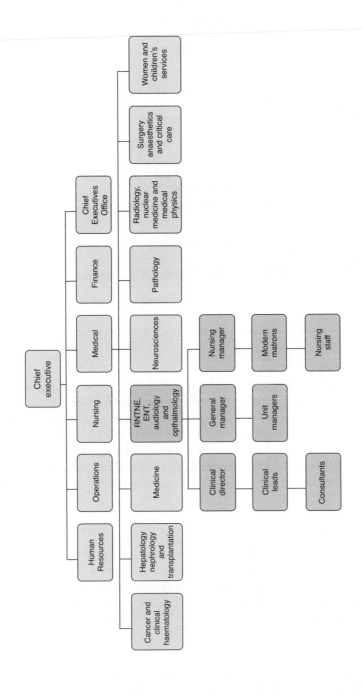

Fig. 20.2 Example of the place of 1 directorate (RNTNE) within the structure of a Trust.

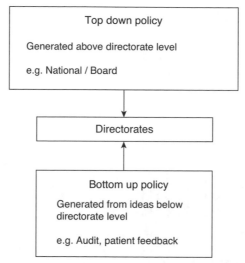

Fig. 20.3 Directorates receive policy from both above and below.

Policies

Policy can be generated at any level: national, regional, or local (see Fig. 20.3).

National level

Political ideology leads to major changes in direction of healthcare management and is often produced around election time. These ideas are fed through the Department of Health (DH) and detailed policy is produced. These policies have included introduction of agencies such as the National Institute for Health and Clinical Excellence (NICE), which produces national evidence-based guidelines (e.g. electrosurgery for tonsillectomy). The DH also provides policy in the form of national service frameworks (NSFs) aiming to improve services in targeted areas (e.g. the management of stroke).

Regional level

Strategic health authorities (SHAs) look at inequalities in healthcare provision and focus on regional needs for healthcare. Healthcare in some areas (e.g. of social deprivation) may dictate policy on provision. Primary care Trusts (PCTs) produce policy to direct local Trust provision of health care, ensuring appropriate services are available for their particular patients.

Trust level

Trusts may produce policy to contend with local issues (e.g. MRSA incidence), or to effect change in the overall Trust strategy.

Service level

Policy may be produced to improve services or safety, or to reach budget targets (e.g. undertake >90% of paediatric tonsillectomies as day cases).

Policy implementation should be a continuous process, with evidence-based policy being monitored with audit and feed back into a change in process. Policy is then regularly updated to reflect current evidence and any new external requirements (see Fig. 20.4).

Top down policies (e.g.18-week wait)

An initial '*idea*' results in an election promise to reduce waiting lists.

The DH produces a policy stating there should be a maximum of 18 weeks from receipt of referral to treatment. Funding is allocated for the PCTs to support the extra work load required in the short term to reduce waiting times. Rules are set so that commissioners know the required time scale and loopholes are avoided.

A Trust Board then plans implementation, and often pilots changes in one directorate. They set dates for both the pilot, and full introduction, allowing leeway within the DH policy to account for delays and problems. They must allocate funds to make the changes.

A directorate level working party implements and audits the process, e.g. 18 week wait team/IT resource, training etc. This multidisciplinary team may consist of out-patient, ward, and theatre managers and clinicians (e.g. surgeons and anaesthetists) with patient involvement. They identify:

◆ Needs: by detailed audit of the present position

◆ Bottlenecks in the system

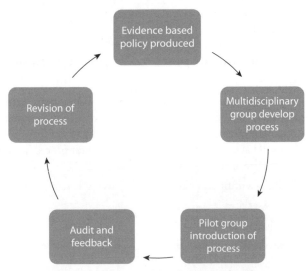

Fig. 20.4 Policy should be regularly updated on the basis of evidence.

◆ A time limit within which to achieve targets

Potential changes are multiple but might include:

◆ Increased number of appointments available, possibly requiring an extended working day

◆ Extra resources for clinical investigations

◆ Waiting list initiatives to reduce the backlog in clinics and theatres

◆ Introduction of one stop clinics to improve efficiency in the system, e.g. avoid patients making multiple trips for outpatient visits and investigations

This 'pilot' directorate can then feed back to the Trust board prior to Trust-wide introduction.

Bottom-up policies: e.g. clinical wish to reduce failure to attend rates

The clinical team observes a problem, e.g. high rates of did not attend (DNA) for in-patient treatments or out-patient review.

A directorate decision is taken to decrease such DNA rates on theatre lists. Clear aims are set out, including the degree of reduction in the measure to be achieved and specific timescales.

The patient pathway is audited along with a patient feedback questionnaire, or walk through with an expert patient.

Key areas for improvement are pinpointed (e.g. difficult admission process). Changes to this can then be instituted (e.g. process bookings and admissions in a single area).

Re-audit of the problem is necessary as part of an improvement cycle (see chapter 19). This may need several audits and improvements before effective changes are identified. Finally, a change in departmental policy (e.g. admission policy) can be instituted. If it proves successful, other services might decide (or be required) to implement a similar change in their area.

How processes are put in place to implement policy

Working groups

This is the managerial equivalent of a clinical multi-disciplinary team (MDT), i.e. a group of individuals with different skill mixes including managers, clinicians, paramedical staff, and non-clinical ancillary staff.

Any such group will have many different ideas of the best process to implement the policy in question. Approaches may include:

◆ Research, utilizing scientific and clinical studies to guide practice

◆ Investment in new services

◆ Strengthening existing services

◆ Education of staff and patient groups

◆ Training

- Rewarding staff for improvements in service
- Feedback to patients on the impacts of their actions on the service they receive

Different individuals in a working group often have fixed ideas about initiating a new process. This may cause conflict. However, if a balance can be achieved, it strengthens the chance of success. The key to this is:

- A clear idea of policy/action points with goals on what is to be achieved and by when
- Leadership skills from the manager, including effective delegation
- Involvement of all groups affected by the process
- Listening to feedback
- Allaying fears and preconceptions from individuals regarding change
- Using information technology and audit departments to their full potential
- Providing incentives to all groups working in the process
- Training all staff involved in the process
- Effective financial management

Quality control of policy and process

Change for change sake is disruptive. It is necessary to demonstrate that change is worthwhile to ensure staff engagement. This will include:

Audit: results of both national and local audits with formal outcome assessment can highlight both positive and negative features.

Patient feedback (see Chapter 38): Usually more informal than audit and often neglected, it is however very useful. Patients will often have a very clear understanding of what would improve their hospital experience.

Clinician involvement: Clinicians are universally keen to provide good services for their patients. However, they often don't know how to get involved or feel excluded from policy aimed at service development. Getting involved is often felt to be only for clinical leads and clinical directors but ground level involvement is a vital component of a successful and effective department.

To engage effectively with managers, clinical staff need to:

- *Listen to politics*: This will provide a good idea of where government policy is heading and some warning of change
- *Keep up to date with current research*: Using databases such as the Cochrane library (i.e. practice evidence based medicine). Some will wish to perform research themselves to improve process or change policy
- *Attend department meetings*: Keeping up to date with changes
- *Become involved in audit*: A very important way for clinicians to influence the process, and a GMC requirement for all doctors. If something is not working, audit it and feedback to effect change.

The problems

Mahatma Gandhi once said: 'A policy is a temporary creed liable to be changed, but while it holds good it has got to be pursued with apostolic zeal.' This mantra would make changes in policy and process easy to introduce, but unfortunately there are often problems.

Resistance to change from established clinicians

Clinicians often feel that medicine is moving towards an evidence-based approach, but that this is not also applied to health policy. A clinician who has managed patients in one way with good results may feel alienated by change. This is appropriate if supported by good evidence. Such individuals should be involved in the process to encourage compliance with change (e.g. bare below the elbows policies, to reduce cross-contamination).

Institutionalization

As healthcare delivery is rationalized across regions, many units providing the same service are being merged. Often the units have a different approach to patient management based on strong cultural and historic influences. Prior to any merger, very careful planning must be undertaken to prevent the merging units continuing to use their old processes independently, creating confusion and increasing risk.

Confusion because of inadequate communication

Clinicians are used to making independent decisions on patient management and may inadvertently (or otherwise) violate changes in policy. Information about reasons for change is often poorly explained, and many clinicians are left feeling that change has not been instituted to improve either patient outcomes or staff working conditions. Clear explanations of policy and process, avoiding frequent changes, can circumvent this. Introduction of too many policies at the same time causes confusion, resulting in none being followed.

Psychology of the doctor–manager relationship

Managers and senior doctors have very different career structures, which can lead to differing approaches. Managers are often appointed to fixed-term contracts (perhaps of only 2 years). They may feel the need to institute change quickly after appointment, so as to see immediate results, creating an impressive curriculum vitae necessary to gain their next appointment. This along with the long-term appointments of senior clinicians can lead to psychological differences as illustrated in the Table 20.2.

Table 20.2

	Doctors	Managers	Doctor-managers
Doctors view of	Guardians of standards Planning for long-term sustainable improvements	Only interested in meeting deadlines, reducing cost and improving efficiency	Potentially 'working for the enemy'
Managers view of	Resistant to change Interested only in individual patients, regardless of costs	Working to provide high quality efficient care within sustainable budgets	Potentially 'working for the enemy'

If these differences are accepted then communication may be helped.

Clinicians talking to managers could phrase their ideas in terms of efficiency and improved quality, rather than emphasizing the new (and often expensive) equipment and drugs that will be needed.

Managers might choose to explain changes to clinicians in terms of improved patient satisfaction, facilities, and equipment, whilst minimizing the budget implications. Such changes might be expected to enhance the potential for effective change being instituted.

Summary

Well-functioning clinical service delivery units contain both clinical and non-clinical staff, working together to achieve a common goal. Policies or processes may originate at or above service level, but all should aim to enhance the safety and quality of patient care.

Further reading

Sutherland, K., Dawson, S. (1998). Power and quality improvement in the new NHS: the roles of doctors and managers. *Quality in Health Care* **7**(Suppl), S16–S23.

Solesbury, W. (2001). Evidence Based Policy: Whence it Came and Where it's Going. *Planning Policy and Practice*. October 2001.

The King's Fund website. www.kingsfund.org.uk (last accessed May 2010).

Chapter 21

Improving quality and safety

Heather Shearer

Key points

- Repetition of the same thing will lead to the same results.
- Most branded improvement approaches are adaptations of more fundamental principles that are common to many approaches.
- Most quality improvement tools originated in industry and have variable applicability to healthcare.
- Measurement presented visually, over time, helps individuals to assess the impact of improvement efforts.
- Service improvement is a complex social intervention that needs to be evaluated appropriately.

> Insanity: doing the same thing over and over again and expecting different results.
> – Albert Einstein

When things don't go as well as we would like, we try harder, work faster and 'just sort it'. These exhortations may have a short-term benefit but can also have adverse effects: for example, rushing can lead to errors. In order to make a better, and lasting improvement, the concept of system or process redesign is important.

A brief history of quality improvement

Systematic quality improvement approaches often originate in the manufacturing world and are more recently being adapted to healthcare. Many of the factors are similar; it is possible to liken an operating list to a production line. However, most practitioners recognize the distinct challenges in healthcare; it is not possible to simply discard a bad 'package' for example when that package is a human body.

Much of the language around quality improvement is used sloppily and influenced by the commercial desires of organizations and management consultants. For these reasons, this chapter will focus upon the work of two original 'gurus' and three widely recognized approaches that are underpinned by the work (Table 21.1).

Statistical process control

Shewart (1891–1967) is credited with much of the mathematical underpinning to statistical process control (SPC). This is a measurement method that can be applied to

Table 21.1 Gurus of quality improvement and their approaches

	Guru	Approaches
1920s	Shewart	Statistical process control (Shewart)
1950s	Deming	System of profound knowledge (Deming)
1980s		Lean (Toyota) Six Sigma (Motorola)
1990s		Model for improvement (Langley et al.)

different types of measure, including both count (attributes), and measurement (discrete and continuous) data.

Shewart classified two types of variation: common and special cause. An illustration of these would be to consider a regular commuting journey.

Common cause variation can occur normally when using the same system and combination of transport (e.g. train, bus, and walk). The exact length of the journey usually varies slightly, one day taking a few minutes more than another day (perhaps all the traffic lights were at red).

Special cause variation occurs under unusual circumstances, e.g. the journey takes twice or three times as long as normal because the train breaks down.

Similarly, the time between prophylactic antibiotic and incision will have both common cause (e.g. slower paced porter, or longer to position the patient before incision) and special cause (e.g. finishing the previous case later than expected, or the lift used to transport the patient from the ward is broken) variation.

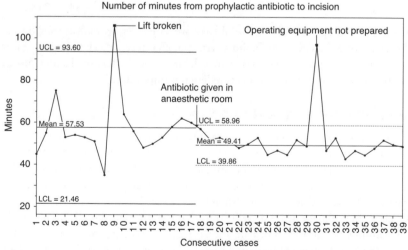

Fig. 21.1 Control chart of prophylactic antibiotic timing. The time of administration of antibiotic prior to operation is displayed. For the first seventeen consecutive cases the antibiotic was given on the ward. From case 18 the antibiotic was given in the anaesthetic room thereby reducing the common cause variation making the process more reliable and predictable. (UCL = Upper Control Limit, LCL = Lower Control Limit).

SPC uses charts to record the measures in a time sequence. Process limits are added using a mathematical formula that describes the upper and lower expected limits of the current process. The chart then displays the statistically expected performance of the current system. The control chart then permits easy visual identification of any impact a change makes upon the system (Figure 21.1).

System of profound knowledge

William Edwards Deming (1900–1993) was a U.S. statistician who went to Japan after World War II. The subsequent success of Japanese manufacturing was attributed to the implementation of his ideas. Deming's *System of Profound Knowledge* can be considered as an over-arching framework that emphasizes four perspectives:

1. Appreciation of a system
   Most products, services, or outcomes result from a complex system of interaction between people, procedures, and equipment. Recognizing this permits questioning and understanding of the interdependencies and inter-relationships between components of the system. For example, understanding the emergency admissions system would help to recognize the impact of a 4-hour admission target upon wards, diagnostics, and discharges.

2. Understanding of variation
   Systems continually exhibit variation, and being able to understand variation is necessary to be able to answer questions about the impact of changes.

3. Psychology
   People play essential roles in the running of systems and delivery of services. Recognizing the way that humans learn, err, and are motivated is core to the success of any improvement challenge. Current thinking emphasizes the importance of human dynamics, commitment, and leadership to implementing and sustaining improvement.

4. Theory of knowledge
   In order to effectively test changes, it is important to have an underlying theory of how the change might produce the desired outcome. This may be rooted in the other components of the System of Profound Knowledge and/or from clinical evidence. The key is to generate a prediction and ask whether the tested change has the predicted outcomes.

Individual improvement methods or approaches may emphasize one or some of these four perspectives.

Measuring improvement

Measurement is crucial to understanding the impact of changes. Three types of measure can be helpful: outcome, process, and balancing.

1. Outcome
   Examples of outcome measures related to improvement activity include: the number of blood stream infections or patient satisfaction. They can be hard to

measure, and also distant in time from the improvement activities (e.g. the definition of surgical site infection includes infections up to 30 days post discharge).

2. Process

Process measures focus upon compliance with procedures that are predicted to have an impact on the outcome measure. For example, when trying to reduce surgical site infections, one process measure would be the number of minutes between prophylactic antibiotic and incision (evidence shows this should be less than 60 minutes).

3. Balancing

As healthcare is a complex system, it is important to ascertain how changes made to certain processes affect others. For example, introducing a falls assessment checklist may have an impact on available nursing time for other activities. Thus, balancing measures are crucial. Balancing measures can also be used to measure the concerns of colleagues (e.g. it'll take too long, it'll cost more, it'll make our job more difficult).

Lean

Lean is one of the best known quality improvement methodologies and originated in car manufacturing world at Toyota. Lean most commonly focuses upon identifying and eliminating waste. The original seven wastes identified in the Toyota approach are given in Table 21.2.

One of the tools in the Lean toolkit is referred to as 5S (Table 21.3). Carrying out these five activities reduces waste. They have been described as 'housekeeping' for quality and safety.

Table 21.2 Waste categories in lean

Waste type	Toyota example	Healthcare example
Overproduction	Production ahead of demand	Patients brought in for procedures before they want
Waiting	For next production step	For test results prior to intervention
Transport	Moving products not required to perform the processing	Using a nursing escort for fit competent patient transfers
Inappropriate processing	Poor tool or product design causes extra work	Repeating tests that have been done too early or where results lost
Unnecessary inventory	Not requiring all components for work in progress to complete finished product	Packaging unnecessary surgical instruments in surgical packs
Unnecessary motion	Moving people or equipment more than necessary for processing	Walking around ward to gather equipment required for a procedure
Defects	Unnecessary effort involved in inspecting and fixing deficiencies	Correcting errors such as wrong-site surgery or surgical site infection

Table 21.3 5S

		5S
1	Sort	Classify equipment and supplies by frequency of use and remove what is not used
2	Simplify/ Straighten/Set	Set in order – allocate a place for equipment and supplies, standardize locations with labelling
3	Shine/Scrub	Clean and check
4	Standardize	Adopt standard work and standards
5	Sustain/ Self-discipline	On-going housekeeping audits

Six Sigma

Six Sigma is a redesign approach developed by Motorola in the 1980s, and seeks to improve the quality of process outputs by identifying and removing the causes of defects (errors) and variability in manufacturing and business processes. It uses a set of quality management methods, including statistical methods, and creates a special infrastructure of people within the organization ('Black Belts','Green Belts', etc.) who are experts in these methods.

The term 'Six Sigma' comes from a field of statistics known as process capability studies. Originally, it referred to the ability of manufacturing processes to produce a very high proportion of output within specification. Processes that operate with 'six sigma quality' over the short term are assumed to produce long-term defect levels below 3.4 Defects Per Million Opportunities (DPMO). A defect is defined as anything that could lead to customer dissatisfaction (Table 21.4).

The application of Six Sigma in healthcare is not widespread nor independently evaluated. Some training was provided to the NHS by the former Modernisation Agency, and some believe that the emphasis on data may make it popular with clinical staff. However, a widely held belief is that it is more appropriately applied to production lines, and that the target of 3.4 DPMO is not achievable in a complex healthcare system.

Table 21.4 Six sigma uses structured five steps for improvement tasks

		Six Sigma
1	Define	High-level project goals and the current process
2	Measure	Key aspects of the current process and collect relevant data
3	Analyze	The data to verify cause-and-effect relationships. Include all relationships and ensure that all factors have been considered
4	Improve	Or optimize the process based upon data analysis and experimental design
5	Control	To ensure that any deviations from target are corrected before they result in defects. Set up pilot runs to establish the capability of the process, move on to production, set up control mechanisms and continuously monitor the process

Productive series

The productive series (NHS Institute for Innovation and Improvement) is an example of successful application of lean principles to healthcare. The series focuses upon Releasing Time to Care, which has a strong resonance with the values of healthcare workers. The first in the series was The Productive Ward, and further packs have been produced including community services, operating theatres, and other settings. Tools used include observation and documentation of existing processes, reducing waste, and visual display of information.

The Productive Ward Benefits:

- Increased safety
- Increased morale
- A 10% increase in time for nurses to spend in direct patient care
- Calmer wards and a reduction in patient complaints
- A reduction in barriers between front line staff and managers, and between disciplines

Model for improvement

The Model for Improvement was first applied to health in 1996 by Langley and colleagues. It comprises three questions and the PDSA cycle (Fig. 21.2). The three questions are:

1. What are we trying we to accomplish?
   This question forces the team to articulate a clear aim. This aim should be specific and measurable. This is sometimes referred to as "What, how much, by when?" A good aims statement helps to inspire and focus the attention of those involved.
   e.g. 'We will reduce patient falls on Ward C by 50% by December'.

2. How will we know that a change is an improvement?
   Measurement is a crucial component of all improvement projects.

3. What changes can we make that will result in improvement?
   Sources of ideas are many and varied. Often individuals and teams already have hunches, or knowledge about what they should be trying to create, or the improvement they desire. It is important to note that a core principle of this approach is to start with small tests. This means that ideas can be tested out so that confidence in their value can be refined over repeated cycles of change.

These 'Deming' cycles (Table 21.5) of change are known as PDSAs (Plan Do Study Act), or PDCAs (Check) and represent a formal but flexible approach to developing, testing and implementing changes through learning.

It is crucial that PDSAs should be small in scale. For example, when working to introduce pre-operative washing for all surgical patients, a first PDSA would find out if the healthcare assistant could wash one patient, on one occasion, before surgery. The learning from this would refine the process (e.g. who does the washing? Can a medicated product be provided?). Subsequent PDSAs would, for example, extend to washing three patients, then five, then a whole operating list.

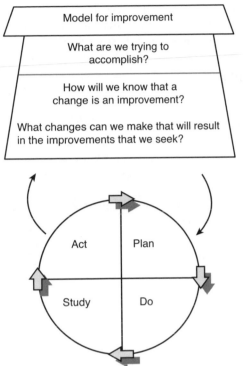

Fig. 21.2 The Plan Do Study Act cycle (PDSA).
Reprinted from Langley et al. 1996, with permission of John Wiley & Sons, Inc.

The Model for Improvement is used by many hospitals to reduce harm events (e.g. infections, falls, drug errors) and improve experiences (e.g. redesign of outpatient clinics, delivery of cancer care).

Table 21.5 The PDSA cycle

The PDSA (Deming) Cycle	
1 **Plan**	Agree the changes to test and implement
2 **Do**	Implement the changes and measure the impact
3 **Study**	Study (or check) the change before and after implementation and reflect on the impact
4 **Act**	Plan the next change or implementation

Summary

The most appropriate evaluation methodology continues to be robustly debated in the quality literature. The most useful evaluation questions are likely to be of the 'Why does X work in this ward, but not that ward?' nature. The traditional gold standard evaluation technique of randomized-controlled trials does not provide an answer to these evaluation questions. This is because randomized controlled trials are designed to control out context-dependent variables (e.g. groups are matched on a wide range of factors such as age, location, physical characteristics). In quality improvement, the desire is to understand the impact of a series of activities in the context in which they were delivered. The evaluation method chosen must reflect this ambition.

Further reading

Books

Boaden, R., Harvey, G., Moxham, C., and Proudlove, N. (2008). *Quality Improvement: Theory and Practice in Healthcare*. NHS Institute for Innovation and Improvement, UK.

Langley, G., Nolan, K., Nolan, T., Norman, C., and Provost, L. (1996). *The Improvement Guide:* A Practical Approach to Enhancing Organisational Performance. Jossey-Bass: San Francisco, CA.

Journals that frequently report quality improvement work
• *Quality and Safety in Healthcare*
• *British Medical Journal*

Useful websites

www.institute.nhs.uk
www.ihi.org
www.institute.nhs.uk/productiveward

Chapter 22

Performance management of acute and specialist trusts

Richard Connett

Key points

- Performance management of clinical governance processes helps ensure high quality care and patient safety.
- Performance management is based on self-assessment, combined with inspections and cross-checking with other sources.
- Performance assessment covers compliance with standards, use of a variety of indicators from across the healthcare spectrum, and the meeting of national targets.
- There have been 4 regulators/inspectors of health care since the year 2000.
- Healthcare regulation is currently undergoing further change and will continue to do so in line with political and social developments.

Introduction

Performance management is an important factor in ensuring high standards of clinical governance, which in turn drives improvement in patient safety. The first national regulator of healthcare was established by the Health Act 1999 and came into being in 2000. There have been three more regulators of healthcare since then, with The Care Quality Commission (CQC) and Monitor being the current ones. Operational performance of organizations is assessed and reported annually alongside financial performance.

Commission for Health Improvement (CHI): April 2000 to March 2004

The Commission for Health Improvement was established in April 2000. It produced the first performance ratings for the NHS covering the year 2002/03. CHI used the star ratings system which has become part of NHS folklore. Script writers such as Jed Mercurio of 'Bodies' fame, use managers blinkered ambition to achieve 3 stars to dramatize simmering manager: clinician tensions. Stars were awarded using the following scale:

- 3 stars – awarded to Trusts achieving the highest level of performance
- 2 stars – awarded to Trusts performing well overall

- ◆ 1 star – awarded to Trusts where there were concerns about particular areas of performance
- ◆ Zero stars – given to Trusts with the poorest levels of performance, or little progress implementing clinical governance

The star rating system was the first ever England-wide performance rating system. Even though the regime operated for just 3 years, people still often refer to star ratings when they talk about performance management. The last star ratings were published for the period April 2004 to March 2005.

Healthcare Commission (HCC): April 2004 to March 2009

In their first year of existence, the Healthcare Commission used the star rating system inherited from CHI. However, the HCC then moved to implement a new performance management regime called the Annual Health Check (AHC). The first AHC was published for the year April 2005 to March 2006. Three more followed covering 2006/2007, 2007/2008, and 2008/2009. The last was published by the Care Quality Commission (the successor to the HCC).

An AHC rating was awarded for each of two main categories of performance:

1. Quality of services
2. Use of resources (later re-titled quality of financial management)

It used a scale of four possible ratings: excellent, good, fair, or weak.

The AHC ratings were published in the October following completion of the previous financial year, thus always lagging 6 months behind the period assessed. The areas, which fed into the AHC, are shown in Fig. 22.1.

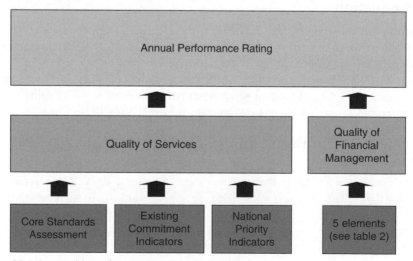

Fig. 22.1 Composition of Annual Performance Rating.

Quality of Services ratings contained three elements:

♦ Core standards

There were 24 core standards with 44 elements. The standards were grouped into 7 domains, and generally covered those areas where compliance could not be measured by recourse to numerical targets:

1. Safety
2. Clinical and cost effectiveness
3. Governance
4. Patient focus
5. Accessible and responsive care
6. Care environment and amenities
7. Public health

These covered disparate areas including clinical and corporate governance, compliance with NICE technology appraisals, safeguarding children, and waste disposal.

Since numerical targets are unhelpful, compliance was measured through a process of self declaration backed by inspection. Some Trusts were inspected on the basis of information received by the HCC indicating a potential risk of undeclared non-compliance. A further group of Trusts were inspected at random.

♦ Existing commitment indicators

These included measures which could be quantified numerically and many related to targets set out in 'The NHS Plan' published in July 2000. For 2008/09 there were 10 existing commitment indicators shown in Table 22.1.

Table 22.1 Existing Commitment Indicators used by the HCC

Indicator type	Measure
Health and well-being	Access to genito-urinary clinics
	Data quality of ethnic grouping
Clinical quality	Time to reperfusion for patients who have had a heart attack
Patient focus and access	Delayed transfers of care
	Total time in A&E departments
	Out-patient waiting > 13 week standard
	In-patients waiting > 26 week standard
	Patients waiting > 13 weeks for revascularization
	Waiting time for rapid access chest pain clinic
	Cancelled operations and those not readmitted within 28 days

* New national targets

These were re-titled National Priority indicators for the 2008/09 year. They reflected changes to NHS performance management, such as an increased focus on MRSA and *Clostridium difficile* infections. They also incorporated the 18-week wait target, marking a move away from separate targets for in-patient and out-patient waits, towards monitoring and service improvement covering the whole of the care pathway. For 2008/09, there were 13 national priorities:

* Survey data:
  * Patient experience – in which patients themselves rate hospitals on a variety of levels, including safety and cleanliness, dignity and respect, waiting times in all areas, standards of care, and good management
  * Staff satisfaction
* Audit data:
  * Infant health and inequalities: smoking during pregnancy and breastfeeding initiation
  * Participation in heart disease audits (evidence of data submission)
  * Engagement in clinical audits
* Quality:
  * Stroke care
  * Maternity hospital episode statistics: data quality indicator
  * Incidence of MRSA bacteraemia
  * Incidence of *Clostridium difficile*
* Patient pathways:
  * 18-week referral to treatment times
  * All cancers: 2-week wait
  * All cancers: 1-month diagnosis to treatment
  * All cancers: 2-month urgent referral to treatment

Patient pathways have been a focus of performance targets ever since publication of the NHS Plan. In the 1990s, it was not unknown for patients to wait up to 2 years for non-urgent surgery. By 2009, 90% of patients were being treated within 18 weeks of seeing their GP. Targets have played an important part in securing (and demonstrating achievement of) this modernization in services.

Quality of Financial Management ratings were made up of 5 elements:

Element	Includes	When assessed
Financial reporting	Preparation of accounts	Once financial position for year known
Financial standing	Balance sheet	
Financial management	In year budgetary control	Performance throughout the year
Internal control	Corporate governance	
Value for money	Planning, efficiency & accountability	

Taken together, these five assessments made up the Auditors Local Evaluation (ALE), overseen by the Audit Commission. For Foundation Trusts, the ALE score was derived from the monitor risk rating. As with the quality of services rating, a 4 point scoring system was used and a rating awarded; excellent, good, fair, or weak.

Care Quality Commission (CQC): April 2009 to present

From 1 April 2009, the Care Quality Commission replaced the Healthcare Commission (HCC), the Mental Health Act Commission, and the Commission for Social Care Inspection. The new organization will focus on outcomes rather than processes, and has taken steps to ensure that the views of service users (including patients, carers, children, and families) are taken into account both when determining policy and when making decisions about service provision.

The CQC has set out the following:

- Outcomes required, in terms of what people who use the service should experience
- What they expect providers to do to meet the outcome

It takes the view that it is up to regulated organizations to determine how this will be achieved in practice. Local involvement of service users will play a key role in pinning down the detail of how outcomes should be delivered. Providers will need to identify evidence in order to demonstrate compliance.

On 15 October 2009, the CQC published the Annual Health Check rating for April 2008 to March 2009 using the same process as its predecessor organization, the HCC (including historical comparisons). However, going forward, the performance management regime for the CQC will be very different from those operated by both CHI and HCC.

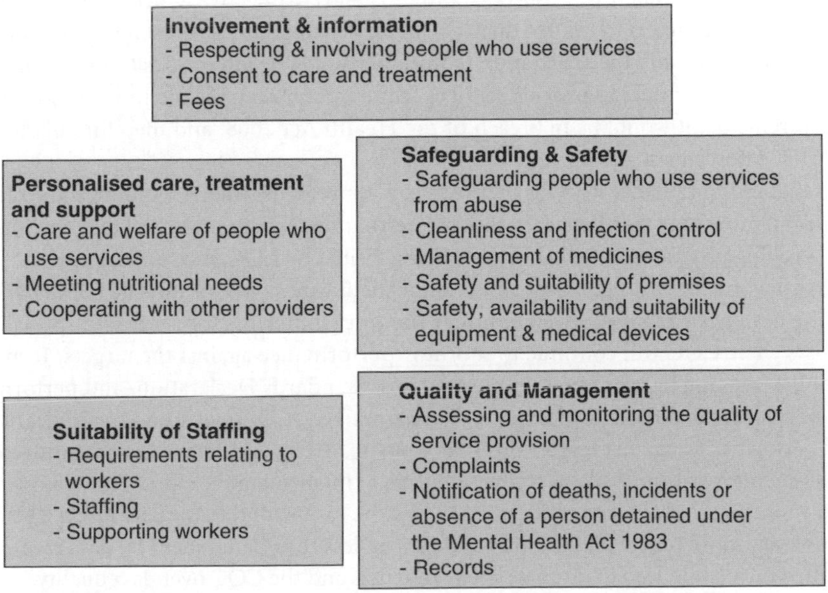

Involvement & information
- Respecting & involving people who use services
- Consent to care and treatment
- Fees

Personalised care, treatment and support
- Care and welfare of people who use services
- Meeting nutritional needs
- Cooperating with other providers

Safeguarding & Safety
- Safeguarding people who use services from abuse
- Cleanliness and infection control
- Management of medicines
- Safety and suitability of premises
- Safety, availability and suitability of equipment & medical devices

Suitability of Staffing
- Requirements relating to workers
- Staffing
- Supporting workers

Quality and Management
- Assessing and monitoring the quality of service provision
- Complaints
- Notification of deaths, incidents or absence of a person detained under the Mental Health Act 1983
- Records

Fig. 22.2 Essentials standards for registration with the CQC.

2009/10 was a transition year. The 24 core standards inherited from the HCC continued to be the performance measures that governed the way trusts were assessed for the whole year. However, an interim declaration against the 24 core standards was made in December 2009 to avoid overlap between the declaring on the outgoing core standards and making applications for registration under the new registration requirements.

Trusts applied for registration with the CQC in January 2010. The registration requirements include a range of essential standards covering quality and safety:

Compared to the core standards, the new registration requirements place a greater emphasis on the quality of personal care provided for all people who use services. The registration requirements will be used to regulate both health and social care providers, helping bridge the health and social care divide.

During February and March 2010, the registration applications were cross checked against various sources of information and additional information was requested from trusts if required.

Trusts were notified of the outcome of the registration process by 1 April 2010. Possible outcomes included

+ registration, without conditions,

+ registration with conditions and an agreed action plan to address areas of non-compliance, and

+ registration refused, in part or in full.

From 1 April 2010, CQC have published the register of providers on their website. The register describes each provider, the date of registration, and any conditions applied.

The new registration system differs from previous national performance management systems in that it is prospective rather than retrospective. Once registered it is the duty of providers to inform the CQC of any changes in circumstances that make them unable to fulfil the registration requirements. If a health or social care organization were to continue to provide services while in non-compliance with registration requirements, it would be in breach of the Health Act 2008, and therefore liable to formal enforcement action.

Ongoing compliance with the registration requirements will be monitored through a programme of inspections. It is anticipated that these inspections will take the form of a rolling programme, with all Trusts being visited by CQC once every 2 years.

At the time of writing, it is not clear what the future holds for targets. For 2009/10 these have been grouped together under the title 'Indicators for acute and specialist trusts'. The CQC will continue to monitor performance against the targets. It may publish a rating based upon the Interim Core Standards Declaration, and performance against the targets, as did the HCC. Alternatively, CQC may move to publication of performance against targets on their website. This would have the advantage of making information available to the public in a timely manner, rather than following a 6-month period for data ratification as was the case with the Annual Health Check. However, more timely publication would mean less time being spent on data ratification, which could lead to disputes between trusts and the CQC over data quality.

Monitor

Monitor is the independent regulator for Foundation Trusts. It was established in January 2004 and is independent of central government and directly accountable to parliament.

Monitor authorizes and regulates NHS Foundation Trusts. Performance is managed using the Compliance Framework. Both the targets within the Compliance Framework, and the indicators used by the Care Quality Commission, are largely derived from the Operating Framework, which is published each year by the Department of Health.

Monitor's functions and powers are detailed in the National Health Service Act 2006. More information about Monitor can be found at www.monitor-nhsft.gov.uk

Internal performance management

Typical information contained within the Trust Board Performance Report might include an assessment of performance against all of the targets published by the CQC. This can be presented using a dashboard or red-amber-green traffic light system. Exception reports follow, explaining reasons behind variances. Where adverse variances exist, effective control measures should be put in place. These are updated on a monthly basis for review by the Board.

Summary

The regulatory system has been in a constant state of flux since the first regulator came into being in 2000. Targets have received a particularly bad press, and are undoubtedly dangerous if allowed to create perverse incentives. However, the general view is that targets have driven up standards in the NHS over the last 10 years. In particular, the access targets have been responsible for reducing the maximum waiting times, which used to run to 18–24 months to 18 weeks, a significant achievement for patients.

Further reading

Commission for Health Improvement. http://www.chi.nhs.uk/Ratings/more_information.asp.

Care Quality Commission. http://www.cqc.org.uk/.

Monitor. www.monitor-nhsft.gov.uk.

Reviews in 2009/10 – Care Quality Commission Consultation Document - Concordat gateway number 157, December 2008.

Guidance About Compliance, Essential Standards of Quality and Safety – Care Quality Commission, December 2009.

Compliance Framework 2009/10, Monitor, March 2009.

The Operating Framework for the NHS in England 2010/1, Department of Health, December 2009.

Section 4

Resource effectiveness

It is tempting to blame all problems in healthcare on the perceived lack of money and investment. High-quality healthcare requires the right people in the right place, at the right time, with the right equipment, delivering the right treatment, to the right patient. This section attempts to demonstrate the importance of a wide range of areas which at first glance might seem unrelated to patient safety. Having appropriately qualified staff in place (*Recruitment and retention*), who are well rested (*Improving working lives*) and up to date (*Revalidation*) is a good starting place for safe care delivery. When things go wrong, or there are concerns about performance then robust and effective support systems need to be activated (*Managing poor performance*). Less obvious, but no less important, is the need for the appropriate tools (*Equipment management*) to be provided in a well-maintained environment (*Facilities – The hidden hospital*), which supports delivery of care and is fit for purpose.

Chapter 23

HR management

Carol Johnson

Key points

- The NHS needs to attract and retain the highest calibre of staff possible to deliver high quality, safe, patient care.
- Key to attracting top talent is employing world class leaders.
- Staff are more likely to remain working in a supportive, progressive culture; providing personal growth and professional development opportunities is crucial.
- Recruiting and retaining staff, and effective succession planning is central to human resource department activity.
- Recruitment and retention initiatives must take account of both national standards, and the Trust's business and strategic plans.

Introduction

Attracting, developing, motivating, and rewarding talent is a continuous and stretching process, but critical for the survival and growth of an organization. Human resource (HR) departments are central to this process. Leading in buoyant economic times can be even more difficult than in a recessionary environment. In both circumstances, making sure the right people are employed for the right jobs, providing an interesting, stimulating, and supportive environment, and ensuring leaders are capable of maximizing the effectiveness of all the resources at their disposal, is a daunting yet essential part of modern day HR management.

HR functions have an impact throughout organizations, significantly affecting both day-to-day operational issues, and longer-term strategic plans. HR directors usually report directly to the chief executive (CEO) and sit as members of the management committee. They will be required to attend all Trust board meetings. Typical HR functions are shown in Table 23.1.

HR makes certain that all necessary processes are followed, ensuring that a Trust is employing its staff legitimately. Thereafter, it is involved in motivating and challenging staff to fully engage in the organization's objectives. They achieve this by instigating effective appraisal systems, and providing staff with support and development opportunities.

Table 23.1

Area	HR role
Recruitment	Work with managers to ensure all posts (medical and non-medical) are advertised and recruited efficiently.
	Advise on appropriate use of ability and psychometric tests.
Payroll and pensions	Responsible for correct pay and pension arrangements for all staff.
Rewards and benefits	Usually arising from staff feedback and may include:
	♦ Implementing flexible benefits programmes (e.g. salary sacrifice in exchange for leave, recognition awards)
	♦ Managing job evaluation programmes (e.g. banding and re-banding posts in accordance with local policies)
	♦ Managing relations with Joint Trust Staff Committees
EWTD compliance (see chapter 24)	Work with managers to ensure EWTD compliance, and documentation of this (e.g. by diary cards).
Occupational health (OH)	Responsible for provision of OH service to ensure:
	♦ Health screening and immunization up-to-date
	♦ Support of staff with work related illness (e.g. work related stress – see chapter 26)
	♦ Provide external support services for staff as necessary
Learning and development	Responsible for on-going staff training and development (see chapters 29–32), both mandatory and developmental.
HR business partners	Advise managers on employee issues (e.g. performance management, criminal records bureau checks).

There are five key areas which the NHS needs to take into consideration when engaging and finding ways of retaining key talent:

1. Attracting and retaining talent
2. Employing world class leaders
3. Providing personal growth and professional development opportunities
4. Succession planning
5. Workforce data and information and its use

Attracting and retaining talent

The NHS must attract and retain the highest calibre of staff possible in order to deliver high quality, safe, patient care, and meet performance indicators from the Department of Health. When selecting applicants organizations report that they use a variety of methods (Table 23.2). However, the 'best' option is remains unclear.

Table 23.2

Methods used to select applicants (%)	
Competency-based interviews	69
Interviews following contents of a CV /Application form	68
Structured interviews	59
Tests for specific skills	50
General ability tests	44
Literacy and/or numeracy tests	39
Telephone interviews	38
Personality/aptitude questionnaires	35
Assessment centres	35
Group exercises (for example role-playing)	26
Pre-interview referencing	19
Online tests (selection)	17
Other	6

Staff like working in supportive and stimulating environments, and feeling valued as part of the organization. This will depend upon the culture of an organization, which may be assessed in many ways.

Common methods of measuring and assessing culture involve monitoring surrogates, such as staff turnover and sickness levels. If the turnover or sickness levels are higher than agreed target levels, then HR should assist managers in addressing the underlying reasons.

Staff surveys (usually web-based or paper questionnaires) can be very useful in assessing culture, and results of annual surveys are closely examined. Whilst many organizations seek the views of all staff, some only evaluate a sample.

The *Sunday Times* publishes the 'Best Employers' survey annually, and it has been used as one indicator of whether an organization is a good employer. Recently, a 'public-sector'section has been introduced and a number of NHS Trusts are participating. The criteria measured (from employee responses) indicate the 'health' of an organization, and companies aspire to be listed in the top 100. Measurement criteria include:

- Leadership – Feelings about senior managers, and company values and principles
- My manager – Views about communications with direct managers
- Personal growth – Opinions about training and future prospects
- Well-being – Feelings regarding stress, pressure at work, and work-life balance
- My team – Judgements regarding immediate colleagues and team-working

- Giving back – Beliefs regarding the positive impact the organization has on society
- My company – Levels of engagement with both job and organization
- Fair deal – Happiness with pay and benefits

Employing world class leaders

The key to attracting, retaining, and making the most of top talent is employing world-class leaders at all levels. World-class leadership can mean many different things, but may include being the best at what you do, demonstrating a passion for excellence, pushing boundaries, being a top-notch communicator, or being an innovator.

Managers play a vital role in motivating, empowering, and developing their staff, ensuring a high-quality workforce (see Chapters 45 and 50). There are however many theories on leadership and management, and many role models to aspire to. Greg Dyke, an experienced CEO, has very interesting insights regarding effective leadership. In response to the question, 'what makes an excellent leader', he replied:

> In short you've got to be who you are. Don't pretend to be anything else. You've got to know how to communicate with the people who work for you, and your customers, but particularly the people who work for you. You've got to care about them. If it's a big organization it's impossible to communicate with everybody one–to–one. Therefore you've got to work out 'how do you communicate.' You have to recognize that leadership is about the stories they tell about you. If you walk into an organization, ignore the security people, ignore the receptionist, are rude to somebody else, that's the story they tell about you. If you go in and know everybody, talk to everybody, that's also the story they tell about you. So you've got to understand that the impact you have on a big organisation is about the stories that are told about you within the organisation.

The need for Trusts to invest in clinical leadership is clear. Not all clinicians will have the ambition, or ability, to become 'top executives'; but finding those few who can, will make a big difference.

Providing growth and development opportunities

The provision of growth and development opportunities with clear, visible progression paths is critical in ensuring the NHS recruits and retains the right people.

Analysing staff turnover statistics over a 2- to 3-year period can give useful insights into problem areas, especially when broken down into departments, bandings, and ages. Identifying high turnover areas quickly can result in enormous financial savings, reduction in stress, and of course, most importantly, higher levels of patient care.

When organizations are polled, the most frequently cited actions taken to address retention are:

- Improving induction processes (e.g. convenience)
- Improving selection techniques (e.g. providing clear reasoning)
- Offering better learning and development opportunities (e.g. time to undertake courses)

- Increasing pay
- Introducing reward schemes (e.g. employee of the month)

Although the majority of organizations believe that improving line manager HR skills is the most effective method of improving retention, only a minority report using this method. One reason for this is that many line mangers show a reluctance to accept 'non-care' activities, feeling it should be left to HR professionals. However, where they can be persuaded to take on more 'people-centred' roles, benefits including increased staff motivation soon follow.

Not all organizations are able to supply turnover data and results from self-selecting responders should be treated cautiously. This lack is surprising given the increased focus on human capital measurement to demonstrate the value of HR and people management. The Association of Chartered Certified Accountants (ACCA) and the Chartered Institute of Personnel and Development (CIPD) have conducted research examining the levels of disclosure of data that UK businesses provide in their reports. The key finding was that many organizations view people as a major driver of sustainability; it is therefore important to develop them.

Succession planning

Effective talent management, and succession planning, enables the NHS to be flexible. The ability to quickly fill a post following new service developments, promotion, or retirement is vital. Considerable cost is involved in recruiting staff (advertising, interviewing, induction, and training), so effective organizations ensure they make every effort to use the investment wisely. They develop a sound knowledge of the potential within their Trust, so that key positions can quickly be filled by high calibre individuals.

For all staff groups, this requires effective appraisal systems, including a personal development plan (PDP). This should ensure staff are equipped (through learning opportunities, secondments, and 'acting-up' opportunities) to take on the more specialist senior roles they aspire to. For trainees within the medical profession this has been undertaken at deanery level by the annual review of clinical practice (ARCP). The NHS now operates a graduate training scheme to similarly equip mangers with the diverse skills needed to become Board-level executives.

Workforce data and information

Accurate workforce planning plays a key part in recruitment and retention initiatives. It provides information to help Trusts put together an HR strategy which forms part of the organization's Integrated Business Plan. Data gathered from various sources (e.g. staff surveys, focus groups, attendance reporting, e-rostering, diary cards) provides useful insight into both levels of productivity and staff engagement and satisfaction indices.

(a) Electronic staff records (ESR)

All Trusts within the NHS use ESR to manage personal, organizational and payroll processes. Both HR departments and accredited managers can elicit a range of reports from this system. Examples of these reports (which may affect both individuals or staff groups) include:

◆ Retirement predictions – providing advanced warning of likely vacancies, to aid in succession planning

◆ Sickness reports – giving an overview of levels of sick leave, allowing recurrent absences to be highlighted. This facilitates early recourse to support services, including retraining, redeployment, counselling or even retirement on ill-health grounds

◆ Ethnicity and gender reports – may give early warning of failure to comply with diversity policies

◆ E-rostering reports – ensuring that staff are working in accordance with EWTD requirements and that requests for flexible working can be accommodated

(b) NHS Performance Indicators relevant to human resources

Trusts must regularly report on a number of key performance indicators (KPI). These are regularly reviewed by clinical governance, risk, and management committees. It is important that action is taken to address areas where performance is sub-standard. In addition to having serious implications for patients, failing to achieve desired targets can put unnecessary pressure on staff, resulting in reduction in motivation and performance. Examples of KPIs and the implications for HR are:

◆ 18-week wait – implications for both patient pathways and staff training. Recruiters must act efficiently to fill vacancies, whilst learning and development teams need to ensure new staff are competent to carry out procedures

◆ Cancelled operations – largely a recruitment pressure, which may impact upon relationships between Trust medical recruitment and deanery staff engaged in training rosters. A close relationship between these parties is vital to ensure junior doctors are available to fill rotas

◆ MRSA and *C. difficile* indicators – impact heavily on OH departments, with responsibility for ensuring staff are appropriately screened prior to starting work. If this system fails, an infection control risk occurs

◆ Mandatory training attendance – learning and developments departments within HR are responsible for organizing this. Failure to achieve mandatory training targets may result in failure of the Trust at the Annual Health Check performed by the Care Quality Commission. This leads to further external monitoring, since mandatory training is in-place to ensure the safety of staff and patients alike. Since attendance at specific times may be difficult, many Trusts have introduced e-learning modules, allowing staff to complete training at their own convenience

The graph below demonstrates (for 1 Trust) the wide range of mandatory training required and compliance levels achieved. Reports can also show which staff groups have most difficulty complying, allowing targeted training to be instituted.

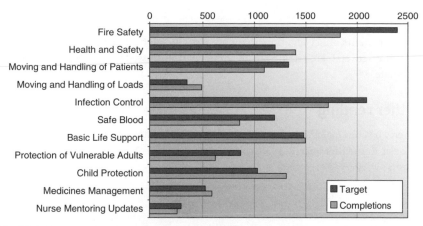

Fig. 23.1 An example of completions aganist targets for mandatory training in 1 Trust in 2008/2009.

◆ Diversity – reports identifying whether discrimination is likely to be occurring. Board strategies should ensure Trusts are equal opportunity employers. An example of how well diversity strategies are accepted in organizations is shown in the table below. The findings from this sample year (2008) suggest that they are most common in the public services sector (of which the NHS is a part).

	Does your organization have a formal diversity strategy? (%)				
	All	**Manufacturing and production**	**Voluntary, community and not-for-profit**	**Private sector services**	**Public services**
Yes	60	45	64	52	91
No	37	50	33	44	7
Don't Know	4	5	4	4	3

The methods used by organizations to encourage diversity include: advertising in specialist publications dedicated to minority groups, promoting development centres, and the use of mentoring and secondment opportunities for those at risk of being discriminated against.

The practice of checking that tests used to detect discrimination are valid, reliable and culture-free has increased over time. Although 84% of respondent organizations say they monitor recruitment, there is still room for improvement. Other activities (such as those described above) to encourage a more diverse workforce, with attendant advantages should be encouraged.

Summary

HR departments are crucial to enhancing patient safety. They ensure appropriate, well motivated, staff are retained by the organization, as well as keeping them safe and up-to-date.

Further reading

Chartered Institute for Personnel and Development (CIPD). http://www.cipd.co.uk/default.cipd.

Brinkman, R. and Kirschner, R. *Dealing with People You Can't Stand*. McGraw-Hill. ISBN 0-07-007838-6.

Chapter 24

Improving working lives

Andrew Rochford

Key points

- 'New Deal' and EWTD were designed to both reduce the risk to patients and improve the working lives of junior doctors.
- Modernising Medical Careers (MMC) was a major reform of postgraduate medical training, devised to improve the quality of patient care through better education and training for doctors.
- Projects such as Hospital at Night and 'Taking Care 24:7' are innovative models of care designed to address the balance between training and service provision.
- Full shift working has a significant impact on clinical governance.
- A major cultural change has begun in the way that the medical workforce is trained, and healthcare is delivered, at both junior and senior level.

Legal requirements

The working lives of junior doctors have changed dramatically over the last decade. The British Medical Association (BMA) negotiated a 'New Deal', which established a contractual limit for doctors in training of 56 hours worked per week from August 2003. The European Working Time Directive (EWTD) was created by the Council of the European Union in 1993 and adopted into British law in 1998 as the Working Time Regulations (WTR). The Directive defines minimum requirements in relation to working hours, rest periods, annual leave, and working arrangements for night workers. The SiMAP and Jaegar judgements in the European Court of Justice clarified the definition of working time (to include all time spent resident on call even if sleeping) and rest. Junior doctors in training were exempt until August 2004 when the WTR were implemented in stages. The last stage, a '48-hour' working week, was made mandatory from August 2009. Junior doctors' working hours are now limited to a shift of no more than 13 hours followed by a break of at least 11 hours.

These regulations formed part of the policies and regulations designed to help the NHS meet the Improving Working Lives Standard outlined in the Government

NHS Plan: a plan for investment, a plan for reform (Department of Health 2000). 'New Deal' and EWTD were designed to:

◆ Reduce the risk to patients and doctors based on the evidence that rested doctors are less likely to make serious medical errors or endanger themselves

◆ Improve the working lives of junior doctors by improving their quality of life and reduce exploitation by NHS Trusts

Evidence highlights the negative effect on health and performance of working long hours, but it should be noted that much of the evidence is drawn from industry and may not be directly transferable to healthcare. Achieving compliance with these regulations has been one of the major challenges that the NHS has faced in recent years. Whether the regulations have achieved their goals is the subject of on-going debate.

Flexible working

The NHS workforce is now more diverse than ever before, reflecting social and demographic changes in the United Kingdom. Women make up over 70% of the NHS workforce, many staff are parents (some are single parents) or may have carer responsibilities, and the demand for flexible working is increasing. There are significant benefits to an organization with mature flexible working policies, including improvements in:

◆ Recruitment and retention of staff

◆ Staff morale

◆ Skill mix availability

◆ Productivity

Promoting flexible working has been a priority of the Improving Working Lives initiative. Flexible working exists in many forms, including the obvious part-time working, but also return to work schemes, career breaks or sabbaticals, and job-sharing. These practices are reinforced by employment legislation including the Employment Relations Act (Amendment 2005), the Employment Act 2002: Flexible Working, and the Work & Families Act 2006. It has been estimated that over 20% of female doctors may be working on a part-time or flexible basis within 7 years of their graduation from medical school and another 6% may have taken career breaks. This has important implications for not only the delivery of healthcare, but also for the number of women represented in leadership roles.

Medical education

Modernising Medical Careers (MMC) was a major reform of postgraduate medical training, devised to improve the quality of patient care through better education and training for doctors. It was launched in 2003 following the Chief Medical Officer's Report *Unfinished Business*, and was introduced with recruitment to the Foundation Programme in 2005 and recruitment to Specialty Training in 2007. The aim of MMC was to provide a 'transparent and efficient career path for doctors'. It included increased accountability for trainees and trainers and nationally agreed specialty training standards leading to more competency-based practice and career progression.

MMC also promised a 'fair, equitable and transparent' recruitment process, the centralized Medical Training Application Service (MTAS). MTAS caused a national migration of junior doctors and collapsed under a media furore in Spring 2007. An independent inquiry, the Tooke Report, was commissioned by the Secretary of State for Health and MMC/MTAS was subsequently scrutinized by a Health Select Committee. The Committee published its report in May 2008 and was highly critical of the way in which the reforms were managed, highlighting failings in leadership, governance, and policy development.

There is an increasing demand on NHS performance to provide a more patient-focused service that delivers 'value for money'. The ideals and subsequent implementation of MMC highlighted core tensions in the NHS: achieving a balance between achieving key performance indicators and training junior doctors (Fig. 24.1).

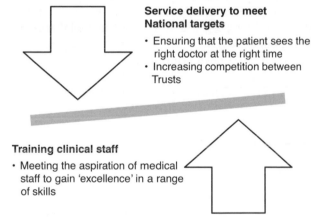

Service delivery to meet National targets
- Ensuring that the patient sees the right doctor at the right time
- Increasing competition between Trusts

Training clinical staff
- Meeting the aspiration of medical staff to gain 'excellence' in a range of skills

Fig. 24.1 There is an inherent tension between service and training, for which an acceptable balance must be achieved.

Innovative models of care

The modern NHS strives to provide high-quality care for all, and needs to adapt to the changing health needs of society. This was summarized by the Junior Health Minister, Lord Darzi in High Quality Care for All – NHS Next Stage Review as:

- Rising expectations
- Demand driven by demographics
- The continuing development of our 'information society'
- Advances in treatments
- The changing nature of disease
- The changing expectations of the health workplace

The medical workforce is responsible for delivering a safe and effective patient experience within the training structure of MMC and constraints of the WTR. This has led to a number of initiatives which have challenged the traditions of medical training and service provision.

Hospital at Night

Hospital at Night (HaN) was a new method of working developed by the Joint Consultants Committee (representing the BMA and the Academy of Medical Royal Colleges) and the NHS Modernisation Agency. It was piloted in four acute Trusts in 2003–04. The programme's original aim was 'to reduce dependency on training grade doctors for providing cover at night, in order to reduce their working hours and eliminate sleep deprivation without damaging their training'.

HaN was a clinically driven, patient-focused change programme. It adopted a multi-professional and multi-speciality approach to deliver care at night and out of hours. Information gathered about workload out of hours revealed that a considerable amount of work could be undertaken by nonmedical staff, and demonstrated a significant discrepancy in the activity levels between different specialties.

Clinical staff were working in isolation (often termed 'silo' working), many tasks were unnecessarily duplicated, and much of the work could and should have taken place during routine hours. Consequently, the 'routine' working day was redefined and extended to maximise education and training as well as increasing hospital productivity (see Fig. 24.2). Clinical staff rotas were redesigned and realigned to ensure

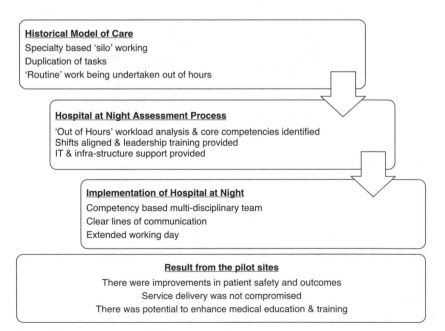

Fig. 24.2 A summary of Hospital at Night implementation.

EWTD compliance, and documentation and handover practices were reviewed and improved. It was acknowledged that the composition of the HaN team would be bespoke for each Trust, but there was significant investment in training to ensure that the HaN multi-professional team had the core competencies and skills required to deal with immediate patient care out of hours. Specialist services were available to be called in from home if required.

There was considerable resistance to change reported by the pilot sites; the model required medical and nursing staff to work very differently and represented a significant cultural shift. However, the pilot sites demonstrated:

♦ Improvements in patient safety and outcomes

♦ No compromise in service delivery

♦ The potential to enhance medical education and training

The project was encouraged throughout the NHS but took time to take effect. A 2006 survey revealed that only 48% of NHS trusts in England had started to, or had implemented HaN. However, a more recent study (the Hospital at Night 2008 UK Implementation Survey) has shown that almost 80% of NHS trusts across England, Wales, and Scotland have adopted the HaN method of team working. Interest in adopting the HaN model has spread beyond the United Kingdom, with active implementation in Hong Kong, Australia, and New Zealand, and increasing interest across other EU member states.

HaN should not be seen as a quick or easy solution to meeting EWTD requirements. Successful implementation requires:

♦ Careful data analysis

♦ Thorough competency and skills assessment

♦ A whole systems approach to change

♦ Strong clinical leadership

Many hospitals are now examining whether this model of out of hours care can be adopted into aspects of daytime working with the 'Taking Care 24:7' project launched across five sites in 2006. The sites have been examining specific aspects of patient care and are supported by grants from the NHS Workforce Projects team. The projects are on-going.

Shift patterns and patient safety

Both HaN and 'Taking Care 24:7' employ junior doctors working in full shift patterns. The reduction of the working week from 56 to 48 hours in 2009 resulted in a further 12% fall in daytime availability of junior doctors in the average rotation. Consequently, juniors will not be present for the shifts where they receive most of their active teaching. It has been estimated that for surgical trainees the combination of EWTD and MMC has reduced their training by 50%. The overall working hours may have reduced, but for the majority the proportion of out of hours working has increased. This is a cause for concern as evidence from both healthcare and other industries demonstrates that the capacity to learn overnight is significantly impaired, and that sleep is required to consolidate new learning. Furthermore, juniors have expressed significant dissatisfaction with the changes: a survey of ENT trainees (BMJ 2005) revealed that 71% of trainees would be prepared to opt out of the WTD to 'safeguard care for patients and their training', and a survey of Specialist Registrars (Royal College of Physicians 2004) reported high levels of fatigue and poor performance on the night shift.

The reduction in hours and associated move to full shift working patterns has led to a decrease in continuity of care. There is a complex relationship between

* Patient safety
* Continuity of care
* Fatigue in healthcare providers

A reduction in fatigue will certainly lead to an improvement in patient safety measured against a variety of task-based activities. However, this leaves the question of whether discontinuity of care adversely affects patient safety. Unfortunately, many of the studies in this area differ in various aspects; there may be publication bias against negative studies and there are no clinical trials.

In the NHS it has been said that continuity of care has been progressively eroded. In acute care, the decline commenced with altered training patterns instituted by Calman in the mid-1990s, when the two-tier registrar grade was unified into a single 'specialist registrar' grade, and training to consultant level shortened. It has been compounded first by the 'New Deal' and then EWTD. There is some evidence to show that a lack of continuity of care leads to an increase in task-based errors. It is worth exploring what defines continuity of care. In its purest form, one would seek for a 'cradle to grave' philosophy with a strong bond and relationship between patient and clinician. However, improvement in information technology and education structures has developed, acknowledging that in a modern NHS no single person can be expected to know everything that an individual patient might need.

	Continuity of care model	Single intervention model
Example	General practitioners in UK	Anaesthesia
	This is undermined by emergence of large health centres and out of hours co-operatives	Accident & Emergency
		Radiology services
Provision by	Junior doctors working on a medical 'firm'	Consultants
	This is significantly challenged by the need to comply with EWTD	
Requirements	Long hours	Effective systems & processes
		In particular, IT infrastructure, standardised handover, peer review, continued medical education

Patient safety remains the most important priority of all healthcare workers and evidence from the United States suggests that the [American] public believe that limiting working hours will improve patient safety. Of course, this should be taken in the context of the American Healthcare system where junior doctors routinely work long hours. There is no such comparison with EWTD and patient care in the United Kingdom. The assumption of at least one of the Royal Colleges has been that the general public would prefer continuity of care over less fatigued doctors.

Handover

In the United Kingdom, there has been a focus of attention on handover highlighted by the General Medical Council's *Good Medical Practice* (2006), which makes clear the expectation that 'sharing information with other healthcare professionals is important for safe and effective patient care'. Evidence suggests there has always been a weakness in the medical handover process that has been increasingly exposed by the reduction in continuity of care. Certainly, the move to shift working and formal handover has been a major cultural challenge for both junior and senior doctors in most clinical areas, and has been acknowledged as a 'critical element' of HaN. Guidance has been issued by the Department of Health and the BMA, in their document *Safe Handover: Safe Patients* (2004) which acknowledges that 'continuity of information is vital to the safety of our patients'.

The evidence from the HaN pilot sites suggested that good handover enhanced the education and training of the junior doctors. Senior leadership and role definition is identified as crucial to success yet the process has never been formalised and remains highly variable. SBAR (Situation, Background, Assessment, Recommendation) is a communication tool developed in the United States, which has been adopted by many healthcare organisations (see Chapter 46). It is an easy-to-remember and reliable framework that can be used for any communication, especially critical ones, which require a clinician's immediate attention and action. It is again being recommended to NHS organisations as part of the National Patient Safety Campaign.

Summary

Clinical governance must underpin changes to work patterns of doctors. Risk assessment and patient safety are paramount to service provision, whilst the need for competency-based multi-professional working requires continued professional development. Shift working may lead to an erosion of continuity of care unless there are robust handover and communication practices in place. It is recognized that responding to the current changing healthcare environment requires strong clinical and organizational leadership supported by clinical audit that is embedded as a cultural norm within the NHS.

It has been argued that HaN has been strongly endorsed by Postgraduate Deans, Royal Colleges, and the BMA because it seems the best way of reducing the adverse impact on training of the inevitable introduction of full shift rotas and achieving compliance with EWTD and 'New Deal'. Medicine has changed and methods of training and service provision which were appropriate 25 years ago are less so now. It is likely that the way in which many NHS services are provided in the future will be significantly different from today: we need a workforce that is both 'fit for purpose' and capable of adapting to change.

Further reading

NHS Next Stage Review: A High Quality Workforce Department of Health, June 2008.

The Future of the Medical Workforce NHS Employers, October 2007.

Fletcher, K.E., Davis, S.Q., Underwood, W. et al. (2004). Systematic Review: Effects of Resident Work Hours on Patient Safety. *Ann Intern Med* **141**, 851–857.

Ahmed-Little, Y. (2007). Implications of shift work for junior doctors. *BMJ* **334**, 777–778.

The implementation and impact of Hospital at Night pilot projects. An evaluation report Department of Health, August 2005.

Safe handover: safe patients. Guidance on clinical handover for clinicians and managers. British Medical Association, 2004.

Chapter 25

Revalidation

Judith Hulf and Kirstyn Shaw

Key points

- Revalidation aims to improve patient safety by raising the standards and quality of practise, as well as identifying poorly performing doctors.
- Revalidation is for all licensed doctors working in the United Kingdom.
- Doctors will be required to provide evidence demonstrating that they are fit to practice. This should present little problem for most doctors.
- Strengthened appraisal will be the key process through which doctors will demonstrate their practice against standards.
- The GMC decisions regarding revalidation will be based on recommendations from a local Responsible Officer.

Introduction

The purpose of revalidation and medical regulation is to provide a positive affirmation of a doctor's practice and to encourage the ongoing development of standards and quality in medical care.

Revalidation is a process where *all* licensed doctors will be required to periodically *demonstrate* their continued fitness to practise, both clinically and in terms of professional conduct. In addition, specialist doctors will need to *demonstrate* that they meet the standards that apply to their particular medical specialty. In the event that a doctor's practice is questioned, then an *evaluation* of supporting information would be required, progressing to an *assessment* if deemed necessary. For most doctors, the provision of such information is based on what they do and should present little problem.

A secondary outcome of the process is the identification of doctors whose performance is not of a sufficiently high standard. However, it is important to highlight that the vast majority of doctors practicing medicine in the United Kingdom are doing so to a high standard.

The implementation of revalidation for all medical specialties is expected to begin in 2011. The process will be regulated by the General Medical Council (GMC) who issued licenses to practice throughout 2009. Revalidation will be divided into two elements: relicensing and recertification.

	Relicensing	Recertification
Who	All doctors in the UK	Doctors undertaking specialist practice
What	Reaffirm right to practice	Demonstrate own level against standards set by the relevant Medical Royal College or Faculty
How	Take part in satisfactory annual appraisals:	Methods set by relevant Royal College or Faculty
	◆ Multi-source feedback from peers ◆ Patient feedback ◆ Personal Development Plan ◆ Recorded concerns (practice or conduct)	Likely to require specialty specific information about practice, including: ◆ Continuing Professional Development ◆ Clinical audit ◆ Knowledge assessment ◆ Clinical outcomes

Standards and supporting information for relicensing and recertification will be discussed at appraisal on an annual basis and reviewed every five years for revalidation.

The scope of revalidation

The scope of revalidation includes the following aims:

- To improve patient safety by raising the overall standards and quality of clinical care
- Identify poorly performing doctors
- To require doctors to demonstrate that they are up to date and fit to practice
- To be a five-year process *not* a fifth year process – doctors should be reflecting on their practice and collecting supporting information on a regular basis throughout the five years leading to revalidation
- It should not be burdensome for the profession (or the service) but attempt to harness the tools employed in working life
- Standards should not vary according to geography or speciality
- Standards and supporting information should be clearly defined for each specialty
- Early identification of doctors with difficulties is essential as they will need access to remedial support within the 5 year cycle; not at the end of 5 years

Since revalidation is only now being developed across the United Kingdom, it cannot be a static process. There will be a phased roll-out of revalidation rather than a big bang start date. Following a period of development, piloting, and evaluation, each element should be implemented when available, but will continue to develop over time to fit with local processes, service delivery, and professional ownership. The first cycle of revalidation may, in itself, be a pilot. Whilst the specific details and processes associated with the ultimate implementation of revalidation in each nation of the

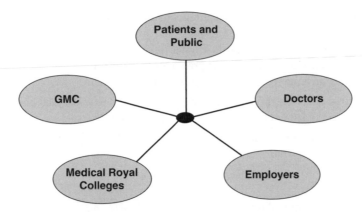

Fig. 25.1 Stakeholders.

United Kingdom may vary, they will all maintain national standards. Electronic systems of recording and support are likely to be essential to avoid gross disruption to clinical service.

The General Medical Council (the sole regulator for the medical profession) (Fig. 25.1)

The role of the GMC within revalidation will be to:

- Issue licenses to practice
- Hold and update the general, specialist and GP registers
- Provide some quality assurance of the revalidation process
- Take the decisions about whether an individual doctor will be revalidated

The Medical Royal Colleges (non-members will need to be in contact in order to revalidate)

The Academy of Medical Royal Colleges and Faculties will ensure the consistent development and implementation of revalidation across the different medical specialties. The Colleges and Faculties, in association with their specialist societies, will:

- Set educational, professional, and clinical standards for their medical specialty
- Develop methods and supporting information to allow doctors to *demonstrate* that their level of practice reaches the specialty standards. This will include both the doctor's conduct (measure of professional behaviour) and their clinical competence
- Be responsible for quality assurance of a recommendation that an individual doctor has demonstrated meeting the appropriate standards for specialist recertification (providing specialty input), i.e. minimising the risk of both false positives and false negatives

The Employers (will be required to appoint a Responsible Officer)

In many cases, the responsible officer will be the existing medical director. They will:

- Oversee the development of clinical governance systems to support the implementation of revalidation. Such clinical governance systems will include:

- The establishment of enhanced appraisal based on the standards defined by the GMC
- Complaints and incident reporting systems
- Training and education around appraisal and revalidation
- Any other governance processes required for revalidation

- Be required to review the supporting information and to make recommendations about the revalidation of individual doctors to the GMC

- Contact the appropriate Medical Royal College or Faculty when they need specialist support, advice, or information

Individual Doctors (will need to ensure that they establish a link with a responsible officer)

Doctors will be required to:

- Demonstrate that they are up to date and fit to practice, i.e. undertake relicensing and recertification leading to revalidation

- Ensure they have all the required supporting information to demonstrate that they are compliant with both generic and specialist standards appropriate to their practice. Supporting information will, in most cases, be directly related to the specific practice of the individual

For those working in the NHS, the most likely relationship is to the responsible officer in the acute or primary care Trust (PCT). Doctors working in the independent sector, private practice, or as locums will also need to be linked to a responsible officer who will be responsible for overseeing and implementing revalidation.

Patients and the public

They will be involved in:

- Patient feedback questionnaires for individual doctors relating to quality of care for relicensing

- Setting standards for revalidation (via the GMC and the Medical Royal Colleges)

- Developing methods for revalidation (represented at the GMC and Medical Royal Colleges)

Standards

The standards for revalidation have been developed by the General Medical Council based on their publication, *Good Medical Practice*. The standards include four key domains:

1. Knowledge, skills and performance

2. Safety and quality

3. Communication, partnership, and teamwork

4. Maintaining trust

Each of these domains is further broken down into a range of attributes with associated generic standards and criteria. Doctors should demonstrate compliance against all attributes using a range of supporting information. This has been developed by the medical Royal Colleges, but is likely to be refined in the future for sub-specialist practice.

Appraisal

Annual appraisal is one of the key elements of revalidation, which all doctors will be required to undertake. This will include a discussion of their practice throughout the previous 12 months. A standardized module for 'strengthened' appraisal, based on the GMC standards framework, will be incorporated into the appraisal interview of all doctors. The framework should encourage doctors to reflect on their work and how it relates to the standards outlined for generic and specialist practice. Most doctors should therefore be fully prepared for revalidation when it is required; thus a formative activity (appraisal) will be developed into a summative process (revalidation). The challenge is to avoid losing the developmental purpose and focus of appraisal.

Supporting information and evidence: What should be in the appraisal folder

Information should be related to current practice and is intended to show the work a doctor does on a regular basis and the standard to which it is delivered.

Common forms of supporting information for doctors will include:

- Multi-source colleague and patient feedback
- Continuing professional development – courses and conferences attended
- Complaints and incidents
- Information about any non-clinical work activities which might include:
  - Teaching: e.g. of undergraduates, postgraduates, and paramedical staff, occurring locally, regionally, nationally, and internationally
  - Research – intended, in process and completed
  - Medical management – at a range of levels, both within and without their own Trust

Clinical work (the main focus of revalidation)

Examples of specialty specific types of supporting information that could be used include:

- Clinical audit
- Clinical outcomes
- Knowledge assessment
- Case based discussion

Most medical care is administered by teams and the quality of care is intrinsically linked to the infrastructure and support available including the:

- Facilities available (see Chapter 27)
- Access to investigations and interventions
- Competencies of other members of the team

Therefore there is growing recognition that revalidation will not be able to consider the practice of an individual in isolation, but that appropriate supporting information may also include information about the performance of the team or the unit. Any supporting evidence should if possible address both individual and team based practice. There is a growing recognition that 'service accreditation' is likely to develop as a parallel and complimentary process to revalidation.

Non-clinical work

The majority of doctors also undertake a range of non-clinical work as part of their regular activity. While revalidation will largely focus on the clinical skills and standards of clinical practice, those doctors who undertake non-clinical work will also be required to provide supporting information for such activities. Many of these activities already involve a form of appraisal or performance evaluation and it is proposed that the satisfactory completion of such evaluations may be sufficient information for revalidation.

Remediation and support

Revalidation is likely to identify a number of doctors who may be struggling. This could range from something as simple as being unable to locate or collect the required supporting information, to significant concerns being identified about a doctor's behaviour or delivery of care. Confidential remedial support should be made readily available to all doctors at any stage of the revalidation process, from the little 'r' of needing advice and guidance to the bigger 'R' of requiring formal remediation and/or retraining. A number of organizations and avenues for remediation are already available to doctors and these will continue. In addition, new forms of remediation and guidance are being identified and developed to provide doctors and appraisers with a range of options to support the revalidation process.

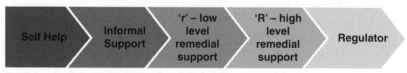

Fig. 25.2 Range of Remedial Support.
Reproduced from Academy of Medical Royal Colleges (2009). Remediation and Revalidation: report and recommendations. Available at: http://www.aomrc.org.uk. London: AoMRC, with permission.

Summary

The regulation of doctors, across the world, has evolved rapidly with the: development of standards of practice, implementation of appraisal, establishment of clinical governance frameworks, and planned introduction of revalidation. Revalidation should prove non-problematic for most doctors (who will be able to prove they are up to date and fit to practise) whilst protecting patients from the small minority of under-performing doctors, thus increasing public confidence in the quality of the medical profession and heath care.

Further reading

General Medical Council. (2007). *Good Medical Practice*. London: GMC.

Department of Health. (2007). *Trust Assurance and Safety: the regulation of health professionals in the 21st Century*. London: Stationary Office.

Chief Medical Officer. (2008). *Medical Revalidation: Principles and Next Steps*. London: Crown Copyright.

Chief Medical Officer. (2006). *Good Doctors, Safer Patients: Proposals to Strengthen the System to Assure and Improve the Performance of Doctors and to Protect the Safety of Patients*. London: Stationary Office.

Academy of Medical Royal Colleges. (2008). *Revalidation*. http://www.aomrc.org.uk/revalidation.aspx

Chapter 26

Personnel: Poor clinical performance

Jeremy Mitchell

Key points

- Poor clinical performance affects quality of care.
- Clinical performance is affected by personal and organizational factors.
- Approximately 1:200 doctors are referred to the National Clinical Assessment Service (NCAS) every year for poor performance.
- The performance of approximately 15% of doctors is affected by ill-health at some point during their working life.
- The performance of at least 5% of doctors is affected by drugs or alcohol at some point during their working life.

Introduction

Poor clinical performance may impact on the quality of care given to patients and may be related to behaviour, conduct, or health issues. Performance of individual staff may be affected by a variety of personal and external factors highlighted in the box:

Possible causes of poor clinical performance

- Deficiencies in clinical knowledge and skills
- Physical illness
- Mental illness, including alcohol or substance abuse
- Cognitive problems
- Recent life events
- Recent promotion
- Workload changes
- Team difficulties
- Organizational changes

Deficiency in knowledge and/or skills

Clinicians are faced with an ever-expanding range of clinical issues throughout their career. Their knowledge and skills will be based on initial undergraduate and post-graduate training, increasingly supplemented by continuing medical education. As careers progress, it is common to focus on increasingly narrow aspects of medical practice.

Some clinicians will have an encyclopaedic knowledge, others will be good crafts-men. A relative deficiency in knowledge may be masked by development of clinical skills (and vice versa). This may not be a problem provided the individual recognizes their deficiencies and does not attempt to practice outside their abilities. However other issues (e.g. mental illness, recent life events) may impair judgement and cause a relative deficiency in knowledge or skills to become more obvious.

◆ *Knowledge*: Traditionally tested at undergraduate and postgraduate levels. The effectiveness of testing is questionable, but nevertheless there is a systematic proc-ess. However, as time passes, it is possible for clinicians to fail to retain knowledge in relevant areas.

◆ *Skills*: Likely to be increasingly honed with appropriate experience as a senior doc-tor. Traditionally very little, if any, assessment of skills has occurred. Often doctors who consider that they work in teams perform their clinical skills in relative isola-tion (consultant surgeons may rarely operate with senior colleagues), and it can be difficult to compare skill levels. Clinical outcome measures (e.g. mortality) are often used as indirect assessments of skills in some groups (especially surgeons). However, these may reflect the whole treatment process, rather than surgical skills alone.

Physical illness

There is a substantial population of clinicians (United Kingdom > 100,000) and in line with the general population a significant number have physical illnesses. It is some-times difficult for clinicians to accept that they too can become unwell and may need treatment. Provided an individual clinician recognizes the possible impact of illness and treatment, making appropriate arrangements to deal with this, it should not impact on patient care. However, on occasion, individuals fail to recognize this impact due to poor judgement or lack of insight. This may be difficult to manage, especially if the individual is a senior clinician. It is important that staff do not attempt to treat their own illnesses, allowing others to make appropriate treatment decisions.

Mental illness

Mental health issues are more common in health service professionals compared to those in other employment. Problems include stress, depression, alcoholism, and drug dependency. All may lead to problems with:

◆ Concentration

◆ Attention

- Memory
- Irritability

As with physical illness there may be a reluctance to seek help before the problem impacts on patient care. For some doctors, barriers in following a chosen career pathway can lead to mental illness and drug dependency, and in others the working environment may precipitate such problems.

Cognitive problems

Cognitive impairment may occur at any age, consequent upon a range of disorders, including head injury, intracranial tumours, alcohol dependency, dementia, and as a medication side effect. Those affected may have poor concentration, confusion and memory loss. Cognitive testing may reveal:

- Diffuse cognitive problems involving attention span, immediate recall, and memory
- Focal issues involving:
  - Frontal lobes (e.g. disinhibited behaviour, disordered abstract thinking)
  - Temporo-occiptal regions (e.g. disordered ability to repeat motor tasks sequentially)

Dementia affects 10% of patients aged over 65, and a smaller proportion under 65. Alzheimer's disease is the commonest cause, with an insidious onset in middle age. It is more likely in those with a family history, or following a head injury. Identification can be difficult in the early stages where there may be mild behavioural problems and depression. More obvious clinical deficits will usually result in prompt diagnosis by colleagues, and appropriate action.

Recent life events

Any significant event in clinicians' personal lives can impact on performance. In particular, bereavement and matrimonial issues may have a prolonged negative effect. Grieving may be prolonged and associated with depression, disordered sleep patterns, and poor appetite. Matrimonial disputes and other issues may be concealed, with problems taking some while to become apparent.

Recent promotion

Following promotion, new responsibilities are acquired, either clinical, managerial, or both. New consultants may find that there are unexpected demands in terms of clinical responsibility, and limited opportunity to seek advice and support from colleagues. It is important for clinical directors and those in similar posts to support newly appointed colleagues.

Those taking on clinical managerial responsibility in addition to clinical duties may find there are unexpected demands in attempting to meet both the expectations of managers and the needs of consultant colleagues. This may detract from clinical performance. Senior members of the Trust must ensure that job plans for those with significant clinical managerial responsibility are constructed allowing an appropriate balance between clinical and non-clinical demands.

Workload changes

Excessive workload, including increased out-of-hours activity (especially with circadian rhythm disturbance), may lead to fatigue. This is a subjective feeling of the need to sleep and a state of decreased alertness, reducing the ability to perform routine tasks (e.g. diagnosis and procedures). There may be spontaneous short periods of unresponsiveness ('microsleeps') potentially impacting on patient safety (e.g. during anaesthesia). Fatigue may be worsened in those with poor general health, hypoglycaemia, or substance abuse. The European Working Time Directive (EWTD), now being fully implemented throughout the United Kingdom, is intended to improve both the health of doctors and patient safety.

Fatigue reduction

Minimize sleep disturbance – ensure adequate sleep before and after work periods
Avoid alcohol, caffeine and nicotine immediately prior to sleep
Napping – sufficiently long enough to allow one cycle of deep (non REM) sleep (i.e. over 90 minutes); ongoing need for appropriate rest areas for shift workers

♦ Regular rest breaks

♦ Adequate refreshments

♦ Bright lighting in work areas

♦ Proper use of annual leave as holiday

Team difficulties

Each clinician is part of a team. Some teams work together better than others. Difficulties may occur due to:

♦ Inadequate team leadership

♦ Poor delegation of duties

♦ Unequal workload

♦ Inadequate engagement in performing allocated duties

Sometimes these difficulties may lead to dispute between team members and a withdrawal of one or more colleagues from one or more functions of the team. This is likely to impact on the clinical performance of individual members and the team as a whole.

Organizational changes

It is increasingly likely that there will be mergers of healthcare organizations and changes in service provision. Mergers of clinical services from different organizations with different systems and working arrangements can lead to rivalry and difficulties in communication and working relationships. This may well affect performance of the clinicians involved. Organizations embarking on restructuring should recognize the potential impact on clinical services, and provide strong leadership and support for all grades of staff during the transition, ensuring that all staff are dealt with in a fair and equitable fashion.

Identifying poor performance

Poor performance by staff should be identified by the relevant service or educational lead. This may follow direct observation or concerns raised by, sometimes junior, colleagues. It is often very difficult to set out what constitutes poor performance in distinction to the expected variation in performance across a range of colleagues. The views of nursing and paramedical staff should be taken carefully into consideration, and organizations should have a process allowing concerns to be raised appropriately by all staff (sometimes referred to as 'whistleblowing'). It is important however to ensure a balanced response to malicious gossip.

How does poor performance come to light?

- Concerns from colleagues
- Whistle blowing
- Patient safety incidents
- Complaints
- Litigation
- Clinical audit

The current annual appraisal system for consultants may not reveal poor performance. It is hoped that the enhanced appraisal process, as part of revalidation will assist in the earlier identification of problems. Poor performance by locum staff may be difficult to deal with, especially if the locum undertakes a succession of short-term locum posts scattered around a number of healthcare organizations.

Each organization should have adequate audit processes in place to assess clinical performance. Clinical audit databases require sufficient resources to establish robust data entry, so outcome data is accurate and meaningful.

Signs of poor performance

- Anger
- Defensive attitude
- Pattern of sickness
- Blaming others

Signs of poor performance *(continued)*

- Obstructive in every meeting
- Dress
- Failure to attend meetings/teaching/other professional or managerial activity
- Frustration amongst colleagues/juniors/seniors
- Long-winded response to perceived criticism

Responding to concerns about poor performance

The response to problems will be different in each setting, but organizations should have established processes to assist in dealing with potential poor performance. The needs of the staff under review should be carefully reviewed, with appropriate support being given. Obviously patient safety should be the primary concern. Support must include:

- Ensuring appropriate continuing professional development (see Chapters 31–33)
- Treating illness – both mental and physical
- Ensuring appropriate services and facilities are available – to avoid fatigue and issues associated with team working
- Mentoring – to help staff through life events (including positive events e.g. promotions)

Some cases can be dealt with informally, but it is important that systematic, detailed, and unbiased investigations into concerns raised occur, irrespective of whether formal or informal processes are used. Investigations should focus on demonstrating accountability for actions, but avoid apportioning blame.

Organizations may decide to respond to concerns locally, with or without external assistance in the assessment or response. Speciality-based assessments are becoming more formally a responsibility of Royal Colleges. Sometimes, it will be appropriate to refer concerns to the National Clinical Assessment Service (NCAS), or rarely, the General Medical Council's fitness to practice panel.

The role of the Royal Colleges in reviewing poor clinical performance

Most Royal Colleges have a system for providing local review of individuals or clinical teams within a healthcare organization (e.g. the 'Invited Review' mechanism at the Royal College of Surgeons of England). The response to a request for a review will depend on the severity of the issues and whether other external organizations have been involved.

The National Clinical Assessment Service (NCAS)

NCAS was set up in April 2001 by the Department of Health following several high-profile cases that significantly reduced public confidence in doctors (e.g. Harold Shipman, paediatric cardiac surgery problems at the Bristol Royal Infirmary).

It is now part of the National Patient Safety Agency (NPSA), and covers all four home countries within the United Kingdom.

NCAS aims to promote public confidence in doctors and dentists by addressing concerns about performance. NCAS acts by:

- Responding to requests for help
- Providing educational services to help organizations improve local management of concerns
- Undertaking research and development to improve understanding of performance concerns
- Increasing its scope to cover associated practitioners (e.g. pharmacists)

Requests for help usually come from employers (e.g. a senior member of staff in a Trust). Occasionally the request for help comes from the individual practitioner or from a 'whistleblower'. Members of the public cannot make a referral directly, although NCAS will help direct their concern to the correct regulatory body.

Sometimes performance concerns are serious enough to warrant consideration of suspension, or exclusion of the practitioner. If an employer is considering exclusion of a practitioner they have a duty to contact NCAS prior to making a 'formal exclusion' order. Practitioners may be placed on 'immediate exclusion' for up to two weeks before the formal stage is reached.

Requests for help will be handled by a member of the casework team, who are the first point of contact within NCAS for both referrers and practitioners. They will pass information to an advisor, who will be a senior clinician or manager with experience in dealing with performance issues. The figure shows how requests for help are dealt with by the NCAS.

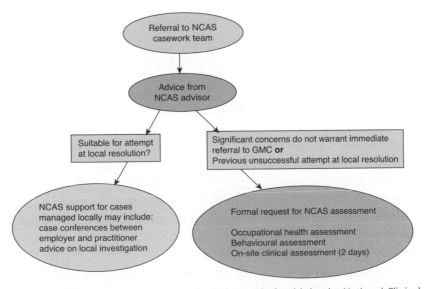

Fig. 26.1 Mechanism by which requests for help are dealt with by the National Clinical Assessment Service (NCAS).

Assessments cover a range of aspects of practice including clinical performance, behaviour, health, and work context. They are intended to:

- Provide an independent review of performance
- Identify areas of concern and factors contributing to these
- Make recommendations for addressing identified difficulties

Reports usually identify recommendations both for practitioners and employers. NCAS will then work with the employer and practitioner to establish a structured action plan, possibly involving a series of meetings between the practitioner, employer, NCAS case manager, and advisor. If a training placement is needed, this will usually be arranged through Deaneries or Royal Colleges. NCAS will follow up the case after 6 and 12 months.

Analysis of NCAS referrals

About 1 practitioner in 200 is referred to NCAS annually. There is little difference in the rate of referral of career grade doctors in primary or secondary care. Analysis of NCAS referrals from 2001-2005 demonstrates that:

- The risk of referral for hospital career grade doctors is about 1.1% per year
- Concerns about behaviour alone:
  - Men (31%) > women (22%)
  - Decreased with age (34% if < 35, 21% if > 65)
  - More likely in groups where clinical failings are harder to observe and measure (e.g. psychiatry)
- Concerns about clinical capability:
  - Increased with age (46% if < 35, 72% if >65)
  - Higher in specialities undertaking technical interventions (e.g. surgery)
- Health concerns were:
  - Unrelated to age
  - Commoner in women (28%) than men (18%)

The General Medical Council

The General Medical Council (GMC) has set out standards for good clinical care in its guidelines *Good Medical Practice* (2006). The fundamental condition is that clinicians must *'recognise, and work within the limits of their competence'*.

The GMC may review a doctor's fitness to practise if:

- *A doctor's performance has, or could have, harmed patients*
- *A doctor has shown a deliberate or reckless disregard of responsibilities towards patients*
- *A doctor's health is compromising patient safety*

Anybody may refer any registered doctor to the GMC. Referrals can be made electronically on the GMC website.

Where a complaint does not itself justify action by the GMC, they will refer the complaint back to the organization where the doctor was working at the time of the incident. They will not usually investigate a complaint that has already been investigated locally and gave no concerns about fitness to practice.

If it is obvious an investigation is required, the GMC investigation staff will obtain documentary evidence, including witness statements from: the doctor, employers, the complainant, and others. They may commission expert reports on clinical matters, and order an assessment of clinical performance and/or health.

Once the investigation is complete, the case is considered by two case examiners (one medical and one non-medical), who can conclude the case with:

◆ No further action

◆ Warning issues

◆ Referral to a 'Fitness to Practice Panel'

◆ Agreement of undertakings

If the case examiners cannot agree, the case will be referred to the Investigation Committee to arbitrate. At any stage, the doctor can be referred to an Interim Orders Panel, which may suspend or restrict a doctor's practice while the investigation continues.

The Fitness to Practice Panel is the final stage in deciding whether a doctor's fitness to practice is impaired. Each panel comprises:

◆ 3–5 medical and non-medical 'panelists' taken from a pool of about 300 appointed by the GMC

◆ A legal assessor

◆ One or more specialist advisors

The panels meet in public to hear evidence and decide whether allegations have been proved, and the doctor's fitness to practice is impaired. The panel may decide to: take no action, accept undertakings from the doctor about future practice, place conditions on the doctor's registration, suspend the doctor's registration, or erase the doctor's name from the Medical Register. The GMC provides guidance to each panel to ensure that decision-making is consistent.

Doctors have a right of appeal to the High Court against any decision to restrict or remove their registration. A doctor whose name is erased from the Medical Register cannot have their name restored for five years.

Council for Healthcare Regulatory Excellence

The Council for Healthcare Regulatory Excellence (CHRE) was set up in 2002 to review annually the performance of the various health professional regulatory bodies, including the GMC. It reviews the decisions made by Fitness to Practice Panels, and may refer cases to the High Court if it considers the decision is too lenient and fails to protect the public interest. It also advises the Secretary of State and Health Ministers about regulation of the healthcare professions.

Summary

Poor clinical performance of medical staff affects the quality of care. It is becoming increasingly likely that performance issues will be recognized and acted upon. Local review of performance should be undertaken systematically and fairly, with appropriate cases referred to NCAS or the GMC, to enhance patient safety.

Further reading

Understanding performance difficulties in doctors – NCAA report (November 2004). Available at http://www.ncas.npsa.nhs.uk/resources/publications/erd/ (accessed 1 November 2009). The information is also available in a paperback: *Understanding Doctors' Performance*. Eds. Cox J, King J, Hutchinson A, McAvoy P. 2005, Radcliffe publishing: ISBN 1 85775 766 1.

National Clinical Assessment Service Handbook (2010, 5th edition). Available at http://www. ncas.npsa.nhs.uk/resources/publications/key-publications/ (accessed 1 November 2009).

Fatigue and Anaesthetists (July 2004). Association of Anaesthetists of Great Britain and Ireland. Available at http://www.aagbi.org/publications/guidelines/docs/fatigue04.pdf (accessed 1 November 2009).

Good Medical Practice (November 2006). General Medical Council. Available at http://www. gmc-uk.org/static/documents/content/GMC_GMP.pdf (accessed 1 November 2009).

Chapter 27

Facilities organization: The hidden hospital

Maria Cabrelli

Key points

- Facilities management (FM) ensures buildings are designed, maintained, and operated in a safe fashion.
- Hard FM are essential physical support structures, e.g. the built environment.
- Soft FM service activities are essential for safe and efficient activity, e.g. cleaning services.
- FM services may be operated by a Trust itself, or outsourced, or a combination of the two.
- Effective FM impacts significantly on clinical outcomes and business continuity.

What is facilities management?

Broadly speaking, facilities management (FM) is concerned with providing and operating buildings that are fit for purpose and safe to use. At best, hospital buildings enhance the user experience, whilst at worst they should avoid doing their occupants any harm.

FM may be usefully divided into 'hard' and 'soft' services, examples of which are shown in Table 27.1.

Table 27.1

	Hard FM		Soft FM
Examples	Power supplies, heating & water supplies, cooling, medical gases	**Examples**	Cleaning services, portering, & catering services, linen services, waste management
Brief description of power supplies	Mains electrical supplies to the building and the electrical distribution networks within the buildings. Oil fuelled generators which take over the provision of electrical power supplies in the event of a electrical mains power failure.	**Brief description of cleaning services**	The provision of a cleaning service to clinical and non – clinical areas within the hospital by staff trained in: ◆ Infection control procedures ◆ Methods of cleaning ◆ Preventing spread of infection ◆ Providing aesthetically pleasing environments

A typical FM structure can be seen in the Fig. 27.1.

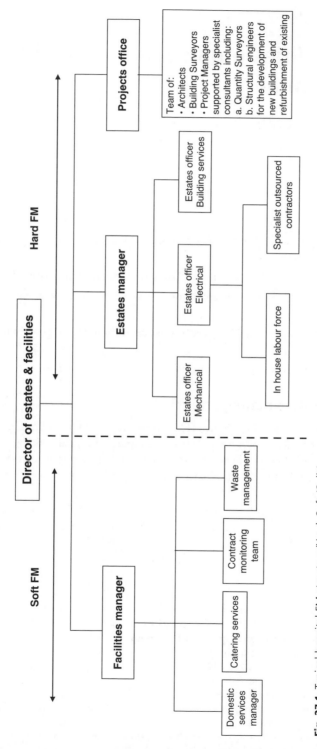

Fig. 27.1 Typical hospital FM structure/Hard–Soft 'Split'.

History: The driving force behind the FM agenda

In the 1980s and 1990s, the FM agenda was mainly led by a cost cutting, competitive culture. It is only more recently (in no small part as a result of this former approach) that public pressure for the NHS to literally 'clean up' its act, has again placed quality at the forefront of the agenda.

'Tip of the iceberg' issues initially drove a change in thinking within the NHS, serving to raise the profile of FM Services and their impact on risk. A huge media response to the public outcry on issues including lack of basic cleanliness and inedible food forced healthcare organizations to seek to address these shortfalls and inadequacies. Initially this consisted of bringing in FM professionals at a senior level to advise on how these now high-profile matters might be improved. Central Government set targets for Trusts to achieve in the area of FM, in addition to those in the clinical arena. By introducing measures of performance including cleanliness, patient feeding and the hospital environment, the Government has brought FM to (or very close to) the top table.

In recent years, therefore the FM agenda has not been led by issues that are of highest risk to patient safety, but rather those which are most visible, and can and do hit newspaper headlines. Patients most easily judge what they can see for themselves, and a dirty hospital and inedible food are easily seen and judged. Even without a public outcry, it would seem to be a basic right to expect to be treated in a clean hospital and be offered appetising and nutritionally balanced food whilst confined to bed.

In reality, the bigger risks to patient safety, wellbeing, and business continuity are not these visible risks, but those which lie just under the surface and come to our attention less frequently (see Fig. 27.2). Unfortunately, on the rare occasions that they surface they do so with a vengeance.

All medical facilities include a range of functions which are important in their own right and carry varying degrees of 'risk'. The highest risks are found predominately in the hard FM areas of:

◆ Infrastructure

◆ Building maintenance

Hard FM are the essential services that support hospital functions, but are 'hidden' out of sight behind closed doors. They are often in obscure, dimly lit basement areas, roof spaces, voids, service ducts, and plant rooms; essentially those places nobody except men in boiler suits ever dare enter!

Since hard FM issues are the highest risk elements in facilities management, one would expect these to have led the agenda for FM services in the NHS. Unfortunately this has not been the case, because they are not seen by the organization or its patients.

Cost cutting cultures

Often ill understood in terms of the contribution toward core business activity, both hard and soft FM functions, have been and continue to be, relentlessly targeted for

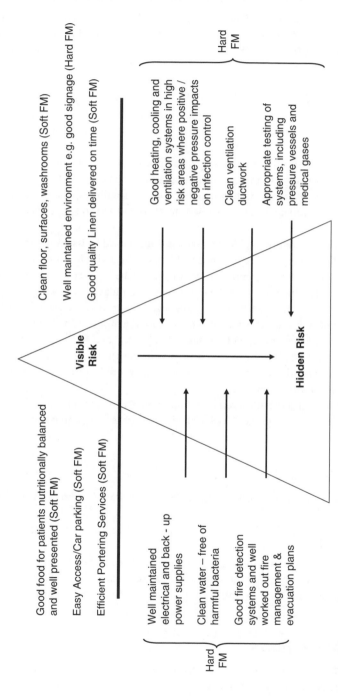

Fig. 27.2 The FM Iceberg.

cost reduction and efficiency improvements. Seen as easy targets by those lacking real understanding of the services and how they operate, decisions are all too often taken for short term gains.

Cutting FM budgets across the board occurs when managers are faced with a savings target from the Trust. Having already negotiated the best tariff for utilities, and pared back the in-house labour force to barely within safe limits, other aspects of FM are targeted. Unfortunately, this may impact at a variety of levels. Examples are found in the table:

	Hard FM	Soft FM
Safety	◆ Does adequacy of water purity really need testing every month or can it be reduced to 6 monthly (thus saving money)? ◆ Does the water tank really need replacing or will it stretch another year without significant bacterial growth?	◆ Can the cleaner on the ward work harder and perhaps take on food service duties? ◆ We have excellent patient food, meeting all nutritional targets. Why not substitute a cheaper option?
Quality	◆ Should the painting programme for the hospital be cut altogether?	◆ Closing the hospital kitchen in favour of cook-chill solutions costs less and saves space, but often leads to less appetizing food.
Service continuity	◆ Should a less rigorous approach to the testing of the back up generator functions be considered? It is very disruptive to clinical services every time a mains power failure is simulated, and the back-up generators do inevitably kick in most of the time (don't they?).	◆ Should we accept the cheapest tender for cleaning services? It's up to the contractor to deliver the service they contracted with us for (isn't it?)

It is important to appreciate the pressures on the FM manager of a cost cutting culture. They may place their own position at risk by failing to meet cost reduction targets; face a poor performance rating at their next appraisal, or be accused of not behaving corporately. It is vital that competing demands on limited finances are resolved in an open and efficient manner. The effect of cutting cost in one area can transfer costs and risk into another.

Outsourcing strategies

Outsourcing strategies have occurred in both the hard and soft FM areas. Early cost reductions were realized as the private sector bid to provide services at the cheapest possible rate by providing staff with less favourable rates of pay, terms and conditions, then those offered to the NHS. This can no longer occur since the NHS insists that firms providing such services pay in line with NHS rates. Savings now only occur if a specialist/private provider can 'manage' its services more effectively than the NHS.

Table 27.2 Potential advantages and disadvantages of PFIs

Advantages	Disadvantages
Private sector meet up-front costs (including of over-runs and over-spends)	Trust may accept higher running risks than usual, since the major driver is the new build.
	The private sector (not the end users) decides the level of risk of failure it is willing to accept for a given cost.
All FM is outsourced	Trust negotiates an inadequate penalty structure for failure of services and so can effect little change if provision is inadequate.
Private sector required to maintain standards throughout lifetime	

Unfortunately this may lull Trusts into a false sense of security as outsourcing is seen as a way of passing on a risk. Is it any less risky for Trusts to pass on problems to others than to know what risks they as a Trust own?

Despite its faults, outsourcing brought the realization that managers needed to examine, understand, and account for costs and services. Service requirements should be specified in written form and performance measured against this. This has brought a far more commercial approach to a set of services previously run unchallenged and under the protection of Crown Indemnity. Each round of competitive tendering results in lessons learnt, with specifications improving, and a clearer understanding of the balance between cost and quality.

The most recent form of outsourcing in hard FM occurred under the Private Finance Initiative (PFI). This is a method by which the NHS procures new hospital buildings by having them designed, built and operated by the private sector.

An important question is then raised 'Why is it that the NHS can afford, and is prepared to set aside proper allocations for, maintenance under a PFI arrangement where investment is not guaranteed, but is unwilling to ring fence similar levels of funds to support buildings in its direct ownership?'

Healthcare facilities are high-risk environments and FM is responsible for ensuring that they are clean and well maintained. It is important that the building infrastructure is sufficiently robust to cope in any eventuality. However, in circumstances when it does not cope it is important to demonstrate that appropriate actions have been taken to mitigate against each risk. Quite a charge, given the high percentage of hospital buildings not designed for modern medicine, which have also suffered decades of under-investment. Maintenance budgets and investment plans have frequently been more about historical allocation, than real estimates of life cycle cost with few plans in place to maintain standards that reach those laid out in legislation. Examples of some of the challenges follow.

Fire

Fire both endangers life and destroys buildings immediately. However, in the medium term it also leads to a loss of capacity for treating patients, who may be in urgent need of a service not readily available elsewhere. A series of hospital fires in the United Kingdom serve as stark reminder that these things can and do happen. Important questions regarding this 'hidden' issue are being raised:

♦ How up-to-date are Trust fire risk assessments?

♦ How much has been spent on fire detection systems?

♦ How often are fire detection systems tested?

♦ What procedures and policies are in place regarding fire-risks?

♦ Is fire safety one of the Trust's risk management priorities?

Power

In the event of a mains failure it is vital that back-up generators take over essential loads. Potential risks include a suite of operating theatres being in full flow with nothing but emergency lighting and 20 minutes battery back up on essential equipment. Whilst it may be disruptive to clinical staff for back-up generators to be regularly tested, the safety aspect cannot be denied; a balance of risks and benefits must be made.

Water supply

A Legionella outbreak in a hospital with imunosuppressed patients could be fatal. Regular testing of water purity and appropriate investment in pipework, water tanks and infrastructure ensures water temperatures are maintained at levels that do not encourage bacterial growth.

Medical gases

Many areas, including theatres, recovery and high dependency units (HDU) rely on the delivery of piped medical gases. Loss of pressure or purity of supply clearly results in the potential for fatal events.

Food

A food poisoning outbreak can be fatal. Mechanisms for ensuring food is stored, prepared, and served hygienically must be in place.

Managing the FM risks: A way forward

NHS organizations rarely know the true cost of their FM services. When calculated under the PFI model, it is found to be significantly higher than current allocations. It should therefore come as no surprise that FM Services often fail to meet best practice requirements.

In addressing this problem, it helps if an FM professional is directly employed by the Trust; preferably having a voice at Board level but at the very least on the executive. This enables a reasonable allocation of Trust capital to be utilized supporting the ageing infrastructure, rather than being allocated disproportionately to only new developments. Such representation encourages proper asset management and benchmarking. It ensures that an overview is taken of all FM costs, starting with major premises costs, essentially the big ticket items including: rates, utilities, and space allocation and utilization. FM then no longer sits in desperate isolation as a drain on precious resources, but:

◆ Informs core business planning for the clinical services

◆ Provides solutions to questions of space

◆ Develops improved new facilities

◆ Enhances use of existing facilities

This opens up opportunities for cost reduction and efficiencies at a level that does not place the maintenance manager in an impossible position as regards savings in either infrastructure or staffing. Income growth is enabled, strengthening the organization, and making it more viable and less likely to seek desperate cost saving measures.

This level of engagement has begun, more successfully in some instances than others. Much has been learnt in the past decade about the risks of always seeking the lowest cost solution without proper regard for quality. It has now been realized that value for money does not always mean the cheapest. Many services remain outsourced, and may lend themselves well to being run that way. However, these are increasingly being evaluated on quality as well as cost. Best outcomes are usually achieved by a multidisciplinary approach, as shown in Fig. 27.3.

The key to moving forward is the development of organizations with an open and honest approach to the management of risk. Such organizations take collective responsibility for the impact that a decision taken in one area will have on another. They are big enough to not perpetuate the blame culture that all too often surfaces when an unfortunate incident occurs. This approach allows for open and honest debate on the relative merits of all risk, clinical, non clinical and FM alike.

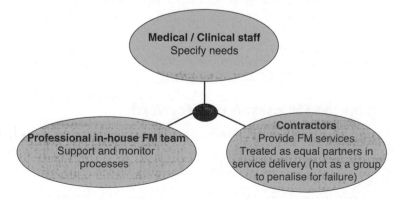

Fig. 27.3 A multidisciplinary input is necessary to ensure effective facilities management.

Summary

In an increasingly risk driven culture, the potential impact of FM can no longer be ignored – it is a core service. It is increasingly recognized that FM has to be managed in the context of a much bigger and wider picture, and not left to its own devices. Despite immense technical knowledge and dedication, the 'man in the boiler suit' cannot pre-empt and plan proactively for the future because of his limited ability to influence policy and decision making at the right level. FM must fill this role.

Further reading

Facilities Economics. Bernard Williams Associates. ISBN 0904237168.

Rational Analysis for a Problematic World. Jonathan Rosenhead & John Minger
    ISBN 0471495239.

Chapter 28

Equipment management

Stephen Squire

Key points

- Equipment in the healthcare setting has a major impact on patient safety.
- Equipment management is: the selection, procurement, installation, training for use, maintenance, and replacement of an organization's equipment fleet.
- Equipment inventories are essential for effective equipment management and the financial management of assets in a limited funding setting.
- Equipment standards are set out by statutory bodies including the International Electrotechnical Commission (IEC), the International Organisation for Standardization (ISO), and the Department of Health (DH).
- Hospitals must demonstrate at audit that all risks associated with their equipment are effectively managed.

A high-tech environment packed with medical equipment is a defining attribute of a medical centre. Clinical staff expect their equipment to be safe, available, and ready for use when needed, but this state can only be achieved with active equipment management. This is recognized by the Department of Health, in their *Standards for Better Health*.

Meeting the standards for better health

These require that Trusts have, and follow, an equipment management policy endorsed by the Board. Effective policies ensure that:

- Equipment is suitable for its intended purpose
- The entire inventory is available and in a safe and serviceable condition when needed
- Users are trained to understand and effectively use the equipment
- Devices are replaced to meet changing clinical needs and standards of safety and care
- Funds are spent wisely, and equipment managed as a financial asset
- Incidents involving medical equipment are resolved in a timely manner

Trusts are audited against these standards and must demonstrate that they are following their own equipment management policy.

Governance and corporate responsibility

The Chief Executive (CEO) has overall responsibility for the safety and welfare of all Trust staff, patients, and visitors. This includes responsibility for the safety and effectiveness of the Trust's medical equipment. All users have responsibility for some element of equipment management, but Trusts must appoint an equipment manager with a clear line of responsibility to the CEO to operate the equipment management policy.

Responsibility for medical equipment management is shared between equipment users (clinical staff) and one or more asset managing groups:

- Clinical technologists
- Biomedical engineers
- Medical physicists
- Electro-biomedical engineering (EBME) technicians
- Medical equipment management technicians
- Estates officers
- Technicians (e.g. anaesthesia or ICU technicians)
- Commercial service providers

Staff maintaining equipment should be registered with a body (e.g. voluntary register of clinical technologists, VRCT) to demonstrate their competence and maintain their professional standards. Registration requires a minimum of three years experience and completion of registered training.

A department that manages equipment may also hold ISO9000 accreditation to independently demonstrate that there are monitoring processes in place to ensure:

- Effective record keeping
- Checking processes for defects
- Appropriate, corrective action is undertaken
- Regular review of processes for effectiveness
- Continual improvement

Equipment management

Equipment management is a series of processes to manage the equipment lifecycle. It is generally accepted that medical equipment has an operational lifetime of 7 years. Commonly, devices will be used for much longer, which is acceptable provided they are well maintained and meet current clinical and regulatory standards (Fig. 28.1).

The equipment inventory

Equipment management starts with a good inventory, identifying the make, model, and serial number of every item of medical equipment, to which is allocated

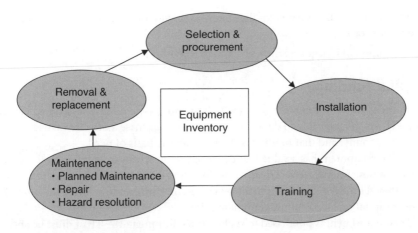

Fig. 28.1 The equipment lifecycle.

a unique asset number. Using the inventory the equipment lifecycle is managed including:

◆ Service history

◆ Asset value

◆ Training record

◆ Risks

Creating a good inventory from scratch is a long job that, if done well, makes everything else possible. The inventory must be comprehensive; any device you can touch should be identified on it (including equipment nobody can remember the source of). There are many computerized systems to assist in creating and managing a complete inventory, which should make it possible to know where each item is in its lifecycle. The inventory informs the Trust's fixed asset register, essential to good financial management and securing future capital funding from the DH.

Selection and procurement

Equipment replacement can be a lengthy process and should be planned in advance. In practice this can be compromised by constantly changing priorities. There are always more pressing demands for new equipment than there are funds to meet them. However, a co-ordinated approach to procurement can stretch limited funding further. Trusts should have a capital committee to oversee allocation and spending of funds for equipment purchases. An understanding of the basic principles of finance as it relates to equipment can explain some of the goals of equipment management, and provide an understanding of the role of the capital committee.

Sources of funding

All funding is accounted as either capital or revenue. Definitions are difficult, but in general, they can be as follows:

◆ Capital outlay results in the *increase* or acquisition of fixed assets of a Trust

- Revenue outlay is necessary for the *maintenance* and upkeep of fixed assets in a fully efficient state

Most equipment is acquired through capital expenditure.

Capital funding

Equipment with a purchase value of £5000 or more is generally classed as a capital asset. Trusts must be able to demonstrate at audit that these assets are managed with financial probity, and that funding is allocated on the basis of need.

Capital equipment has a value that depreciates linearly over its theoretical lifetime from purchase price to zero. Trusts receive funding equal to the value of depreciation from the DH to spend on equipment replacement. This funding forms the bulk of a Trust's capital replacement programme funding.

If new equipment is purchased to replace old equipment, the Trust must be able to demonstrate that the old equipment has been disposed of and removed from its asset register (inventory). Trusts are required to demonstrate at annual audit how capital funding is spent. In effect the auditor will need to be able to resolve the:

- Business case for expenditure
- Purchase order to buy the equipment
- Asset purchased

Commonly a Trust will operate equipment assets after their theoretical value has reached zero. This allows the funding allocated for replacement to be spent elsewhere. In the long term, problems can build up when replacement becomes necessary for safety, clinical, or support reasons.

Revenue funding

Single items of equipment of value below £5000 cannot usually be purchased as part of a capital programme, unless they can be seen as part of a system, e.g. syringe pumps as an infusion management system. However, it is possible to acquire new equipment with revenue funding by:

- Managed services
- Leasing
- Charitable funds

Managed services

Trusts can buy a complete service from a company, including all elements required to deliver the service, paying for it out of revenue on the basis of treatment episode.

> e.g. Trusts may provide haemofiltration services by the paying for individual treatments. The supplier provides all elements required to deliver the service, including supplying and maintaining all equipment (including fluids) and providing user training.

There is a potential cost reduction (by a VAT saving on the service element) but Trusts should check carefully the specific details of their agreement with H M Customs and Excise NHS Administration Team.

Care should be taken to understand the implications of the contract entered into and the costs of any future changes in demand. Moreover, if the service is ended by either party the Trust will need to re-provide the equipment and systems to operate and manage it.

Leasing

Leasing can be used to acquire capital value equipment with revenue funding. Leasing is a method of borrowing money secured against the value of the equipment purchased. Leases typically run over 3–7 years during which time the equipment is owned by the lease company.

Over the whole duration of a lease, a Trust will typically pay 125% of the capital value of the equipment, but in small payments. At the end of the lease period, the Trust does not own the equipment but must either purchase it for the residual value or re-lease it.

It is essential that leased equipment is carefully managed to ensure lease payments are stopped or re-negotiated at the end of the lease period. The lease terms will require that the Trust keep the equipment in good condition, managing the equipment, including paying for maintenance and resolving hazards.

The financial benefit of leasing is subject to changes in taxation law, which can make it more or less attractive to Trust finance departments. Purchases that are wholly self–finanacing though increased revenue are good candidates for leasing as the higher costs can be accounted for in the business case.

> e.g. Acquiring an X-ray room funded via leasing. The increased cost of lease procurement can be allowed for in the business case. The higher cost can be paid for by the increased activity and resulting increased income. Without a lease purchase this acquisition might not otherwise be possible if all normal capital funding was already allocated.

Charitable funds

Most Trusts have access to charitable funds. These have the extra advantage that medical equipment purchases made using these funds are exempt from VAT. This must be agreed with the supplier and stated clearly on the purchase order.

The capital committee

This committee decides upon how Trust capital funding is spent. The purchase of any equipment must be justified by the impact upon income (through changes in clinical activity) including loss of income if it is not replaced. Departments submit requests for new equipment to the Trust's capital programme.

A business case for new or replacement equipment should briefly outline the costs, benefits, and opportunities, if possible tied to an income stream, risks, and

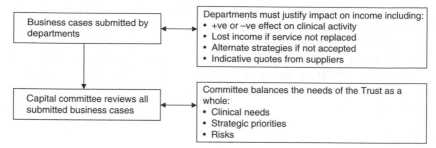

Fig. 28.2 Cartoon demonstrating the way in which business cases are managed.

alternative strategies. One conundrum of making a capital bid is in knowing how much equipment will cost without pre-selecting the solution. It is advisable to talk to a range of suppliers and ask for indicative quotes. Always include VAT in the bid and allow for all the likely costs, without pricing the bid so high that it no longer looks a rational project. Under-valuing bids can seriously disrupt capital programmes.

When submitting a business plan, the entire cost of owning the equipment over its life cycle, or 'cost of operation' must be calculated including:

- Purchase cost including servicing any loans or leasing: this determines the funding source
- Installation
- Integration/interfacing with other systems
- Training
- Licences
- Consumables and disposables
- Maintenance contracts
- Additional parts
- Breakdown repair
- Warranty arrangements
- Software upgrades
- Decommissioning and disposal

An example of how a Trust might prioritize needs and major risks is shown in Table 28.1. Clearly, low need and high risk figures will result in high priorities.

Procurement process

The actual process of procurement is determined by the value of the equipment to be purchased. The timescale can range from a few weeks (revenue funded) to many months, for more expensive equipment via European tendering.

There may also be nationally or regionally negotiated 'framework' agreements that remove the need for tendering, speeding up processes, and sometimes providing better value for money.

Table 28.1

Replacement equipment	Need	Risk	New equipment
Equipment that must be replaced because it is defunct/near defunct, or continued use will breach legislation	1	5	Equipment necessary for a vital service development
Existing equipment deemed inadequate by an outside non-legislative authority	2	4	
Existing equipment of suboptimal performance or poor service history and with no back-up	3	3	Equipment needed for important service developments
Existing equipment of suboptimal performance or poor service history but has back-up	4	2	
Equipment working well but 'time expired'	5	1	

Selection process

In response to an advertisement, several companies usually tender their equipment and a selection must be made, based on testing against agreed written specifications that suppliers should be given. It should include:

- Meeting the technical requirement (including regulatory and local standards)
- Integration and interfacing with equipment already in use
- Meeting the clinical requirement (clinical effectiveness)
- User reaction during trialling
- Supplier quality (including support, service, reputation and past experience)

The selected solution (preferred supplier) will give the best value for money, most closely meeting the specification, at the best price.

All stakeholders should be consulted when making a procurement selection, not only clinical staff, but also groups whose procedures and infrastructure systems will be affected. This might include: infection control, information technology, equipment maintenance staff, estates, finance, and education. Medical devices are increasingly integrated as part of wider information systems, having impacts that may not be immediately obvious.

Companies competing for the business are entitled to challenge the process of selection and may demand to see how it was made. Therefore, carefully defined and recorded evaluations must be made.

Having selected the preferred supplier and awarded the contract, it is essential to complete the project (equipment delivered) within the financial year. Non-foundation Trusts must complete expenditure on capital programmes or lose the funding (to another bid).

Installation

At the point of installation, equipment becomes an asset owned by the Trust and governance issues apply. New equipment must be tested against the applicable standards (e.g. IEC 60601) to demonstrate initial safety.

Training

The equipment inventory can be used to plan a training programme, ensuring all staff are trained on equipment they use. This can be a mammoth task, so training effort should be targeted at equipment with the highest outstanding risk. Underestimating the cost (both financial and time) of training is almost universal, and a major potential risk. On-going user support is also necessary.

Maintenance

Medical equipment is complex and breakdowns occur. Also almost all equipment requires planned maintenance. This may only be an inspection, or involve regular major overhaul with prophylactic replacement of parts on a planned schedule.

All repair and planned maintenance work must be recorded, with equipment decontaminated (and certified as such) before work is carried out. Work undertaken should at least meet standards recommended by the manufacturer, and be carried out in a suitable environment by maintenance staff with appropriate recorded training, using standardized procedures. Spare parts must be of a suitable standard and test equipment must have a scheduled traceable calibration.

Equipment hazards

Medical equipment (like all electronic goods) can go wrong because it is poorly designed or maintained. Various systems are in place to minimize the negative effects of this. *CE marking*, applied by the manufacturer and verified by an independent certification body, is required before a medical device can be marketed in Europe. This indicates that the device meets the relevant regulatory requirements and, when used as intended, works properly and safely. Problems inevitably arise after marketing and these must be communicated to equipment users.

The Central Alerting System (CAS) (formerly known as SABS, Safety Alert Broadcast System) issues reports from the Medicines and Healthcare products Regulatory Agency (MHRA). Manufacturers operate a medical device vigilance system (MDVS). They issue a field safety notice (FSN), detailing field safety corrective actions (FSCA) to be taken by them when a medical device, already on the market, has been involved in an incident that may re-occur. The FSCA may involve withdrawing, replacing, or modifying, equipment, parts, or instructions, to reduce risk of death or serious deterioration in patient health. The Trust's response to medical device alerts generated by MHRA specifies that the CAS liaison officer will contact equipment maintenance staff and users to see if a particular warning notice is important to the Trust.

Internal incidents must be investigated, and malfunctioning equipment directly involved in an incident (or suspected of putting patients or staff at risk) should be immediately withdrawn from service. Discovering the root cause of the incident is more likely if:

◆ Equipment is seen in context

◆ Settings on equipment are unchanged

- Disposables (and their packaging) have been retained
- Nothing is done to overwrite internal event logs

The staff member using the medical device at the time of the incident must report the incident both internally and possibly to the MHRA, noting the make, model, and serial number (and Trust asset number). To minimize risks to patient safety, equipment management staff will hold equipment in quarantine until any fault is corrected, or no fault is found and the cause of the incident was designated as user error.

Removal and replacement

At disposal, assets must be removed from the asset register (to ensure capital charges no longer accrue) and service contracts cancelled. Disposal must be in accordance with the waste electrical and electronic equipment directive (WEEE). The WEEE directive aims to both reduce the amount of electrical and electronic equipment being produced, and encourage everyone to reuse, recycle, and recover it.

Summary

Equipment management is a key element of effective healthcare provision. A successfully managed inventory of equipment should provide sufficient, safe, and suitable equipment for clinical staff to use. By recording technical and financial history, it will secure safe operation and future funding for replacement.

Further reading

"Managing Medical Devices" DB2006(05), MHRA Device Bulletin November 2006.
The Central Alerting System brings together CMO's Public Health Link (PHL) and the Safety Alert Broadcast System (SABS), https://www.cas.dh.gov.uk/Home.aspx.
The Medicines and Healthcare products Regulatory Agency (MHRA), http://www.mhra.gov.uk/index.htm.
The International Electrotechnical Commission (IEC) http://www.iec.ch/.
International Organization for Standardization (ISO) http://www.iso.org/iso/home.htm.

Section 5

Learning effectiveness

The need for all staff to know what is the best thing, at all times, for all patients, in all healthcare settings in which they work, over the course of their whole career is a high aspiration. However, every patient would wish this to be the case for their own care. Thus the requirement for all staff to have appropriate knowledge, skills, and behaviours, is fundamental. Starting in a new position requires both general knowledge and that specific to the environment (*Induction*), and Trusts are expected to be able to show that they provide this (*Training*). Since the knowledge base and mores of society develop over time, this cannot be a one time event (*Continuing professional development*) and will extend both over time, but also over levels of expectation (*Competence*). With the massive expansion of techniques utilized in the healthcare professions, individuals will need help to ensure they can find (*Knowledge management*) and save (*Clinical information systems*) knowledge that enhances patient safety.

Chapter 29

Induction: At an organizational level

Les Gemmell

Key points

- Induction is the formal process of acclimatizing a newcomer to the organization.
- Patient safety is a priority and all staff, especially the newly qualified, must be aware of their limitations and be actively encouraged to ask for help.
- All healthcare organizations must provide an organizational induction programme for their staff, which must contain statutory elements, such as Health and Safety.
- The opportunity to stress the values of the organization at induction must not be lost.
- Departmental induction should include team building and familiarization with the working environment and essential equipment.

Every NHS institution should have an induction programme; at both organizational and local levels. The need for staff induction programmes within NHS workplaces has been clearly recognized and is supported by the British Medical Association (BMA), General Medical Council (GMC), the Department of Health (DH), the Royal Colleges and the Postgraduate Medical Education and Training Board (PMETB). The NHS lifelong learning framework (designed to support the NHS Plan) encourages staff to have an understanding of the NHS and their local organization, as well as working effectively in teams. PMETB have produced generic standards for training which:

- Set out the standards by which all training should be assessed
- Must be applied wherever postgraduate medical education and training takes place, including all service providers (e.g. the independent sector) not only the NHS

PMETB have made induction a mandatory part of the standards of education for all medical trainees. NHS Employers have produced induction packs for new starters in the NHS for all the career groups. These are national resources that can be found on the NHS employer's website, and are intended to supplement inductions carried out locally within NHS Trusts. Domain 6 states: 'Trainees must be supported to acquire the necessary skills and experience through induction'.

Designing an appropriate and cost-effective induction package is a difficult task. However, induction programmes have been developed, and subsequently implemented, in hospitals and general practices throughout the United Kingdom. Induction should be relevant to the role of individuals and teams, and appropriate to the organization. Many induction programmes include mandatory training such as fire safety and manual handling. Although induction is normally associated with staff joining an organization, it is no less important for staff taking over a job from a current postholder.

Induction programmes should also be undertaken by locums, those returning to work after long absences, overseas staff, career grades, and those starting in the organization at the most senior levels. Locum practitioners are seen as a "high risk" group, often missed out on induction programmes. This can be rectified utilizing innovative ways to reproduce the programme (e.g. DVD or web-based). If locums are secured through an agency, the contract with the agency should require that an induction similar to the Trust's programme be provided by the agency. In situations where a locum is engaged on a personal basis, the doctor should be in a position to demonstrate that they have covered the required elements of induction.

The benefits of induction programs may include the following:

Potential benefit	Means of producing benefit
Create a good impression	Formal process of acclimatization
	Ensure staff feel welcome and valued
Team building	Reinforce importance of seeking assistance from senior colleagues
	Assurance that assistance will be forthcoming
Reduced recruitment costs	Reduced turnover with motivated and committed staff
Influence current staff	Increased involvement in the organization

Induction should be considered as part of an inter-linked system, starting with recruitment and linked with appraisal and assessment of the individual. Induction programme advice specifically for doctors is widely available. The GMC gives advice to doctors at the earliest stage of their career in its publications *The New Doctor* and *The Early Years*. Publications on the arrangements for foundation training have reiterated this advice and both are intended as induction to practice advice. The guide to specialist registrar training covers induction for more senior trainees and the Departments of Health have issued guidance for consultants and overseas doctors.

Induction is defined by the *Oxford Dictionary of Human Resource Management* as 'the formal process of acclimatizing a newcomer to an organisation'. An induction programme has to provide all the information that new employees and others need. However, participants must be able to assimilate this information without being overwhelmed, or diverted from the essential process of becoming part of a team providing healthcare. Induction is not expected to repeat large portions of the undergraduate or postgraduate curriculum.

Duration of induction will vary, lasting from several hours to a week, depending on the complexity of the work, organization, and job responsibilities. By including statutory and mandatory training, a high-quality induction will ensure that new employees are practicing in a way that ensures not only the safety of patients they care for, but also their own. The process of induction begins on recruitment when the job applicant forms their first impressions about the Trust. Increasingly, central recruitment and selection are being utilized for medical staff, thus the first impression of the organization is through the organizational induction programme, and only then through the workplace orientation. As part of this process, there must be opportunity for new employees to build up working relationships and find roles for themselves within their new teams. It is important when designing the course to make it both participative and learner centered. Staff members should be allowed to critically appraise the programme's content and make suggestions for improvements, including induction. Induction will usually consist of both statutory and other elements.

Statutory elements

The Health and Safety at Work Act 1974 requires NHS Trusts to provide training to safeguard, so far as is reasonably practicable, the health and safety at work of its employees. This was expanded by the Management of Health and Safety at Work Regulations 1999, which identified situations where health and safety training is particularly important. This typically includes:

- Health and safety
- Control of infection
- Control of substances hazardous to health (COSHH regulations define these)
- Waste disposal
- Fire prevention
- Manual handling
- Security
- Violence and aggression

Non-statutory elements (which may nevertheless be mandatory within a Trust)

The principles of the induction process are to make newly appointed staff feel welcome and valued, and to provide them with the development they need to fulfill their role.

- *Physical orientation*: describing where facilities are. Should include a tour of the workplace

◆ *Organizational orientation* should include an introduction to co-workers, showing how:

- The employee fits into the team
- Their role fits with the organization's strategy and goals
- Organizational history, including its services, culture and values

◆ Explanation of *terms and conditions*

◆ Completion of *employment documents* including payroll, pension, occupational health etc.

◆ A clear outline of the *job/role requirements.*

Induction should not be delegated entirely to the human resource departments. There must be contributions by senior clinical staff and postgraduate tutors. Individual clinical and educational supervisors have the primary responsibility for ensuring induction takes place in their relevant area. It may not be feasible or desirable to provide the total induction package on the day of commencing work. However, there are some elements that need to be covered as priority information required at the beginning of work. Major features should be:

◆ Programmes designed so that elements critical to patient safety are presented on the first day in a face-to-face manner

◆ Avoid overload of induction programmes, particularly on the first day, so important messages are not lost

◆ Stress the importance of working as a member of a multidisciplinary team

◆ Acknowledge the importance of good individual practice (as *per* the GMC)

As a member of a team, the items shown in Fig. 29.1. should be introduced early in the programme:

Stressing the importance of good individual practice as advocated by the GMC will include:

◆ Clear medical record keeping

◆ Safe prescribing and transfusion practice

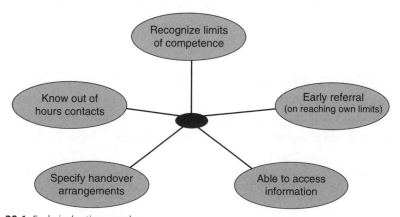

Fig. 29.1 Early induction needs.

- Dealing with concerns of patients, relatives and carers
- Cardiopulmonary resuscitation arrangements
- Safe use of equipment
- Awareness of how to deal with patient safety incidents

Induction should also stress quality control procedures. These will cover patient, Trust and staff domains. Quality assurance for patients will include ensuring effective consent and protection procedures, whilst adverse clinical event and coroner's reports will also help protect the Trust. Staff will need to be involved in appraisal as part of their ongoing development and should be aware of what mechanisms are in place to protect them from bullying or harassment.

There must be an appropriate mechanism in place to monitor the induction programme, ensuring that all doctors have taken part and have grasped the relevant information. The appraisal process provides a means of documenting a doctor's effective involvement in induction.

Summary

The induction program at organizational level is an essential constituent of the employment process of every doctor. There are statutory and non-statutory elements that should be included in the program. The induction program can be used to set out the values of the employers' organization. The importance of a patient safety ethos must be a part of all induction programs. It is essential to audit this process to ensure the effectiveness of the induction process.

Further reading

General Medical Council. (1997). *The New Doctor*. London: GMC.

Evans, D.E., Wood, D.F., and Roberts, C.M., (2004). The effect of an extended hospital induction on perceived confidence and assessed clinical skills of newly qualified pre-registration house officers. *Medical Education*, **38**(9), 998–1001.

Ward, S.J., (1998). Improving quality in hospital induction programmes. *BMJ*, classified supplement, 21 Feb.

The NHS employers website. www.nhsemployers.org.

Chapter 30

Training and organization

Lesley Bromley

Key points

- The aim of training in healthcare is to improve outcomes for patients.
- Training should result in individual learning and enhanced educational performance.
- There are both statutory and mandatory components to training.
- Organizations must be able to demonstrate that they train and supervise staff in an ongoing manner.
- Individuals should be given time to undertake training, but professionalism also implies self-directed development.

Training should result in individual learning and enhanced organizational performance

This generic description of training sums up beautifully the all round benefits of training in healthcare organizations, and why training needs to be organized and effective. All organizations train, and effective organizations train more than less effective organizations. We can see examples of this all around us:

- Retailers Marks and Spencer and John Lewis are well known for the high levels of service given by their staff. To achieve this, they open later one morning a week to undertake staff training. They value their staff and develop them, their management traineeships are highly sought after, and they see money and time invested in training as well spent. They see the returns in reputation and profit.
- Airline industry training has revolutionized air safety. In the 1960s and 1970s, a series of fatal crashes were found to be due to 'human error'. Listening to the black box recorder conversations from the cockpit, it became obvious that the recurring theme was poor communication between crew members, particularly communication from junior to senior members of the crew. Crew Resource Management (CRM) is a training programme designed to instil:
  - Appropriate behaviours
  - A shallow gradient of authority
  - Enhanced situation awareness

Its introduction has been associated with vastly improved air safety. Regular refresher training is required to keep ideas fresh in crew members' minds, and to move forward a massive cultural change.

Where clearly identified rewards are seen (more profit/fewer crashes) the value of training is acknowledged.

There are very few healthcare organizations in the public sector that do not have education and training as part of their mission statement. Furthermore, almost all health care professionals, if asked, say teaching and training is one of the more positive aspects of their job. On the other hand, those who are involved in training and education in healthcare frequently feel that the provision of service, and the achievement of targets, pushes the training agenda to the back of the queue:

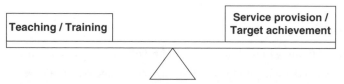

Fig. 30.1 Tension may exist between the demands of service and training needs.

Responsibilities of both the organization and the individual are set about with rules and regulations. In the following sections, the responsibilities and requirements of the organization and the individual will be considered.

The organization

An organization that provides healthcare (be it a hospital or a primary care trust) is bound by legislation to ensure that it maintains acceptable standards. For many years after the founding of the NHS, local management committees made up of the great and the good 'oversaw' the running of the hospital, encouraging training as a method of attracting good staff to the institution. In the twenty-first century, a different carrot is used. The Clinical Negligence Scheme for Trusts (CNST), now known as The National Health Service Litigation Authority (NHSLA) is a Special Health Authority set up under the 1977 NHS Act, to provide indemnity insurance for negligence claims against Trusts. In order to reduce the premium paid to the NHSLA Trusts have to demonstrate that they:

- Carry out basic training
- Supervise trainees at work
- Maintain records of training undertaken over a period of employment

To get off the mark with the NHSLA, an organization must provide a comprehensive induction for all individuals that it employs (see Chapter 29). In addition, they are required to undertake both statutory and mandatory training programmes. In many Trusts, there is a training department, who will organize the provision of such training. Individual posts in the Trust will be subjected to a training needs analysis and the training required will be defined.

Statutory and mandatory training needs to be delivered before the organization does anything about training its employees in how to actually deliver healthcare.

Statuary training: Required by law for all employees

This includes fire safety, manual handling, and basic health and safety. Whilst these do not sound particularly thrilling, they are of course very important. Fires, which are thankfully quiet rare in hospitals, can break out at any time. As the hospital is largely manned by junior doctors and nursing staff at night, this group needs to be particularly targeted for fire training. Despite its obvious importance, fire training has a bad name, as being boring; in large part because it is delivered in lecture form. Where simulation centres with ward areas are set up, practical fire training based on scenarios is much more effective and memorable. E-learning may also be an effective method of delivering this training.

Mandatory training

This falls into two categories, training mandated by:

◆ External bodies (e.g. Care Quality Commission, NHSLA)

◆ The Trust itself

The Care Quality Commission (previously the Health Care Commission) is a non-departmental public body with a statuary duty to inform the Health Secretary and the National Assembly of Wales of the performance of the NHS. It acts as the NHS watchdog. External bodies require Trusts to provide 22 different areas of training. The NHSLA and the Care Quality Commission define which staff groups need to attend which training (and this can be summarised within training needs matrices). Many Trusts run health and safety update days to deal with the continued training and updating of staff. They may be run as infrequently as quarterly or as often as twice a month depending on the size of the workforce.

In order to deliver this training each Trust needs to write and approve a strategy and policy for each of the mandatory training topics. Much of the mandatory training is of course very valuable, and impacts greatly on patient safety. Unfortunately, it has often not been made terribly relevant to bedside delivery of care to individual patients. New approaches are being sought to make its delivery more effective. Many training courses now have competency assessments incorporated into them, particularly blood transfusion, basic life support, and medical devices training. This helps to make the learning relevant, changing behaviour in a positive way. Using competency assessment as a test at the end is also valuable to the trainers, focusing the content and the style of teaching towards the practical aspects of the subject.

Roles and responsibilities

In the past, organizations seem to have concentrated on delivering this generic training to all staff groups except doctors. Post-graduate medical training is commissioned by:

◆ The Deaneries

◆ The Foundation Schools (first two years of training)

◆ Specialist Schools

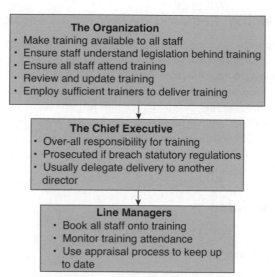

Fig. 30.2 All levels of the organization have some responsibility for training.

◆ The Postgraduate medical education and training board (PMETB): the independent regulatory body responsible for all postgraduate medical education and training. From April 2010, PMETB merged with the GMC but will continue to regulate postgraduate training from within the GMC.

Their stated vision is to:
• Achieve excellence in postgraduate medical education, training, assessment and accreditation throughout the United Kingdom
• Improve the knowledge, skills and experience of doctors and thus the health and healthcare of patients and the public

All of these authorities have become much more interested in how statutory and mandatory training is delivered to trainees. Foundation training has a defined curriculum, and much of the mandatory training is included in it. Deanery, PMETB and Royal Colleges have now combined their training inspections, and any PMETB/GMC visit will require detailed description of the induction programmes, and continuing and update programmes for, amongst others, infection control, transfusion practice, and resuscitation training as mapped onto the curriculum.

Making learning these statutory and mandatory subjects more effective

The first opportunity that the organization has to deliver this training is at the beginning of an individual's employment. Most trainees complain about induction, particularly in relation to 'boring lectures and irrelevant information, which takes up too much time when there are jobs to be done'. Having a captive audience, is no excuse for poor delivery of training, and much of the information is not well suited to delivery as face-to-face lectures.

The effectiveness of induction programmes is mainly unknown; feedback from them is very variable. Generally however, induction is seen more positively by non-medical staff than by medical staff. This may be in part due to the more frequent rotation of trainee doctors with repeated exposure to similar, but slightly different, programmes. Using innovative methods of pre-employment education (e.g. web-based and other e-learning methods) with a testing of knowledge on arrival in the organization may be more effective. Most importantly, for it to be retained, the induction information (statutory, mandatory, or just essential to working in the organization) needs to be personally relevant and interesting.

For many organizations achieving universal attendance at induction is a constant challenge, but induction is only the beginning of the training process. For all groups of staff the organization needs to provide time and opportunity to update and extend their knowledge and skills. This may be provided in-house, or may involve study time to attend external courses. For medical staff there are preset study leave allocations. This is not so for other staff groups and the ability to access study leave is very variable across the professional groups.

The most important principle for organizations is that training should produce better outcomes for the patients. If good clinical audit demonstrates improved patient outcomes when training is regular and effective, individuals are more likely to commit themselves to the process and encourage others, producing cultural change.

The individual

Healthcare professionals are just that: professional. Implicit in being a member of a profession is the obligation to maintain the standards thereof. What should patients be able to expect of their health care professionals? A professional is defined as some one engaged in, or suitable for a profession, who conforms to the standards of that profession, and shows great skill and expertise: Characteristics of professional practice include.

- ◆ Expertise
- ◆ Knowledge
- ◆ Skills
- ◆ Ethical behaviour

Therefore, maintaining current knowledge is a prime responsibility of any professional.

A high proportion of NHS staff are undertaking post-graduate or post-basic training, and have undertaken courses and programmes to acquire their current levels of knowledge and skill.

Training medical staff in the NHS

The postgraduate education of doctors has undergone significant change in recent years.

• *Medical schools* – produce graduates following their own curricula. The General Medical Council has a role in inspecting medical schools and sets down recommendations for the content of the curriculum.

• *Foundation Schools* – loosely based on the medical schools geographically, but whose primary relationship is with the post-graduate deanery in its area. These provide a two-year programme incorporating a year of post-registration training and a year of SHO-equivalent posts. The curriculum is set out by PMETB, who aim to ensure that postgraduate training for doctors is of the highest standard.

• *Specialist Schools* – commissioned by deaneries to provide training in broad subjects into Specialist Schools (e.g. the London School of Medicine, the North-West School of Surgery). These schools have taken responsibility for the core training years (ST1/ST2) in their subjects. Higher training years are still largely organized in training programmes, with individual training programme directors (TPDs), for each sub-speciality (e.g. cardiology, ENT, surgery). These TPDs are part of the specialist school management board. Schools commission Local Education Providers (LEPs) such as acute or primary care Trusts, to provide training posts in the speciality. Core training may be provided entirely within one Trust, or involve rotation between Trusts, but higher training inevitably involves posts in several Trusts.

The formal process of governance of medical education is complex and the relationship of the key players is shown in Fig. 30.3.

Post-basic training in nursing

Increasing numbers of nurses are specialising in particular areas. This is usually by means of part time courses combined with a specific post. Many universities have a faculty of nursing, and offer postgraduate diploma and master's degrees. It is now an essential requirement to have a higher degree for specialist senior nursing posts.

Managing continuing medical education for an individual specialist

Once specialist training is complete and the individual is working in a post as a practitioner, the need for training and education does not cease. For some individuals, their area of work will remain general, and they will need to maintain a wide range of skills and knowledge. Continuing professional education and development will be necessary and should be included in job plans. In many cases, professional bodies will need to see evidence to allow an individual to maintain registration. For medical staff, this function is usually carried out by the Royal College who has issued the certificate of completion of training (CCT).

Some individuals may find that over time they become highly specialized in their work, and they would not be in a position to maintain skills in all areas of their speciality. Maintaining log books, which is now expected as part of appraisal and job planning, can inform:

• Individual educational needs

• The need for speciality rotas

• Departmental policy

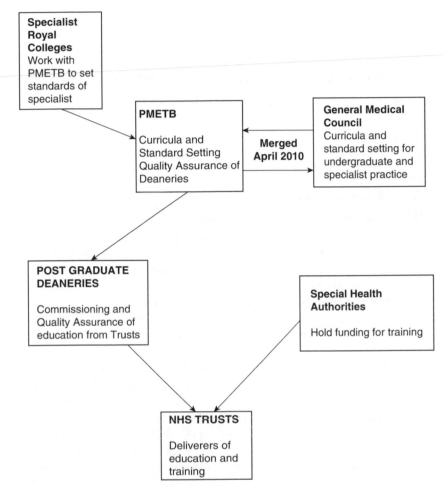

Fig. 30.3 Relationships between organizations in the provision of post graduate 'medical' education.

Good audit should ensure that specialists are performing sufficient elective cases to ensure skills for the out of hours emergency work.

Study leave, internal and external meetings, teaching and training others, and examining for the Royal Colleges and European Diplomas, all help to keep individuals up to date. However for most specialists, once they have finished training, they rarely work with their peers. Using professional education time to work with another specialist can be very instructive and allows individuals to review their own practice in a positive way.

An organized approach to maintaining education is essential. Keeping up to date is also about keeping interested in what you do. 'Burn out' is a real phenomenon in healthcare. One of the ways of avoiding this is to make long-term plans for professional development to ensure continued challenges and growth as a professional. Part of continuing education is to spend time reflecting on past performance, and planning future activity to ensure this.

This kind of career management is of value to both individual and organization. A workforce that is interested, challenged, developing, and educated will provide better care to patients.

What the individual can expect the organization to provide

A well-managed organization will provide the individual with opportunities, including the time to:

- Reflect and plan, as part of appraisal and job planning
- Undertake instruction in new knowledge and skills
- Maintain existing skills
- Work with peers and review practice
- Undertake individual and departmental audit

The resources for these activities, IT, time, and financial support for courses and study are an investment by the organization in maintaining a productive and motivated workforce. Frequently, Trusts put enormous effort into individual initiatives related to imposed targets or external visits (e.g. from the Care Quality Commission), which raise standards for a short time and are followed by a decline back to the status quo once the spotlight has moved elsewhere. It would seem much better to really invest in individual education, changing behaviour in a long term and sustainable way.

What the organization cannot provide for the individual

No amount of courses, study time, or work place based training can improve outcomes for patients unless individuals are prepared to match this input by their own private reading and study. Professionalism is a way of life, and maintaining reading of professional journals, and keeping general knowledge up to date is up to the individual. Caring about what we do and being proud of our work is something that comes from each person, and is happily a widespread experience amongst healthcare professionals.

Summary

Organizations can and do provide opportunities for training of their staff. However, as professionals it is vital that all staff are aware of their own responsibilities as regards training, which is crucial to enhancing the safety of patients.

Further reading

Fundamental Human Factors Concepts. UK Civil Aviation Authority Document ref CAP719 February 2002.

NHSLA. www.nhsla.com.

The Health and Safety at Work Act. (1974). Her Majesty's Stationary Office.

Health Care Commission. www.healthcarecommission.org.uk.

Post Graduate Medical Education and Training board. website including results of National Trainee Surveys, www.pmetb.org.uk.

Chapter 31

Continuing professional development

Siân Jaggar

Key points

- Why – the primary aim is enhanced patient safety and care.
- Who – All practitioners should expect to undertake continuous professional development (CPD) throughout their career.
- What – CPD should be regarded as an uninterrupted range of activities the aim of which is to allow a practitioner to reach a more advanced level of practice.
- When and How – CPD is a never-ending lifelong professional activity, which should be undertaken in a wide range of areas, using a variety of means.
- The barriers to undertaking effective CPD – time, energy, and finance need to be recognized and addressed by all individuals and organizations.

The quality of care provided to patients is presumed to be related to lifelong learning. Continuous professional development (CPD) is therefore a requirement for all those who profess a commitment to competence. This is true in all areas of life – holiday-makers would be surprised if the pilot and crew of their aeroplane had learnt their trade on a DC-8 (last manufactured in 1972), but were now working in an Airbus (which had its first flight in 1992) with no further training! It is no less true for all staff working within the medical environment.

Definitions

- *Continuing* – uninterrupted in time or sequence
- *Professional* – connected to a vocation or calling
- *Development* – evolution to a more advanced stage

Thus, CPD can be regarded as the ceaseless evolution to a higher level of clinical competence. It should be undertaken by all practitioners in order to ensure they work at the highest level possible.

Members of a profession historically differ from society in that they are granted the following:

- *A monopoly over the use of a body of knowledge*
  Whilst modern technology has made this more available to the whole of society, much of it remains complex and difficult to interpret. Thus professionals should

ensure that they not only keep up to date with the knowledge base, but also transmit it effectively to patients, relatives and other practitioners. This will inevitably require effective knowledge management (see Chapter 33).

- *Autonomy* (a right of personal freedom and self-government)
  The historical right of medical staff to self-regulation is rightly reducing, with greater society (and therefore patient) representation on both regulatory and association bodies being state sanctioned. It is still however the case that professionals will be regulated to a great extent, by their peers.

- *Prestige*
  Doctors still have a greater range of influence than much of society: a simple example being that of the right of a doctor to sign passport and identity forms.

- *Financial rewards*
  In all western societies, doctors' salaries remain within the top 10%.

In return for this, they are expected to do the following:

- *Provide altruistic service*
  Physicians should place the interests of their patients and society, above their own. Thus, they must be aware of how to protect individuals in (or potentially in) their care, in ways that are not necessarily interesting to them. Some of this is mandatory and enshrined in legislation, but this should not lead staff to view it as unimportant.
  For example, be able to respond effectively should a fire occur in their place of work (a rare, but not unknown, occurrence which poorly responded to causes unnecessary disability and death).
  For example, understand and undertake the current best practice to avoid transmission of infection (known to be a major cause of mortality in hospitals worldwide).

- *Conduct their affairs with morality and integrity*
  Thus, doctors must be able to distinguish right from wrong and act honestly. This may seem obvious, but societal standards do change over time and this is reflected in law. Failure to maintain knowledge in this area can lead to great distress.
  For example, the organ retention scandals of the late twentieth century would have been unthinkable earlier in the century, and failure to recognize the changes that had occurred in the outside world led to much anguish for both the doctors involved, and their patients.

- *Be accountable for their actions – 'duty of care'*
  Staff are clearly accountable to the patients they treat. But, all decisions will have a wider impact (in terms of resource allocation) on other patients, and the ethics of this should be taken into consideration. Many decisions will also have wider societal implications, and doctors must be mindful of this. Doctors should therefore maintain some knowledge of major developments in areas outside their own area of special interest.

Thus, whilst many individuals perceive CPD as a medical knowledge acquisition event (and this is clearly important), an ongoing understanding of the other aspects of professionalism as currently accepted by the society in which they live, is also vital.

What lifelong learning should involve

Training programmes worldwide currently emphasise competency. Society should perhaps be able to expect more than this of their professionals; we would all want to be treated by an expert and so do patients. This requires everyone to undertake on-going development of practice and expertise (Fig. 31.1). This difference is well understood in a variety of areas of life:

For example, amateur musicians (fond of the pastime) practice until they get it right, whilst professionals practice until they cannot get it wrong. As in medicine, this 'musical training' process involves knowledge (of the particular pieces to be attempted – even if recently composed), skills (in manual dexterity) and attitudes (an ability to transmit meaning in addition to particular notes).

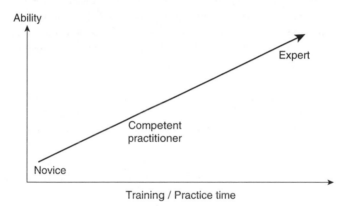

Fig. 31.1 Training and practice over a period of time are required to become an expert.

It might be argued that the areas of primary importance in CPD are learning and practicing:

◆ *Distinguishing important information* from amongst the overwhelming amounts now available. This is of particular importance if doctors are to be able to help patients with access to vast numbers of 'facts' gleaned from Internet pages of various quality and provenance. An understanding of the practice of evidence-based medicine is thus crucial.

◆ *Critical appraisal skills* – often taught in the context of journal clubs.

◆ *Identification of own educational needs* (i.e. self-assessment).
This is particularly problematic, as it requires effective self-assessment; evidence suggests that doctors are poor in this regard, when compared to supervisors, externals tests or audits. This holds true over a wide range of activities:
For example, technical skills – ranging from an awareness of how often one actually washes hands between patients to the ability to perform interventional procedures at first attempt.
In this doctors are no different to other professional groups, including lawyers, engineers, and psychologists. The current appraisal system required for all doctors in the NHS can be regarded as a first effort to improve this.

- *Ethical decision making* – often assumed, rather than actively discussed. Both trainees and senior staff consistently report this as one of the most difficult areas of practice.
- *Team working* – to include aptitude in both leadership and followership (which clearly require different skill sets). Important areas will include communication skills (with patients, relatives and other staff members), coping with uncertainty and 'failure', and improving quality of care. Of particular importance are the non-technical skills including feedback, leadership and the like.

Time and duration of CPD

Doctors (and indeed all professionals, both within and without the medical environment) should expect to undertake continuing professional development. Following completion of undergraduate training, a professional can expect a career lasting in excess of 30 years. During which time huge changes in technology, diagnostics, pharmacology and research-based evidence should be expected to occur, in addition to general social mores.

Some development will be expected to occur within the supporting professional activity (SPA) time funded within the contract. However, professionals have an obligation to maintain their own levels of knowledge, and it is important that doctors realize this does not end at completion of final professional examinations. It is inevitable, and individuals should expect, that they will undertake some of this development in their own time. Thus time management will be crucial if a sensible work–life balance is to be reached.

Why undertake CPD

CPD is necessary because

- Basic post-graduate education is focused on competency
  This has been mandated to ensure that all staff reach a basic minimum level of practice – a laudable aim, since any system is only as strong as its weakest link. However, it has been associated with a shortening of training time, in terms of both hours and duration. Since expertise requires practice, the corollary is an even greater need for lifelong training and development in both technical and non-technical skills. This will include the ability to teach others.
- Time changes understanding of cause and best treatment options:
  An example is the treatment protocol for peptic ulcer disease (Fig. 31.2).
  A doctor who fails to keep up to date with these changes will impose extra unnecessary risks on their patients either through unnecessary surgery, or withholding of important interventions.

Of course, with the ever-increasing amounts of available evidence, doctors may have difficulty locating information crucial to their area of interest. Utilising IT alerts and advisories to locate pre-examined issues (e.g. NICE guidance) may help to keep track of information about factors impacting on safety of patients.

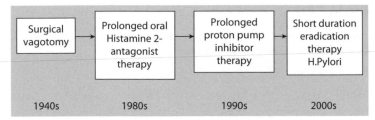

Fig. 31.2 'Best practice' changes over time with new developments.

How to undertake CPD

Historically, this has usually occurred by means of lectures, at regional, national, and international meetings. However, the mere acquisition of new knowledge and novel skills is unlikely to be enough to optimize practice. A range of evidence demonstrates that passive educational activities are poor at changing the behaviour and practices of clinicians, even in a manner that they know is supported by a strong evidence base. Change in practice is most likely to be achieved if the learning is:

- Active, e.g. action learning sets
- Multiple, i.e. occurs on a repeated basis
- Meets a perceived need by the
  - Organization – most likely to provide systematic support
  - Team – any change requires the whole team to be motivated
  - Individual – individuals need to believe in change before engaging in further learning
- Addressing barriers to change

Thus, the most commonly undertaken CPD activity (attendance at lectures) is actually, by design, quite unlikely to change practice within a unit. A simple example of how this might be altered to enhance change as compared to traditional conference attendance is that of the provision of appropriate post-operative analgesia within 1 hospital ward:

	Traditional	In the workplace
Knowledge provision	Passively via lectures	Interactive discussion involving all staff groups on ward round
Occurrence	Usually single events	Weekly
Use to staff	Knowledge acquisition by 1 individual	Treat and avoid pain in actual patients on ward
Barriers addressed	Lack of individual staff knowledge	Lack of knowledge of all staff in multi-disciplinary team
Outcomes	Rate of reported errors in prescription (vary widely) but >50% not unusual (despite all doctors being trained in this)	Prescription levels requiring some change (including addition of an analgesic) ↓ from 70% to 15% over duration of junior staff attachment on 1 ward

Barriers to CPD

In general, staff are keen to improve their knowledge and skills, but barriers may prevent attendance at events. These include:

+ Time
+ Energy
+ Finance

Time

Doctors, like all professionals, are time-poor and thus it can be difficult to plan for learning outside of the workplace. Where possible, this challenge is met by bringing the process into the ward, clinic or theatre and this also increases the likelihood of bringing about change. Of course, this is the basis of training programmes, but has several problems. It:

+ Is generally restricted to non-career grade posts; this issue might be addressed by using supporting professional activity (SPA) time. An example could include visiting units undertaking similar work to learn from peers. This will inevitably require negotiation and agreement to undertake SPA work outside the Trust.
+ Will tend to increase the time taken for regular practice (with concomitant impacts upon waiting times) – a possible mechanism used to overcome this is designating some work times as 'training' sessions, with fewer patients booked.

Thus, time management skills are crucial to effective CPD; indeed the need for them is so great that many Trusts now provide training specifically in this area. When successful, combined with good knowledge management (see Chapter 33) barriers may be effectively broken down.

Energy

Health service staff are, in general, extremely committed to their work. Where this leads to long extra hours of work (clinical or self-development) it can lead to burn out. Under these circumstances, taking time out to work in novel places can be helpful.

For example, medical conferences can be useful in this regard despite the fact that the learning environment is often passive. Meeting with colleagues between formal sessions is frequently perceived to be the most useful part of a conference: unsurprising, since active discussions regarding how each have met their personal challenges of improving care, would be expected to change practice most efficiently.

Evidence suggests that multi-disciplinary training is particularly effective in changing practice. Unfortunately, even where hospitals provide these programmes, medical staff show poor levels of involvement. Cited problems include the following:

+ Organizational – difficulty in releasing staff from clinical practice
+ Personal – worries regarding the pace and approaches to teaching and learning, in addition to differing levels of background knowledge

Where all staff groups can be persuaded to take part in good quality multi-disciplinary activities major changes can be observed. This reflects the fact that a team is only as good as its weakest member (not as many would like to believe, its' strongest).

Walking through patient pathways as a team is a potential mechanism for addressing these issues, since the team sees the ways practice may effect change that is helpful to all. Whilst often viewed as management activities, these may highlight issues for all team members, leading to new learning and practice change.

Finance

Educational activities are rarely free (even if they appear so to the individual undertaking them). Monetary support may be provided from a variety of sources:

♦ *Internal* – where the *individual* pays for their own development. Under such circumstances, the cost may be tax deductible, if shown to be required for continuation of practice.

♦ *External* – which may be local, regional, or national.
  Trusts generally provide a source of study leave funding for permanent medical staff. As with the deanery supplied funding for trainees, this is rarely enough to support all necessary development costs. However, within most consultant contracts there is funded SPA time that is designed to aid professional development activities.
  Traditionally, a high proportion of the financial burden of continuing medical education (CME) has been carried by *private companies* both pharmaceutical and equipment manufacturers. Whilst these companies frequently provide high-quality education, and indeed, undertake (or support) a high proportion of new research, they are businesses and their aim is eventually to change behaviour (prescribing or otherwise) in their favour.
  For example, a company might be more likely to spend time providing information on how to treat asthma (perhaps utilising their new drug), rather than how to diagnose the condition effectively.

Summary

Lifelong learning and development is integral to the working practice of any professional. Whilst it may be tempting to limit CPD to 'interesting and novel factual' conferences, this alone is not the mechanism most likely to ensure appropriate changes in patient-centred practice. It is important to recognize barriers to development, to ensure ever improving patient safety.

Further reading

Driessen, E., van Tartwijk, J., and Dornan, T. (2008). The self-critical doctor: helping students become more reflective. *BMJ* **336**, 827–830.

Davis, D., Evans, M., Jadad, A., et al. (2003). The case for knowledge translation: shortening the journey from evidence to effect. *BMJ* **327**, 33–35.

Shaughnessy, A.F., and Slawson, D.C. (1999). Are we providing doctors with the training and tools for lifelong learning? *BMJ* **319**, 1–3.

GMC guidance on continuing professional development. http://www.gmc-uk.org/education/continuing_professional_development/cpd_guidance.asp.

DH publication. 'Working together, learning together: a framework for lifelong learning in the NHS' (2001). http://www.dh.gov.uk/en/Publicationsandstatistics/Publications/PublicationsPolicyAndGuidance/DH_4009558, Last accessed May 2010.

Chapter 32

Competence

Ian Runcie

Key points

- Formal competencies are prescribed at all levels of training in an attempt to improve patient safety.
- Competencies often fail to scratch the surface of true professionalism.
- Ultimately, competence is the responsibility of the individual doctor.
- Training institutions must administrate competencies whilst recognizing their limitations.
- Major problems exist due to reduction in working hours of junior doctors, making protected time for education vital.

Definition

Competence implies the knowledge and wisdom to decide on the correct course of action within a field of activity, and the technical skills to carry this out.

Pillar of competence	Time when traditionally gained	Stage where should be gained
Knowledge	Medical students	
Skills	House officers/Foundation years	Throughout medical student time and whole career as a doctor
Wisdom	Specialty registrars	

In contrast, a substantial body of evidence clearly indicates that *expertise* (in many spheres, within and without medicine) is a function of experience; i.e. it is a function not only of how much an individual knows about a given area but also how much practice in that area has been acquired.

There is a danger when introducing competency-based training that achievement of competencies themselves becomes the main goal. There is an even greater danger that some vital areas may be seen as unimportant, purely because they are difficult (or even believed to be impossible) to measure. Ultimately the aim of any system of official assessment should be to equip the learner to become good at self-assessment.

Knowledge

Gaining knowledge

This occurs via a mixture of

♦ personal perusal of books and information technology,

♦ formal and informal teaching by peers and seniors - often pedantic but improved by use of resource based methods, interaction, conversation, and example, and

♦ experience of patients and their ability to educate staff.

It may be necessary to pass an exam or two along the way and there is no doubt that these can be important motivators.

Higher professional training is the traditional method of maintaining up-to-date knowledge, and thereafter doctors decide on their own pathways. Requirements agreed by National bodies include:

♦ Auditing personal practice against nationally agreed standards

♦ Clinical governance activity, examples include:
  • Attendance at morbidity and mortality reviews
  • Clinical incident reporting
  • Self reporting of errors, e.g. Incident reporting to Trust management

♦ Appraisal

Assessing knowledge

Knowledge is in theory the easiest of the components of competence to measure. Examining bodies produce learning objectives that must be attainable and measurable. Both attainment and failure must be accompanied by effective feedback.

It is argued that a core of knowledge is essential to carry out a job, and that this core can be measured by traditional methods (e.g. 'clinicals', 'vivas', essay questions MCQs, OSCEs, and their many variants). The utilization of computers has made statistical analysis of results simpler, but the extent to which this produces a competent doctor is unclear. It should come as no surprise that when experienced doctors take examinations they do no better (and often worse) than their less experienced trainees.

Skills

These may be sub-divided into physical and cognitive skills.

Gaining physical skills

Physical skills include, for example, clinical examination, diagnostic, and therapeutic or surgical abilities. Students and trainee doctors have a range of competencies to achieve; a process that is now formalized and institutionalized. The Modernising Medical Careers (MMC) process assumes that there is a necessity for basic abilities to be gained and assessed, and that doctors should not be placed in a position of having to carry out procedures for which they have not been trained.

The increasing use of tick box style competencies is useful for indicating which basic skills must be attained, but rarely come near the actual requirements of medical practice. They leave a gap in organized training crying out to be filled by the reconsideration of an apprenticeship system, and increased appreciation of the importance of dialogue between teachers, trainees, and peers. However, the completion of competency tasks (that are assessed) can be learning activities, provided that feedback and assistance are available. This particularly applies when the learner gets into difficulty or needs guidance. Investment in designing measurable tasks therefore has the dual role of training and competence assessment.

Assessing physical skills

Designing robust measurements to assess competence in physical tasks may require more effort than testing for knowledge, but where feedback and assistance are available may fulfill a dual training and assessment function.

The early assessment tools required by MMC, and now the post-graduate medical and education training board (PMETB) are the following:

♦ Case-based discussion (CbD)
  CbD is used to assess clinical reasoning and decision making (i.e. the application of knowledge to patient care). The trainee presents a case to a senior colleague, who should explore why the trainee acted as they did, provide feedback and make suggestions for development.

♦ Directly observed procedural skills (DOPS)
  DOPS is a structured check list for assessing clinical procedures. It includes not only knowledge and technical skills but also, for example, aseptic technique and the willingness to seek help where appropriate. It is important that the skills observed are sampled from the curriculum.

♦ Mini-clinical evaluation exercise (mini-CEX)
  The trainee is observed during a clinical encounter and rated on a number of technical and professional dimensions. Feedback is given, mapped to the general medical council's Good Medical Practice.

♦ Mini peer assessment tool (mini-PAT)
  Mini-PAT aims to assess the professional behaviour of trainees in the work setting, by those who regularly work with them. The original research showed that for many trainees as few as 8 assessors could provide consistent evaluation. The views of a range of co-workers are collated and the information used to reinforce or improve performance. It is of note that the NPSA would not accept so few as 8 ratings as being valid and, as yet, there is no hard evidence of long-term changes in trainees behaviour. However, in some specialities this 360° appraisal has already been added to the annual review of clinical practice (ARCP) required of all trainees.

Any assessment of practical experience should clearly include:

◆ Number of procedures successfully performed

◆ Clinical outcomes

◆ Efficiency (or speed)

A good example from the literature is the assessment of competency in performing colonoscopy, which was investigated in a multi-centre study. Perceived wisdom was that 100–200 colonoscopies are required to reach technical competence (as defined by reliable visualization of the caecum). The researchers wanted to factor in efficiency as well as clinical outcome.

	Experienced gastroscopist	Trainee < 150 gastroscopies	Trainee > 150 gastroscopies
Time taken (min)	< 20	> 20	< 20
Visualization rate of caecum (%)	90	90	90
Polyp detection rate satisfactory	Yes	Yes	Yes

Polyp detection rates remained satisfactory throughout the study but with increased time and supervision requirements in the early stages. The researchers suggested the minimum threshold number of procedures for clinical competence in screening and diagnostic colonoscopy to be more than 150, which happily coincided with accepted wisdom. Such evidence-based studies, rather than achievement of competencies themselves (that may be introduced for managerial or political expedience) should remain the basis for recognition of skills training by the profession.

Even if the official bodies fail in this respect, the maintenance of professional standards require that the individual and his or her trainers should be aware of the true nature of the requirements for clinical competence. Educational processes in medicine need to be ultimately designed to encourage the individual to set their own personal aims accordingly. Hopefully this will be reflected in their personal assessment and appraisal process.

Gaining cognitive skills

Cognitive skills include, for example, interview skills, decision making. These have historically often been regarded as 'common sense' and left to the trainee to acquire, or not. Evidence from other high-risk industries (e.g. nuclear and oil) suggests that these skills can be learnt, and training should be available. The anaesthetists' non-technical skills (ANTS) system is a behavioural marker system developed by industrial psychologists and anaesthetists, whilst NOTSS (non-technical skills for surgeons) defines the cognitive and interpersonal skills required by a competent surgeon. These non-technical skills are divided into principal skills (for ANTS: team working, task management, situational awareness and decision making), which can then be sub-divided into observable elements. The systems are intended as a framework to discuss behaviour and provide examples of good and poor practice to aid development. Such formative assessment is crucially dependent upon effective feedback to trainees and allowance for development in areas of weakness in a constructive manner.

Assessing cognitive skills

In addition to the formative component of behavioural marking systems (now being developed in paramedical arena, e.g. scrub practitioners list of intraoperative non-technical skills [SPLINTS]), summative assessment reports are possible. Observable elements are graded on a 4-point (4=good, 3=acceptable, 2=marginal, 1=poor) scale, or noted to be not observed. This then provides an overall score for non-technical elements observed during a particular case.

Training and assessment in interpersonal communication, leadership, and decision-making is now mandatory for most of the aviation regulating bodies. It seems likely that clinicians will also be expected to move toward a more formal process of assessing these areas of activity.

Wisdom

The attainment of wisdom does not stop at an exam and most doctors find that learning is a career-long requirement. The how, when and why to apply the knowledge and skill gained can be regarded as the higher facility of clinical wisdom and judgement. 'Attitude' or 'behaviour' is frequently cited, and the ability to deal effectively with colleagues and patients can be regarded as one of the basic requirements of the wise doctor. How to impart this to trainees and include it in their assessment remains a considerable challenge. Sadly there is ultimately no substitute for experience when faced with difficult decisions.

Gaining wisdom

◆ Apprenticeship and reflective learning

Compared with modern educational methods that are increasingly concerned with measurement, an apprenticeship process may seem too tentative. It requires that the mentor is of good professional standing and is able to pass on significant, value-based experiences to the learner. Feedback from the trainees is an important way of maintaining this. Historically, the senior doctor acted as a guide, and counselor in relation to aspects of medical practice that encompassed professionalism. This process remains necessary as competencies alone (no matter how wide ranging) do not themselves make a fit doctor.

The apprenticeship system may no longer be workable at foundation level but at higher levels trainees and trainers should be able to negotiate a working relationship, which takes the trainee up a path of graded responsibility towards autonomous patient care. Progress must be recorded, and agreed graded responsibility individualized.

Somehow procedures need to be agreed that allow for changing shifts and reduced juniors' hours. Protected time for education is a vital ingredient and needs to be maintained with vigilance. This needs to include time for critical reflection, involving discussion and written analysis of both real and imagined clinical situations. The Royal College of Physicians (RCP) has recently recognized that such medical professionalism lies at the heart of being a good doctor.

♦ Personal attitudes

The wise doctor should be aware of how to correctly and effectively interact with staff and patients. In submissions to the RCP, the common themes were that doctors today cannot expect instant respect, and that there was a degree of healthy cynicism amongst non-medical contributors. Even the continuance of the word 'profession' was challenged, although a modern definition of professionalism was substituted. Despite this, it seemed that the medical profession remains the most trusted of professions. How do we keep it that way? Over and over again, the expected requirements involve not just a doctor's knowledge but also their behaviour. Comments submitted included.

'If a doctor has an inappropriate attitude or cannot communicate effectively, patients are likely to consider them lacking in competence' and *'Modern patients are increasingly concerned about the manner in which they are treated, wanting respect and courtesy, as well as kindness, good communication and the understanding of options'.*

Difficulties in these areas are compounded by the paucity of available training, which has traditionally been by example both good and bad. Learning such crucial skills need not be confined to clinical situations. Potential help may be provided by the following:

♦ Training videos

♦ Simulator courses: these may provide courses in:

  • Anger management
  • Team working
  • Crisis management

'What would you do' instances can be used, offering a series of possible actions and follow-up actions, with the reasons for each decision being as important as the decision itself.

Clearly this requires discussion if judgement is to be assessed. In any given situation, trainees may take a different course from the teacher. Only if reasoning is discussed can judgement be assessed. It may turn out that, in consideration of a complex situation, the trainee has taken factors into account not considered by the trainer. These effects have already been observed in non-medical scenarios, such as that described in Box 32.1.

Assessing wisdom

This area has traditionally been the Cinderella of assessment processes. It is an area of professionalism, and development in training that can be seen as intangible and difficult to define. However, the airline industry already uses crew resource management

Box 32.1

Car mechanics considered how to manage a faulty spark plug; there was no correct answer.

Less experienced mechanics tended to offer a replacement. This results in a higher bill for the customer and loss of a potentially useful spark plug, but usually provides a quicker result.

More experienced mechanics tended more towards cleaning, but there were wide variations within the pattern. Considerations, other than cost, included the state of: other spark plugs, the engine, the vehicle in general, and service history. Moreover, the more experienced mechanics wanted to know more about the customer, including:

◆ Was the customer in a hurry to get going?

◆ Was it a regular customer with a known preference?

Immediate profit was a factor, but consideration of what would satisfy the customer and result in a return visits was also considered. Thus variables amongst the experience mechanics soon become immeasurable though perfectly understandable.

(CRM) scenarios as part of their regular assessment of fitness to practice. The medical profession may find similar practices useful.

Behavioural marking systems used to monitor non-technical behaviours that can enhance safety in clinical areas grew, largely from ideas developed by NASA. Research demonstrated as far back as 1979 that human factors were pivotal in aviation safety.

Historically, a doctor might be labeled as not getting on with colleagues but to provide insight and steer the doctor to self understanding and the ability to work in teams, some more concrete descriptors are necessary. Again, the ANTS, NOTSS, and SPLINTS systems list activities that are parts of team working and give examples of how to rate the behaviour of clinicians. They also give examples of appropriate situations in which such assessments could take place. The developers of the systems recognize that markers are limited to the observable at any particular time. This is a criticism leveled at many assessments, which cannot begin to encompass the whole even at one time period, let alone over a prolonged period. At present, training and assessment on non-technical skills is in its infancy and largely confined to junior staff. However, it seems likely that this will spread to career grade staff in the future.

Summary

Competence-based training, including regular assessment, aims to ensure a minimum acceptable level of practice. However, the profession needs to retain the understanding that there are limits to pure measurement. High-quality thinking needs to be disassembled, with doctors learning to explain their decisions and defend them in debate.

Further reading

Archer, J., Norcini, J., Southgate, L., Heard, S., Davies, H. (2008). mini-PAT (Peer Assessment Tool): A Valid Component of a National Assessment Programme in the UK? *Adv Health Sci Educ Theory Pract. May* **13**(2), 181–192.

Bloom, B. S. (1956). *Taxonomy of Educational Objectives, Handbook I: The Cognitive Domain.* New York: David McKay Co Inc.

Fish, D., Coles, C. (1998). *Developing Professional Judgment in Healthcare.* Oxford: Butterworth Heinemann.

Fish, D., de Cossart, L. (2007). *Developing the Wise Doctor: A Resource for Trainers and Trainees (In Practice).* London: RSM Press, ISBN: 978-1-85315-618-2.

Report by Royal College of Physicians of London. December (2005). Doctors in society: Medical professionalism in a changing world. Technical supplement.

Chapter 33

An introduction to the concepts of knowledge management

David Greaves and Peta Jane Eastland

Key points

- Continuing medical education (CME) is a critical knowledge creation activity, which may occur informally. Management should facilitate and foster this, ensuring that its products are shared, since it is likely to enhance patient safety.

- Knowledge is information organised and interpreted in ways that make it actionable.

- Healthcare professionals are knowledge workers, and healthcare is a knowledge creation industry.

- Knowledge management includes restructuring work in ways that facilitate knowledge creation, in pursuit of organizational objectives.

- Tacit knowledge (personal knowledge that individuals are unable to express) is often the most important resource in the knowledge creation organization, and it is frequently transmitted in an informal manner.

In 1988, Peter Drucker, the father of modern management, wrote:

> Twenty years from now, the typical large business will have half the levels of management and one-third the managers of its counterpart today.

This prediction was based on the need for change in response to the emergence of knowledge creation industries. These organizations (or industries) have the construction of knowledge as a major element of their business. They are characterized by the number and importance of their knowledge workers. Healthcare is a knowledge creating industry. Twenty years on, many fields of business have undergone this predicted transformation. Healthcare, however, has lagged behind. Most healthcare professionals have not heard of knowledge management. However, the principles of knowledge management are applicable in healthcare and it is important that doctors understand them. It is first necessary to understand what is meant by 'knowledge' (Fig. 33.1).

The definition of knowledge narrows as it moves into the context of a business or an organization. Here, knowledge is defined as that which assists the company to achieve its aims, be they profit (e.g. supermarkets), excellence in performance (e.g. an opera company), or better patient care (e.g. a primary care Trust).

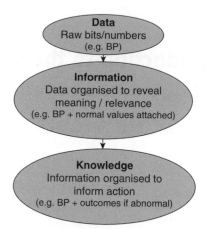

Fig. 33.1 Data, information and knowledge are related concepts.

A knowledge worker is someone employed for their knowledge of subject matter, rather than their ability to perform manual labour (i.e. brain not brawn). Their daily task involves the re-synthesis and creation of knowledge to solve problems in pursuit of organizational aims. It includes those in the information technology fields (e.g. computer programmers and systems analysts) and also those hired primarily for their knowledge of a subject (e.g. doctors, nurses, teachers, and scientists).

Knowledge management is the process by which information and knowledge from within and outside the organization are made available to the teams that are building, creating, and advancing knowledge. It:

♦ Gets the right information, to the right people, at the right time

♦ Helps people create knowledge, and share and act upon information in ways that will measurably improve the performance of an organization

♦ Is the process by which the knowledge an organisation needs is leveraged

  • Knowledge leverage is recruiting, sharing, and stealing knowledge to enhance an individual's, or a team's, capacity to create knowledge and solve problems.

  • Financial leverage is borrowing money to supplement existing funds for investment in such a way that the potential positive outcome is magnified and enhanced.

The 'profession' of knowledge management rests on the idea that it is efficient to have a specialist department (headed by a chief knowledge officer) that facilitates the gathering, capture, storage, and provision of knowledge within a company. Formal approaches may facilitate this process. In small organizations, it is relatively easy to know who knows what and where relevant information can be found. In large organizations, this is less obvious, and efficient development of an idea requires team members to know who knows about what, and where to go for help.

Knowledge management is thus more than books, libraries, and databases, more indeed than information management and librarianship. These are all aspects of efficient knowledge handling, but not the whole story. Successful knowledge management requires:

+ A clear understanding of corporate or institutional objectives
+ Adjustment of working practices to facilitate creative flow, e.g. defining a time when routine clinical work stops and all teams meet to discuss recent adverse events

Introducing the concept of knowledge management to a business may lead to major changes in practice and as with all change there will be winners and losers, enthusiasts, and nay-sayers. There have been examples where the entire business mission of a company has been changed by the introduction of knowledge management systems; e.g. a business review showing that using an organization's know-how to advise other firms as a consultancy is more profitable than manufacturing a product themselves.

What a medical manager needs to know about knowledge management

+ Healthcare is a characteristic knowledge industry
+ The delivery of quality care depends upon the activities of specialist knowledge workers (e.g. doctors, nurses, physiotherapists, pharmacists)
+ Patient treatments and management systems are constantly changing and improving. Specialists work in a multiplicity of changing teams, interpreting expert advice and a range of opinions
+ Healthcare professionals must transmit changes to one another and build new systems of institutional knowledge

Managing knowledge for healthcare professionals is difficult. A fundamental problem in passing knowledge to other teams (or transmitting it down generations of workers) is that experts often do not know how they do the things they do. Much of their knowledge is *tacit* (or 'hidden') *knowledge*, rather than *explicit* (or open) *knowledge* (Fig. 33.2).

Michael Polyani had the important insight that experts often could not explain how they knew what to do – they just knew. This simple observation has far reaching consequences. If experts do not know exactly what directs their decision making it is difficult to pass the knowledge on. Traditionally this has been accomplished by long apprenticeship, with novices learning by watching and being watched. This can be demonstrated to result in learners satisfactorily assimilating the expert process. Only by long experience of watching and trying things out can tacit knowledge be passed on. For example, the amount and range of analgesia required for a patient under anaesthesia, to ensure that they awaken pain free, but with minimal side effects following major surgery varies widely.

The desire for faster learning drives the search for ways to capture, and explicitly teach expert process. Is this search for short cuts to expertise a fruitful endeavour? Some consider that the essential nature of experts is the fluidity with which they take information and clues, re-formulating them in the light of past experience;

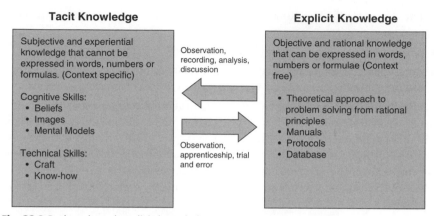

Fig. 33.2 Both tacit and explicit knowledge are important to experts.

and that this intrinsically expert process cannot be explicitly captured, taught, or tested.

Large business organizations often repeatedly undertake complex projects. In the interests of efficiency, they capture and record the decision making processes involved, providing this knowledge to future teams undertaking similar tasks. Whether the task is building an oil refinery (or clinic) or launching a new product (or diagnostic service), much of the knowledge involved falls into the category of know-how and tacit knowledge. There has been some success with a technique of sending observers to watch expert practice and note the knowledge used. This is then explained and refined through discussion with the experts. Much of this – including some previously tacit knowledge now rendered explicit – is then kept as a resource for future projects.

Leaders and managers in knowledge creation industries need to appreciate the value of tacit knowledge and understand how laborious the process its creation and transmission is. This must not be seen as inefficiency and made the victim of cost saving.

Knowledge workers are difficult to manage

Knowledge creation organizations have been driven to change their management structures in order to deal with the working practices of knowledge workers.

Healthcare is an excellent example of a knowledge organization. Specialists (from many disciplines) form teams. Some of these are permanent (e.g. breast cancer team) whilst others are entirely *ad hoc* groups defined by the particular needs of a single patient. Thus teams form, do their work, and disappear as required, without the intervention of middle management.

Mid-level managers of knowledge workers find themselves in a difficult position:

◆ If experts in the field themselves they tend to 'go native' and be subsumed into the project teams. The team recruits them as a resource, a role they are only too happy to undertake. This undermines their management function, leading management to doubt their impartiality and distrust their judgement. In the medical management of healthcare this is a pitfall for the clinical director.

◆ If not an initiate of the knowledge creating processes, it is all too easy for their well-meant interventions to stand in the way of the development of a new better practice, thus perpetuating existing practice. In many fields, real progress comes from some apparently outlandish idea; although many of these journeys off the beaten track will lead nowhere. The manager who is an outsider in the knowledge field will be less able to decide when to let ideas run and when to close them down.

The business answer has been, as Peter Drucker predicted, to drastically reduce the number of middle grade managers in knowledge creation industries. Teams manage their everyday business themselves. In this model the manager becomes a facilitator and sounding board, helping and reviewing the progress of their teams and acting as a conduit to higher management.

	Production workers	Knowledge workers
Industries	Traditional industries	Knowledge industries
	Hierarchical structures	Often *ad hoc* groups
	e.g. production-line workers	e.g. teachers
Features	Often semi-skilled	Individuals with a range of inter-locking abilities
Training	Relatively straightforward	Prolonged
Replacement	Easy	Often time-consuming and difficult
Knowledge loss	Rare	May occur with the loss of a few individuals

What of the NHS? The letter to the Secretary of State that accompanied the 'Griffiths' enquiry into NHS management (1983) stated:

> At no level is the general management role clearly being performed by an identifiable individual. In short, if Florence Nightingale were carrying her lamp through the corridors of the NHS today, she would almost certainly be searching for the people in charge.

The enquiry led to reorganization and the introduction of many new managers. Was Sir Roy Griffiths (previously a supermarket manager) right, or was this a case of a retail trade manager not understanding the management structure of a knowledge industry? Since then there has been an expansion of management as a stand-alone profession in healthcare. Doctors can aspire to be clinical director or medical director, but average consultant participation in managing their own service has been greatly eroded. For many other knowledge worker groups (e.g. nurses, clinical scientists) the ability to participate in knowledge creation teams is even more constrained by management. While knowledge creation industries elsewhere have been shedding tiers of management, the NHS has been attempting to introduce additional middle grades. Seen from the perspective of a knowledge creation organization this is problematical. Perhaps healthcare should look to knowledge creation industries rather than supermarkets for useful models of management practice.

Communities of practice

The formal and informal teams that knowledge workers use to do their work are known as communities of practice. Some are limited to the main workplace, whilst some are extended to like-minded individuals in other institutions with meetings or links forming a virtual community. Communities of practice are important to knowledge workers for a number of reasons:

- Their sources of information and knowledge are extended (e.g. multi-disciplinary teams)

- They can see their particular discipline being undertaken in a different environment, possibly leading to questioning assumptions about work (e.g. directorate groups, sub-speciality networks, specialist societies)

- The community of practice is able to work together to extend the knowledge of each team and each individual (e.g. extended clinical teams, commissioners)

Managers in knowledge creation organizations must understand the role of the communities of practice and should facilitate them. This includes creating suitable informal facilities for meeting and talking. Knowledge workers tend to talk shop, taking their work with them wherever they go, and many businesses have found it productive to encourage these processes. Many managers see staff facilities, coffee rooms, and kitchens as an unproductive expense, but they are mistaken. Knowledge management strategies should include positive creation of informal facilities because many good ideas will be generated where workers meet.

Continuing medical education (CME) is a knowledge management activity

For many knowledge workers, including those in healthcare, an important community of practice is the specialist society or special interest group. It is common experience for doctors to find that managers do not take a positive or constructive view of CME because:

- It takes clinicians away from clinical work

- It costs the organization money (often begrudged)

- They come back with fancy ideas that cost more money

Managers of knowledge workers should be taking a different view. Since the mission of healthcare is to extend the best possible care to the greatest number of patients, then their task should be to see that maximum knowledge value is obtained. Cost containment is a necessary constraint on the real mission of healthcare, not a mission in itself.

In pursuit of their mission, managers should help teams address clinical and organizational issues, and search out examples of good practice by any means possible. Local clinical audit and governance meetings, and specialty societies are all part of this quest. In medical practice these activities constitute CME, and most doctors and managers view these activities as 'personal' learning. An alternative view would be that they are 'organizational' learning. If this is accepted, then individual doctors and their managers have a responsibility to ensure that CME is appropriate to the organization and that efforts are made to capture any new knowledge and make it available to other team members. An organization that eschews knowledge creation and capture makes itself over-reliant on staff turnover for fresh ideas.

The problem of capturing and storing knowledge

When an organization is small and there are few teams it is easy to record knowledge and make it available. This changes as an organization grows.

	Small organizations	Large organizations
Number of teams	Few	Many
Knowledge bank	May be small, but easily accessible e.g. departmental journals	Useful large range of information, but may be remote, requiring specialised assistance e.g. university library
Knowledge management	Easily available e.g. local guidelines	Remote from clinical need e.g. untargeted e-mails

There is a danger that knowledge management becomes remote from clinical need. It is no accident that the majority of Medline 'hits' for knowledge management are found in IT and librarianship publications. When formalizing knowledge management systems, it is inevitable that the focus will turn to these closely allied disciplines. This is not inappropriate, but the danger lies in concentrating on what they know: data storage, retrieval, and dissemination technologies. Knowledge management should also encompass reviews of organizational objectives and practice, ensuring they are aligned so as to maximize knowledge creation. It is important that knowledge custodians and managers work closely with knowledge workers to capture as much valuable knowledge as possible without storing a fund of useless information. Examples of systems available to store and manage knowledge in medical practice include:

- Electronic patient records
- Clinical guidelines
  - Locally developed
  - National (e.g. NICE, specialist societies)
- Procedural protocols (e.g. ALS)
- Evidence-based practice movement (e.g. Cochrane Collaboration)
- Risk management systems (e.g. DATIX, STEIS)
- Specialist journals and search resources (e.g. Medline)
- Intranet and Internet resources
- Blogs, Tweets, Wikis etc

Summary

Knowledge management does not comprise the individual systems for handling data, information, and knowledge. Rather it is the organizing of these resources, along with a management ethos and management systems that facilitate the creation of knowledge. Information and knowledge management systems should be designed so as to be useful to the clinical teams. These should include informal areas where individuals meet, enhancing the dissemination of tacit knowledge.

Further reading

Collison, C., Parcell, G. (2004). *Learning to Fly: Practical Knowledge Management from Leading and Learning Organizations.* Oxford: Capstone Publishing.

Drucker, P.F. (1999). Knowledge-worker productivity: The biggest challenge. *California Management Review* Winter, **41**(2), 79–94.

Harvard Business Review on Knowledge Management (1998). Harvard Business School Publishing, Boston. ISBN 13:978-0-87584-881-5.

Polyani, M. (1967–2009 reprint). *The Tacit Dimension.* University of Chicago Press. ISBN 9780226672984.

Rumizen, M.C. (2002). *The Complete Idiots Guide to Knowledge Management.* CWL Publishing Enterprises: Madison WI. ISBN 0-02-865177-9.

Chapter 34

Clinical information systems

Simon Finney

Key points

- When properly implemented, clinical information systems have the potential to improve patient safety and reduce medical error.
- Poor availability and performance of systems impacts adversely upon patient safety.
- Decision support is a powerful tool to reduce errors of omission and commission.
- Clinical information systems can enhance the quality and reduce the burden of clinical audit.
- Unless users can be actively engaged, new systems are likely to fail.

New computer applications including computerized imaging systems, electronic laboratory results, and patient administration systems are implemented in hospitals. Introduced in the hope of improving quality and efficiency of patient care, whilst reducing medical errors, they at times fall short of this goal. Since to some extent all contain clinical data they can be termed 'clinical information systems' (CISs), and are components of an electronic health record. Comprehensive electronic health records are key strategies of both U.S. and UK governments, with estimated costs of $75–100 billion in the United States alone.

Picture archiving and communication systems (PACS) have transformed radiology departments, and are considered essential. They have eliminated the problems of lost films, and the requirement to view certain modalities on specific display stations. Images can be stored and backed up electronically, being immediately available in patient-care locations remote to the image source. The success of PACS systems has been aided by the presence of only relatively few imaging modalities, and the industry driven Digital Imaging and Communications in Medicine (DICOM) standard for file formats and communication between imaging systems. Nevertheless, new modalities such as real-time 3D ultrasound and full field mammography have taken time to integrate into PACS.

A CIS covering an inpatient episode or outpatient consultation contains even more complex data since:

- The range of observations is greater
- Observations are repeated over time
- Items are a mixture of text, images, and numerical values

◆ Interactions occur between data (e.g. electronic prescriptions and records of drug administration)

Examples of the range of data that can be stored in a CISs are included in Table 34.1.

Table 34.1 Examples of data collected in clinical information system

Type of data and examples		Comments
Text		
	Ward round transcript	Enhanced handover
	Discussion with family members	Avoiding unnecessary distress due to poor communication
	Operation note	Essential data if future surgery planned
Selections from a list of options	Grade of laryngoscopy for intubation	Key piece of information for future anaesthesia
	Names of drug hypersensitivities	Documentation known to be poor between clinical episodes on paper records
	Glasgow coma scale	
Numeric		
	Electronic prescription instructions	Clarity in intended dates, dose, frequency, route etc, unobscured by poor handwriting
	Blood biochemistry	Electronically generated, measured repeatedly
	Dose of drug administered	Safety alerts can be imposed
	Heart rate measurement	Electronically generated, measured repeatedly
	Urine volume	Manually input, measured repeatedly
Image		
	Documentation of a wound	Important clinical adverse events, e.g. Decubitus ulcers and surgical site infection
	Description of a rash	Often poorly documented
	Ultrasound or radiology	Usually encompassed within a PACS system

The roles of and functions of a clinical information system

A CIS can fulfil several roles, often simultaneously:

◆ Decision support tool – passive or active

◆ Medico-legal record of patient care

◆ Clinical audit tool

◆ Management tool

◆ Research tool

Passive decision support

Data from multiple sources can be presented together on a single system facilitating interpretation. For example, heart rate, temperature, respiratory rate from monitoring presented contemporaneously with laboratory analyses of C-reactive protein and white cell count to assist consideration of whether a patient has evidence of infection. Whilst relatively simple electronically, this avoids users opening multiple applications and endeavouring to remember (often incorrectly) multiple values.

Clinical care can also be manipulated by prompting with specific questions. For example, it is widely felt that all mechanically ventilated patients should be considered for deep venous thrombosis prophylaxis, gastric protection, and interruptions of sedative medications daily. Junior doctors can be prompted about these issues daily whilst recording the discussions of ward rounds (see Fig. 34.1). Similarly, a safety issue in critical care is the avoidance of bloodstream infections related to intravascular catheters. A CIS form where insertion of catheters is documented can also reveal standards based on evidence that operators are expected to comply with during insertion (e.g. use of 2% chlorhexidine for skin preparation and allowing it to dry).

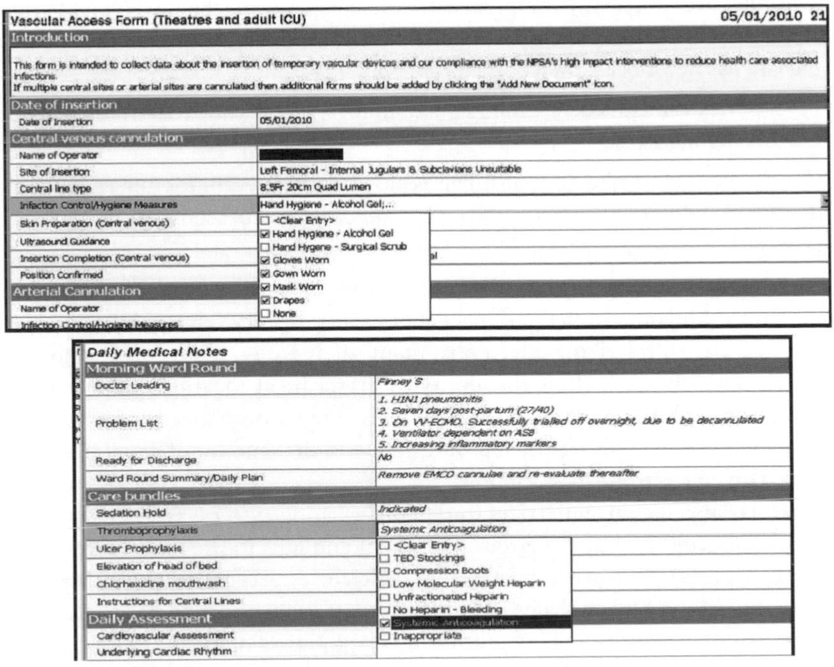

Fig. 34.1 Examples of passive modification of process using a CIS.

Active decision support

This has greater potential, countering errors of both omission and commission, but is harder to implement. If a system contains all vital signs that contribute to an early warning score (e.g. the modified early warning score [MEWS]), it should then warn nurses which patients have high scores and significant risk of deterioration. Similarly, systems can inform clinicians that patients are demonstrating signs of infection by integrating monitoring, laboratory, ventilator, and blood gas analyser data. They can then be advised to consider sending appropriate microbiological samples or review antibiotic therapy.

Pharmacy decision support has probably the greatest potential to reduce errors. Many patient safety incidents relate to drug administration, particularly of injectable drugs. An absolute expectation is that drug sensitivities should highlight warnings to prescribers, e.g. warning that a patient is penicillin allergic when prescribing Tazocin (Piperacillin and Tazobactam). It is also reasonable to expect users to be warned of apparent drug interactions, or abnormal doses in light of current metabolic function. Whether the system should prevent a user from making what it perceives as an unwise prescription (*decision constraint*), or just require users to confirm that they have considered the potential problem and still wish to prescribe the drug (*decision support*), is unclear. Clearly the thresholds imposed on decision support are important to ensure that:

◆ Excessive warnings don't obscure very significant ones

◆ Warnings are sufficiently comprehensive to be dependable. Staff will tend to move towards a perception that "no warning" means "no problem" when it may be that the CIS has never been 'taught' the problem

◆ Level of risk is included, e.g. mild nausea may be inconsequential in the setting of life threatening sepsis

◆ Consistency between institutions. This is particularly relevant for nurses and junior doctors moving between hospitals and expecting (incorrectly) to be warned of events

Electronic prescribing requires careful consideration and has been subject to review in the United Kingdom by the National Patient Safety Agency. Thus, whilst it is widely recognized that e-Prescribing can combat many safety issues, it has potential to create new problems. These include the ability to prescribe at locations remote from a patient, standard prescription dosing being accepted automatically (e.g. for a very small patient on an adult ward), and inflexibility in the amount of detail that can be provided on an electronic prescription.

There are also technical barriers to reliable warning systems (e.g. misspelt drug allergy is unrecognized by the electronic system and fails to provoke a warning to a new prescription). Similarly infrastructure deficiencies preventing timely laboratory data reporting may mean drugs are prescribed at inappropriate doses. Real-time alarms from patient vital signs monitors travel across dedicated networks that are considered as medical devices; similar quality levels are needed for all essential warnings.

Nevertheless, eight studies from two U.S. inpatient institutions suggest that on-screen point of care computer reminders can significantly improve processes of care. This will undoubtedly be a focus of attention for CISs as there is a trend to focus on process, presuming that patient safety will increase in parallel.

Medico-legal record of patient care

Electronic health records can be more comprehensive, accurate, timely, and persistent, than paper; key features of high quality records. Many aspects of patient care are generated electronically (e.g. vital signs from a patient monitor, laboratory results) and many can be input manually by practitioners (e.g. transcript of a ward round or patient discussion, measurement of volume of urine produced, record of a drug administration). These are then stored electronically and provide a permanent record of the care the patient received (see Fig. 34.2). If the security of a system is sufficient and the backup systems robust then these records:

- Cannot be lost or amended
- Contain detail of the source of data (automatic or a specific healthcare practitioner)
- Show timings when data were recorded
- Document alarms generated by monitoring devices
- May show when a practitioner opened a record

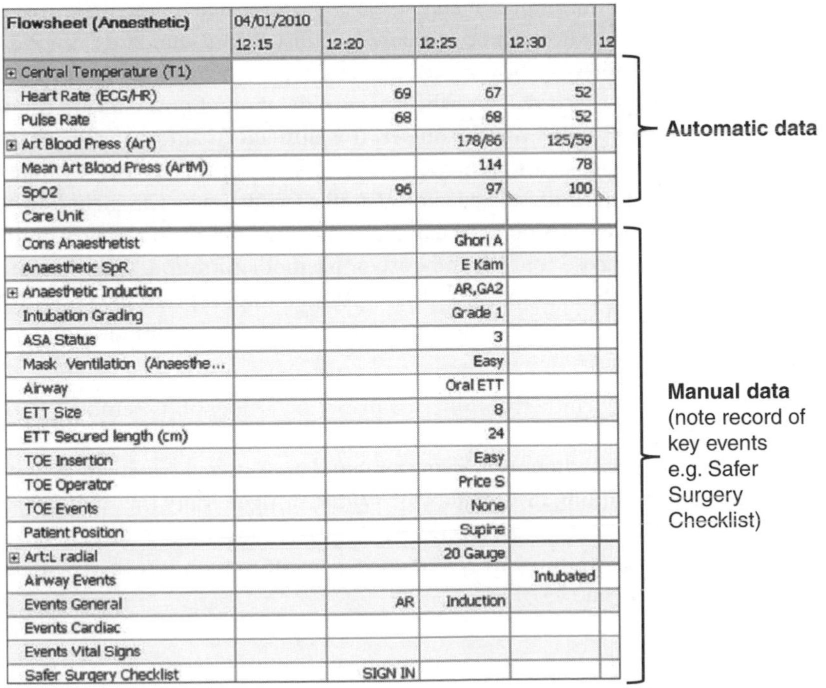

Flowsheet (Anaesthetic)	04/01/2010					
	12:15	12:20	12:25	12:30	12	
⊞ Central Temperature (T1)						⎫
Heart Rate (ECG/HR)		69	67	52		
Pulse Rate		68	68	52		
⊞ Art Blood Press (Art)			178/86	125/59		⎬ Automatic data
Mean Art Blood Press (ArtM)			114	78		
SpO2		96	97	100		
Care Unit						⎭
Cons Anaesthetist			Ghori A			⎫
Anaesthetic SpR			E Kam			
⊞ Anaesthetic Induction			AR,GA2			
Intubation Grading			Grade 1			
ASA Status			3			
Mask Ventilation (Anaesthe…)			Easy			
Airway			Oral ETT			Manual data
ETT Size			8			(note record of
ETT Secured length (cm)			24			key events
TOE Insertion			Easy			e.g. Safer
TOE Operator			Price S			Surgery
TOE Events			None			Checklist)
Patient Position			Supine			
⊞ Art:L radial			20 Gauge			
Airway Events				Intubated		
Events General		AR	Induction			
Events Cardiac						
Events Vital Signs						
Safer Surgery Checklist		SIGN IN				⎭

Fig. 34.2 Screen images of a care records created during induction of anaesthesia using manual and automatic data sources.

Data captured electronically are accurate representations of what the data source was recording at the time. Manual records of vital signs are inaccurate in terms of their temporal resolution, absolute values, and completeness. Automated collected data are usually complete (so long as the cables are attached) and temporally accurate, but have a background error rate in terms of accuracy. For example, many heart rate monitors misinterpret a pacing spike and the ensuing ECG complex as two heart beats rather than one; peripheral oximeters will fail during a period when an automatic blood pressure cuff is inflated. These types of error have been estimated to occur at a rate of less than 0.1% of observations. This can be reduced by asking users to manually filter and confirm automatically collected data, but this step increases the workload for healthcare providers.

A potential advantage of automatically captured data is a reduction in the time practitioners spend documenting events. Time and motion studies have estimated the reduction in time spent documenting as 20–25% for nurses and 15% for physicians. Reductions are greater if data is entered at the point of care rather than a central station, but tend to be less the longer a CIS has been operational. Whether this is due to increasing burdens of a higher level of documentation is unknown. Great care has to be taken to avoid over-burdening staff with recording data not directly related to patient care.

Clinical audit tools

A CIS can facilitate clinical audit as it contains a comprehensive representation of the care a patient received, which can be compared against agreed standards. Since data are held electronically they can be retrieved and evaluated more quickly than a manual examination of paper records. Nevertheless, consideration of how data are entered into a system must be made from the outset. It is difficult to automatically analyse large bodies of text. By contrast, numeric entries or selections from lists lend themselves to analysis. Examples of isolated clinical audits facilitated by CIS include analysis of timings and values of aminoglycoside monitoring relative to changes in drug prescription; blood glucose control; and dose of haemodiafiltration. Quality indices should be generated automatically by a CIS if it stores the appropriate data. Examples include rates of readmission within 24 hours, compliance with care bundles, and rates of nosocomial infections.

Management tools

A CIS can generate large amounts of management data that facilitate many activities (e.g. billing, understanding of workflows). Whilst not generally the focus during implementation of a system, and not a driver for practitioners using the system, CIS generated data can be exploited by senior management to plan future activity and needs (see Chapters 17 and 45).

Research tool

Large quantities of data about patient care stored electronically have great potential for retrospective observational studies. Data sets are often large and comprehensive, and associated analyses can provide valuable observational evidence to support clinical theories. Furthermore, a CIS can be set up to collect important data prospectively, forming part of the case record for specific studies, enhancing persistence, accuracy, timeliness, and audit trails.

The utility of a CIS as a research tool depends on the ability to transfer data stored in the CIS to other analysis software. Since a CIS is rarely primarily a research tool, few are associated with robust statistical analysis tools able to present data in both parametric and non-parametric summary forms. Modelling and regression undoubtedly need to be undertaken on expert statistical systems. Any transfer of patient-related data to a different system should be subject to appropriate information governance measures, ensuring ongoing security and ethical approval for its use by that researcher. Nevertheless, extending the current knowledge base has a clear long-term impact on patient safety.

Other considerations for Clinical Information Systems

Standardization

The success of the PACS has been in part due to the universal adoption of the DICOM standards by manufactures. The standards are less defined for CIS, which encompass more complex data sets. It is important to consider functionality with other health care systems so patient data are freely available. For example, a new finding of a drug sensitivity made by a general practitioner should be transferable ultimately to a hospital inpatient CIS. This level of integration is far from being realized. Attempts to standardize data in CISs from different vendors include SNOMED-CT (Systematized Nomenclature of Medicine-Clinical Terms). This language assists communication between electronic systems. It is a comprehensive, multilingual, hierarchical system that meticulously describes concepts. Thus, differing computers will refer internally to a heart rate by the SNOMED-CT code 364075005, rather than what is displayed to the user, which may be heart rate, cardiac rate, HR, or even Herzfrequenz in an alternative country. Additionally, the HL7 (Health level 7) standard defines how hospital systems send messages between each other.

Infrastructure requirements

Decisions regarding the hardware infrastructure that supports a CIS are of equivalent magnitude to the decisions regarding the CIS itself. Commonly, the two aspects are not considered in conjunction, but rather by different professional groups.

Any system containing essential clinical data must be available continuously. There is risk to patients if previously recorded facts (e.g. drug reactions) cannot be retrieved. Systems that are available 99% of the time are clinically useless, since this equates to 1.68 hours every week when it may be unavailable. By contrast, most would find 99.999% (colloquially referred to as five nines availability) or even 99.9999% (six nines) acceptable. These equate to 5.26 minutes and 31.5 seconds of loss of service each year respectively. To achieve this degree of reliability requires considerable infrastructural investment with: duplication of hardware and network components, uninterruptable power supplies, and system designs that have no single point of failure. Both planned and un-planned periods of down-time should be considered in service level agreements with IT providers. Alternative arrangements can be made for planned downtime, but patients are cared for continuously and how to deal with unplanned service interruption must be clear.

Slow response times by a CIS are perceived correctly by users as effective downtime. Speed is the result of the interaction between hardware, network components, and software. Determining the exact source of poor performance can be challenging. It is worth noting that vendors often stipulate minimum specifications for hardware.

Security

The same standards of security apply to both electronic and paper records, falling under the remit of the Caldicott guardian and data protection officers. It is important to protect both the confidentiality and probity of records. Most organizations accept electronic passwords in lieu of a signature, allowing actions to be attributed to specific individuals. The quality of the audit trail regarding data source and accessing is a key asset to any CIS. Most institutions have policies regarding the complexity and changing of passwords. Paradoxically, requiring users to change passwords frequently can reduce security, as easy to remember systems are adopted. Similarly, 24-hour support for issuing new user names and forgotten passwords is necessary to avoid individuals sharing accounts. Clinical Context Object Workgroup (CCOW) is an emerging standard allowing users to use multiple CCOW-enabled applications simultaneously whilst only providing their username and password for one.

A general Caldicott principle to protect confidentiality is restricting access of records (or parts thereof) to users who require access to fulfil their role. Ideally, a person should only be able to gain access to the records of patients for whom they are responsible, and be granted access to other records by agreement of the patient or the process of referral. Sensitive aspects of a record such as histories of drug abuse, psychiatric histories, and medical records for prisoners should have further restrictions. The use of incorrect patient identifiers (e.g. pseudonyms for the famous) is not safe. Multi-layered security is complex to manage and can prevent timely access to records for valid reasons, particularly in the setting of emergency clinical care. More usually, therefore, users gain access to records based on their role in an organization: doctors, nurses, and administrators having different privileges. Some users may have multiple roles as patient, doctor, manager, or technician. Ideally, the role should be explicit as a record is accessed. The role of a "Super User" with access to everything in a system creates a specific vulnerability. Patients may request that none of their record is kept on a CIS, with the associated problems of multiple systems within an organization.

There are many concerns about the physical security of a record to threats including: fire, theft, hardware failure, and computer viruses. These can be mitigated by multiple back-ups of data both on- and off-site. Transmission of records should remain along trusted routes and be appropriately encrypted. Unnecessary and insecure links to computers external to those of the CIS should be avoided.

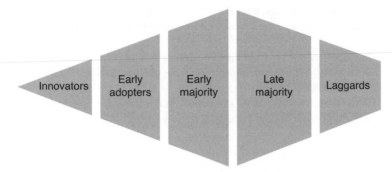

Fig. 34.3 Everett Rogers Technology Adoption Lifecycle model.
Adapted from Rogers, E. (1962) *Diffusion of Innovations*. Free Press, London, NY, USA.

Another key security aspect of electronic records is the concept of persistence. Most electronic records do not allow deletion of data, only updating; thus, the full history of a data item is held. Persistence also relates to the whole record remaining available after a care episode (possibly indefinitely as electronic storage is cheap). Whilst this may be clinically useful it conflicts with the Data Protection Act (UK) which states data should not be kept longer than necessary.

User engagement

Benefit from any CIS is only accrued when comprehensively adopted. A mixture of paper and electronic records is hazardous as neither is complete. Practitioners respond to new technologies at different rates (see Fig. 34.3). Thus, whilst innovators and early adopters will engage and drive the direction in which a CIS develops, the late majority and laggards need to be convinced that there are benefits both personally and for patients. High availability of the system and avoiding overburdening users with non-clinical data presently not recorded on paper are key steps. Facilitating the return of data for personal logbooks, audits, and investigations under appropriate governance rules, allows everyone to gain from other functionalities rather than merely the few innovators.

Summary

Secure CISs have the potential to rapidly impact upon patient safety by both passive and active decision support. However, in allowing the manipulation of large quantities of clinical data they may also allow development of systems and services that enhance healthcare in the longer term. User engagement is vital at all stages.

Further reading

van de Velde, R., Degoulet, P. (2003). *Clinical Information Systems: A Component-Based Approach*. Springer: Berlin.

Gruber, D., Cummings, G.G., Leblanc, L., *et al.* (2009). Factors influencing outcomes of clinical information systems implementation – A systematic review. *Computers Informatics Nursing* **27**, 151–163.

Poissant, L., Pereira, J., Tamblyn, R., *et al.* (2005). The impact of electronic health records on time efficiency of physicians and nurses: a systematic review. *J Am Med Inform Assoc* **12**: 505–516.

National Patient Safety Agency. Guidelines for hazard review of ePrescribing systems. Available from http://www.connectingforhealth.nhs.uk/systemsandservices/eprescribing/hazard_framework.pdf.

Shojania, K.G. (2009). The effects of on-screen, point of care computer reminders on processes and outcomes of care. *Cochrane Database Syst Rev* **3**: CD001096.

Section 6

Patient experience

The NHS was established to provide healthcare free for all at the point of delivery. Over time, it became apparent that there were wide variations provision and access, with very little emphasis on what patients and the public needed or wanted. Modern NHS Policy is focused on placing the patient right at the heart of healthcare provision (*Patient and public involvement*), with patients having opportunities to determine how, where, and by whom their care is delivered. This section sets out the fundamentals of patient and public involvement, illustrating how healthcare is evolving in a way that takes account of what patients want, giving them a voice in determining how it is delivered. To do this, patients and the public need to be consulted about new developments, as well as being involved in specific projects that are likely to impact on the way they use and receive healthcare (*Patient consultation*). Moreover patients are invited to comment on the care received through national surveys, the outcomes of which are used to inform regulators. More recently, the concept of patient reported outcome measures (PROMs) have been introduced to ensure providers understand, and measure, outcomes from the patient perspective (*Patient feedback*). Increasingly, healthcare providers are required to produce appropriate patient information in a range of media to ensure users are informed about services and treatments (*Patient information*), and also to provide support for patients who wish to raise concerns through the *Patient Advice and Liaison Service* (PALS). Innovative approaches to care delivery have included giving patients the opportunity to become expert patients who self-manage their condition, but have access to specialized advice if required (*The Expert Patient*).

Chapter 35

Patient and public involvement (PPI)

Rachel Matthews

Key points

- Patient and public involvement increases the accountability of the NHS to the tax-payer.
- Patient and public involvement requires different approaches depending on the purpose of the activity.
- The experience of patients is a key feature of quality improvement in health care delivery.
- Patient and public involvement can support service improvement and the concept of co-design which draws from patient and staff experience is being adopted in health care settings.
- Section 242 of the NHS Act 2006 requires health services to make arrangements to involve those who use services and the Darzi Review (2008) reinforces this as part of the new national quality framework.

PPI in the NHS

The inquiry into the deaths of children following heart surgery at Bristol Royal Infirmary remains a watershed in shaping public attitudes towards health care professionals. This investigation, together with events at Alder Hey Children's Hospital in Liverpool and the serious crimes perpetrated by Dr Harold Shipman revealed practices, procedures, and behaviours that challenged many peoples' assumptions about what happens in health care settings.

The NHS is based on a set of values, beliefs, and attitudes and what people expect today from health care is very different from what was expected in 1948. Patterns of illness and disease have shifted. People expect to live longer and are anxious about their health and quality of life in later years. Diagnosis, treatment, and care are more complex and reflect developments in science and technology.

The concept of 'user involvement' is not new in public services but the desire to give patients and the public an opportunity to be involved in decision-making about their health and health services is relatively recent and has greater prominence following the review by Lord Darzi, 'High Quality Care For All' which;

• reiterates the need to put patients firmly at the centre of health care, and

• introduces quality measures based on patient experience, safety, and outcome.

These will ensure that patients have a key role to play in determining

• how and where they receive health care, and

• the standards of care they expect to receive.

Why involve patients and the public?

The NHS is funded through public taxation and the public has a right to know how the resources are being used. Collectively and individually, health care professionals are accountable to patients. Most professionals would be unhappy if a decision about their health, treatment, or care did not take into consideration their personal views and this expectation should influence the way they provide care. Fundamental to PPI is the belief that patients, carers, relatives, and the public can offer views and opinions about health care. Not everybody wishes to articulate their experiences but opportunities to do so should be created for those who choose to articulate.

The consequences of not involving patients and the public is the risk of creating and developing services that reflect only the needs and aspirations of those employed to work in them. The part that public opinion can play in commissioning health care and social services is recognized and this is unlikely to diminish in the future. There are powerful emotional reasons for PPI and these should be supported with convincing cases for measurable quality improvement so that patients and the public benefit.

Patient and public involvement or engagement?

Consensus is not always there about the terms used in relation to PPI or what is meant by them. A useful and succinct description of PPI is offered by Kelson:

> Patient involvement encompasses both individual involvement (for example, the central role of patients in decisions about their own health and care) and involvement at a more collective level (patient representatives, for example, actively contributing to NHS policy and planning decisions).

Definitions have developed in recent years and the concept of 'engagement' has reached greater prominence. The Picker Institute Europe and the Care Quality Commission use the term patient and public engagement (PPE) more frequently. It is hard to involve a person or people in decisions if you have not understood what interests and motivates them. Connecting with them to identify this in a way that appeals to them is to engage them. It is not a one-off activity and effective engagement is likely to lead to long-term involvement. Health care professionals and providers need to articulate what they actually do so that patients, carers, and the public can make an informed decision about the role they can play to influence services.

To help people be meaningfully involved in decisions about health, it is important to understand their perspective. For example, to understand what patients expect from an anticoagulation service, it is necessary to approach those with direct experience of anticoagulation. A patient taking warfarin is more likely to help because ultimately any anticoagulation service change will have an impact on such a patient.

Engagement then is a term that reflects the approach that health professionals need to take in order to achieve involvement. Engagement is about recognizing that the person who receives care or uses services may hold a different view or opinion which can inform professional practice. It demonstrates a desire to see things from the patients' point of view and to communicate the purpose of treatment and care in a way that the person who receives care or uses the service can understand. Involvement is about creating opportunities for individuals and groups to participate in decision-making to achieve a specific goal.

Recent legislation and policy

The NHS Plan 2000 set the scene for radical reform of health services and included pledges about

- the availability of information,
- patient choice,
- cancelled operations, and
- regulation of professional standards.

The NHS Health and Social Care Act 2001 was a key influence in the development of PPI in the NHS. Under Section 11 of this act, it placed a legal duty on strategic health authorities and NHS Trusts to involve and consult with patients and the public. New structures were introduced following this act including

- Independent Complaints Advocacy Service (ICAS),
- Overview and Scrutiny Committees (OSC),
- Patient Advice and Liaison Services (PALS), and
- PPI Forums.

The influence of equality and diversity legislation, including the development of single equality schemes is intended to place greater emphasis on listening to those people whose voices have not always been heard including those from black minority ethnic, refugee, and disabled communities.

The challenge encountered by all those involved with PPI is that there has been little stability to allow practice to develop.

- Section 242 of the NHS Act 2006 has superseded Section 11 of the Health and Social Care Act 2001.
- The local Government and Public Involvement in Health Bill was passed in 2007 and from April 2008, the Commission for Patient and Public Involvement in Health (CPPIH) together with PPI Forums were abolished to be replaced by Local Involvement Networks (LINks).

- LINks are intended to provide a voice for the public in health and social care and take a broader approach to engagement and involvement.
- The National Centre for Involvement (NCI), a consortium made up of the University of Warwick, the Centre for Public Scrutiny, and National Voices funded by the Department of Health closed in August 2009 on the completion of its contract.

Getting started

Any PPI activity should have a clear purpose or aim. Initially, this may be about developing process but eventually should have a greater emphasis on achieving a positive impact on the experience of patients and the public. Outcome measures for PPI can be difficult to establish so it is important to start with clear goals. There are a variety of ways to involve people as individuals or collectively. Figure 35.1 summarizes these and the potential for different outcomes depending on the approach taken.

Who to involve?

Who to involve will be determined by what is to be achieved. Health care organizations must identify all those who will be affected by what is planned and proposed.

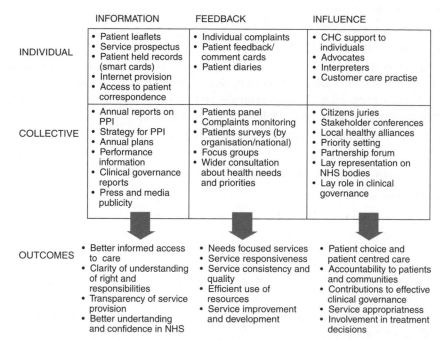

Fig. 35.1 Main dimensions of public and patient involvement – linking initiatives to key dimensions.
Figure reproduced from "Signposts – A practical guide to patient and public involvement in Wales" (2001) with kind permission from the Office for Public Management (OPM) and the Welsh Assembly Government (WAG).

This is called a stakeholder analysis. For this analysis minimum attention to the following questions is vital:

+ Who is likely to be affected by the proposal?
+ Which individuals or groups have an investment (of time, money, resources, and interest) in what happens now?
+ Who is likely to be excluded if they are not kept informed about proposals?
+ Who has influence and authority to act on the experience and opinion of patients and carers to achieve change and improvement?

Box 1 Patient panels

Panels started as an idea to recruit to a central 'pool' of people. Patients, especially those with long-term conditions, associate themselves with specific wards, departments, and clinicians. Recruitment through posters and leaflets often has limited results.

By utilizing staff PPI Champions, nurse consultants, and clinical nurse specialists, personal invitations may be extended to patients and carers to join a panel. This is likely to achieve greater success. Registration to a panel demands no formal time commitment and allows patients to decide how much or little they wish to be involved.

Depending on the distance from their health care provider patients can be contacted by telephone, email, and post. By developing a panel, contacts are ready to be approached for a specific activity or event. Panel membership can be complemented by contacts made through PALS, complaints procedures, and patient-support groups.

How to involve?

It is important to identify opportunities for involvement and to select the appropriate tools and methods to use some of which were outlined in Figure 35.1.

+ Quantitative methods such as surveys can provide valuable, collective, snapshots of patient opinion but need to be carefully designed and administered to achieve meaningful results.
+ Qualitative methods including focus groups and interviews can provide rich data about values, attitudes, and beliefs.
+ A combination of approaches is likely to give the most comprehensive picture of what people think.
+ The Experience Based Design (EBD) approach developed by the NHS Institute for Innovation and Improvement provides a comprehensive toolkit to support patients and staff who want to collaborate to achieve safety, quality, and service improvement.

Any decision about the approach should take into account those who want to be involved. Not everybody will want to complete a survey, some people prefer to work in small groups, and others are intimidated by formal meetings.

Box 2 PPI core groups

A tertiary centre has a PPI core group that consists of staff, patients, and carer representatives. Initially members were frustrated that there was no clear role or purpose and no achievements to publicize. By working together to understand what motivated them to keep meeting four times a year anxieties were confronted and terms of reference were agreed upon.

This group met with the estates and facilities team to learn more about projects that are taking place in the trust and to share their experiences about the hospital facilities and environment. At the end of this one-day event, the estates and facilities director was able to adjust some priorities in the department and focus on work that is likely to have an immediate impact on the experience of patients, for example, improving external signage and upgrading key reception areas. The PPI core group members can see how their views influence decision-making. The estates and facilities team hear at first hand the experiences of those at the receiving end of their project implementation.

When should people be involved?

It is perhaps easier to say when it is not appropriate to involve patients and the public. The National Consumer Council (2008) identifies nine principles of deliberative public engagement (Table 35.1).They refer to a specific approach but these principles form a firm foundation for other types of involvement. If it is likely that there will be difficulties in adhering to them, further preparation and planning is required. If decisions are already taken and there is no prospect of changing them, it is inappropriate to seek views.

Table 35.1 Effective deliberative public engagement: nine principles

The process makes a difference
The process is transparent
The process has integrity
The process is tailored to circumstances
The process involves the right number and types of people
The process treats participants with respect
The process gives priority to participants' discussions
The process is reviewed and evaluated to improve practice
Participants are kept informed

How to measure success?

In the early stages of developing PPI, it is easier to focus on successes with process rather than outcome. It is also important to identify what success means and from whose perspective it is sought. Participants may say that an activity has been successful because they feel as though their voice has been heard but the activity in itself may not have sufficient impact to influence existing practice. The baseline assessment of PPI in England conducted in 2007, and repeated in 2008 and 2009 by the NCI recognized these difficulties.

One of the recommendations is to *'develop clear and practical metrics to measure the impact of involvement activities in a repeatable and comparable way and allow easier evaluation of activities by Trusts and regulatory bodies'*. Until this happens, all PPI activity should at least have agreed aims and objectives against which local success can be measured.

PPI and patient safety

The involvement of patients is a growing debate in relation to patient safety. This area is under-researched and the role of patients in improving safety had been largely ignored until recently. Individuals can play a role in promoting safety and Vincent and Coulter suggest that patients can do this by:

+ Helping to reach an accurate diagnosis,

+ Deciding on appropriate treatment or management strategy,

+ Choosing a suitably experienced and safe provider,

+ Ensuring that treatment is appropriately administered, monitored, and adhered to, and

+ Identifying side effects or adverse events quickly and taking appropriate action.

But do patients want to be involved in promoting safety? Different parties approach patient involvement from different perspectives. Entwistle (author to provide ref) argues that we must draw the distinction between *'relying on* patients to check on the delivery of their health care to ensure their safety and *involving* patients in their care while efforts are made to improve their safety'". Lyons comes from the perspective of safety engineering and describes the pros and cons of involving patients. She argues that patients are *'unlikely to provide a consistent and reliable contribution to the safety process of their own care'*. She concludes that it would be wrong to burden patients with this responsibility but *'increased reliability and transparency would surely foster greater trust and confidence in healthcare professionals'*.

Patients want greater transparency especially in relation to safety incidents but there is little if any evidence to measure the impact of direct patient reporting to safety incident monitoring systems.

Summary

Health care which does not include the perspective of patients and the public is unlikely to sustain their trust and commitment. Perceptive practitioners recognize that they can learn from their patients and be richer in their practice because of this. Emotional arguments for PPI are of limited long-term value unless they can be supported by robust evaluation which influences the development of practice and leads to improved experiences for patients and carers. Patient safety is a key issue in the health care agenda and patients can play a part in reducing risk and promoting safety but this should not diminish the accountability exercised by those with professional training and responsibilities.

Further reading

Bate, P., Robert, G. (2008). *Bringing user experience to health care improvement.* The concepts, methods and practices of experience-based design. Radcliffe: Oxford.

Green, S. (2007). *Involving people in healthcare policy and practice.* Radcliffe: Oxford.

National Consumer Council (2008). *Deliberative public engagement: nine principles.* http://collections.europarchive.org/tna/20080804145057/http://www.ncc.org.uk/nccpdf/poldocs/NCC208_nine_principles_engagement.pdf accessed 14/11/09

Vincent, C., Coulter, A. (2002). Patient Safety: what about the patient? *Quality and Safety in Health Care,* 11, p 76–80.

Chapter 36

Patient Advice and Liaison Service

Eve Cartwright

Key points

- Patient Advice and Liaison Services (PALS) were introduced as part of a government plan to make health care services more accountable to patients.
- PALS is a confidential service with a remit to ensure patients can raise concerns and have them resolved promptly with a minimum of bureaucracy.
- Information obtained through PALS can identify risk and safety issues which need to be addressed as part of effective risk management and clinical governance.
- Key themes raised with PALS include poor communication, appointment delays and cancellations as well as concerns about privacy and dignity, and hospital facilities.

Introduction

The Patient Advice and Liaison Service (PALS) was introduced into hospitals as a result of the government's ten-year plan for the NHS, '*NHS Plan: a plan for investment, a plan for reform*' (2001).

This document sets out in Section 17–19 that:

- When patients are concerned that the NHS is not achieving the desired outcome for them they should have a route for raising their concerns and having them addressed.
- Patients should have an identifiable and easily accessible person to whom they can turn for advice and support if they encounter problems while using NHS services.
- This person or service should be impartial and objective.
- PALS will support/enable patients to make formal complaints.
- PALS will work with organizations in the community to ensure additional support.
- Solutions to problems identified and issues raised should be found informally if possible.

This became enshrined in law in the NHS Act 2002 and PALS was introduced into all hospitals to provide a channel through which patients could easily raise their concerns and have them resolved locally. The core functions of PALS as defined by the DH are to:

◆ Be identifiable and accessible to patients, their carers, families, and friends.

◆ Provide on the spot help with power to negotiate immediate and speedy resolution of problems.

◆ Act as a gateway to appropriate independent advice and advocacy support from national sources.

◆ Provide access to accurate information about the Trust and other health-related issues.

◆ Act as a catalyst for change and improvement by providing the Trust with feedback on problems and gaps in services.

◆ Operate within a local network with other PALS in their area and work across boundaries.

◆ Support staff at all levels within the Trust to develop a responsive culture.

In April 2009 changes were made to the way complaints are to be handled giving more emphasis to personal contact. Previously, if a complainant was not satisfied with the response to a formal complaint they had recourse to Independent Review via the Healthcare Commission. This stage has been replaced by more face-to-face work between the complainant and the Trust to resolve the issue and, if that fails, direct referral to the Parliamentary and Health Service Ombudsman. The purpose of the Ombudsman's office is to provide a service to the public by undertaking independent investigations into complaints where the NHS has 'not acted properly or fairly or have provided a poor service'.

How PALS works with those who raise concerns

◆ Details of concerns are recorded along with contact details of the complainant.

◆ The concern may initially be framed in the form of a complaint (formal); PALS staff members establish whether the patient wishes to use the complaints procedure or whether they would prefer PALS to try to solve the problem informally.

◆ PALS staff establishes an agreed course of action. Verbal consent is obtained from the complainant to contact relevant staff in an attempt to solve the problem. Issues of consent, confidentiality, and recording are explained and documented.

◆ PALS make contact with the relevant staff and assess whether they should deal with the problem directly with the complainant. PALS may need to remain closely involved until they can see that a solution has been found and should undertake a follow-up contact with the patient and/or staff member, to ensure resolution.

◆ If the issue cannot be resolved PALS may liaise with an appropriate senior member of staff.

◆ Where appropriate the PALS staff should check whether the patient is happy with the outcome or whether the patient wishes the matter to be dealt with through the formal complaints procedure.

- If the issue remains unresolved the service user can be offered a number of options:
  - Referral/self-referral to the Complaints Department
  - Referral to an advocacy service
  - Referral to the Independent Complaints Advocacy Service

All information should be documented for future reference.

Although PALS is not truly independent (PALS teams are usually employed by Trusts) there is expectation that they are impartial. PALS staff must consider all aspects of a particular concern and remain objective. PALS staff members require particular skills to enable them to work effectively, e.g. diplomacy, tact, and ability to analyse problems. PALS was not set up to reduce the number of formal (or written) complaints but this has been the effect on occasions. Use of PALS has almost doubled between 2005/6 and 2008/9 and complaints have decreased by more than a quarter.

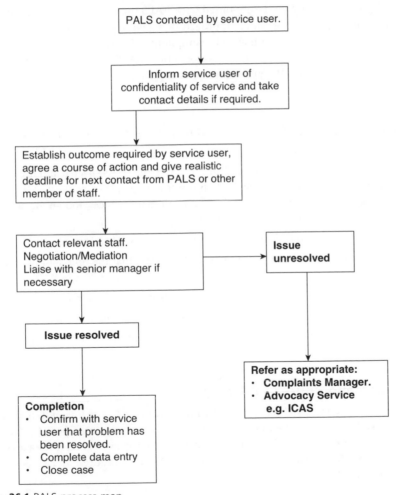

Fig. 36.1 PALS process map.

Feedback from PALS users is almost 100% positive whereas feedback from those who are surveyed about their experience of making formal complaints are largely negative. Reasons for this include:

- PALS is a personal service where patients can discuss their concerns informally and are not expected to write letters.
- Patients have an individual to liaise with.
- If PALS has not resolved the problem to their satisfaction, patients can formalize their complaints with assistance from PALS.

As from April 2009 PALS issues not resolved within 24 hours may be *recorded* as a formal complaint.

As a result of this relationship with patients PALS is better able to understand the patient experience, deal with the bigger picture, and recognize areas where previously unidentified risks to patients may exist. This information can be fed into the Trust clinical governance system. Issues raised with PALS must be viewed as part of the overall 'learning from experience' approach being widely promulgated across the NHS. Trusts must ensure that incidents, complaints, claims, and PALS information are analysed together to identify key areas for action. PALS consider risks not only to patients' health but also the potential risk to reputation of individual health care professionals and the Trust.

PALS within an NHS Trust – structure and organization

Managerially PALS may be positioned anywhere in a trust but usually sits within the governance directorate. The independence of PALS must be respected and the service encouraged to working autonomously but with any support requested. It is not uncommon for PALS to run bereavement and voluntary services, too, in the hospital. This can be beneficial in a number of ways:

- Volunteers can act to make patients more aware of the PALS service.
- Patients may be more at ease with non-staff and feel that the non-staff have more time to listen.
- Volunteers give feedback to the PALS service on areas of concern for patients.
- The skills of the PALS staff are also suited to bereavement management.
- PALS staff can take up sensitive issues on behalf of bereaved families at a time when the families feel unable to raise their concerns.

Location and hours of opening

PALS offices are ideally situated near the main entrance to the hospital in an area highly visible and accessible to patients. During office hours a member of the PALS team will be available and out-of-hours patients can leave voicemail messages on a dedicated line. Most Trusts also have a dedicated PALS email address and a link via the hospital's website.

Leaflets and information

PALS is responsible for providing to patients leaflets produced both internally, e.g. on how to make a complaint and from external organizations, e.g. Independent Complaints Advocacy Service (ICAS).

Links with other organizations

In order to help service users, it is important that PALS is resourceful and able to link people to relevant organizations which may be able to help. This includes:

- Local and national voluntary organizations,
- Social services,
- Cultural and faith groups, and
- Condition specific self-help groups.

Contribution to committees

PALS is in a good position to provide the patient's perspective on a range of issues. PALS may be represented in a number of groups and committees including:

- Complaints Groups,
- Bereavement Group,
- Clinical Practice Committee,
- Patient and Public Involvement (PPI) Champions, and
- Multi-Disciplinary Teams especially for chronic condition, e.g. heart failure, diabetes, and palliative care.

The importance of engendering confidence in hospitals: What makes a difference to patients and why

All patients need confidence in their hospital and all staff involved in their care management. Those who use the hospital, including relatives, visitors, and carers have expectations that they will be treated courteously, will understand what treatment they will receive, how it will be delivered, and why it is necessary. Patients are most likely to complain or raise concerns when their expectations are not met. The most common theme in PALS contacts with patients relates to poor communication.

Communication

Failures of appropriate communication can be the result of a range of factors involving the interaction between staff and patients, families and carers. These include:

- *Lack of Clarity*: The problem of a patient being told one thing and hearing another. Without understanding what is being said, a patient has no basis on which to form a decision about treatment. This is particularly pertinent when seeking 'informed consent' when it is vital to ascertain that a patient has understood the potential

Box 1 Lack of clarity

A patient being treated for heart disease was told, on being discharged, that if there were 'any problems' to return to the hospital. He collapsed at home several days later; so the family returned, as per perceived instructions, to the hospital, the patient sitting in the back of the car. The hospital reception was staffed at night by a security guard who had no experience of dealing with emergencies. When he called the surgical ward nurses they told the family to go to A&E elsewhere but eventually agreed to admit the patient. The patient died the following day. There is no evidence that the patient would have survived had he gone directly to A&E but the family felt that precious time was lost as a result of the miscommunication.

risks, intended benefits, alternatives, and effects of no treatment. Complex information is often delivered rapidly using unfamiliar jargon. Anxious patients find it difficult to retain information and supplementary leaflets can be helpful. There is also a need to be aware that what is commonplace to health care professionals may not be so to the patients. An example is shown in Box 1.

Patients also have a responsibility to be clear when answering questions or giving details of their medical history. The task of health care staff is to help the patient relate their story accurately and PALS can assist with this, acting as an advocate for the patient by giving them time to prepare for a consultation or review information delivered afterwards. Staff can misread what patients want or expect and, therefore, need to explore and understand patients' expectations using this as the focus of any communication. Discharge is a frequent source of problems due to communication failures. Patients are told they may go home the next day but although no specific time is given the patients frequently expect that they may leave after breakfast. There are perceived delays waiting for final blood tests or medications which may result in discharge not taking place until the afternoon.

◆ *Behaviour*: On occasion staff may misunderstand a patient because of their behaviour. While allowances are made for patients and relatives being anxious because of concerns about the patient's health staff may not be aware of other circumstances which may contribute to what may be considered unacceptable behaviour. Patients can be easily considered as 'difficult' due to mental health problems, learning difficulties, or just because they ask lots of questions. Staff need to find ways to manage so-called 'difficult patients' in a manner which keeps communication open, allows treatment to continue, is helpful to the patient, and does not put the members of staff in an intolerable position. PALS can help by getting to know the patient better and ensuring that health care staff members appreciate the patient's perspective. Patients may be reassured by having 'an outside person,' i.e. PALS available while they are in-patients.

◆ *Staff attitudes*: Experience indicates that there appears to be little correlation between a compassionate manner and a doctor's ability. From the patient's perspective being dealt with brusquely may be a reason to find fault and is sometimes interpreted as lacking in thoroughness. PALS experience shows that patients are forgiving of health care professionals if they feel included in discussions and clear explanations are given in a timely manner. Patients will overlook their appointments being delayed, their notes being lost, and their operations being cancelled if they have received an explanation and have been treated compassionately.

• *Honesty and casual remarks*: It may appear that patients expect doctors to provide answers to everything. In the experience of PALS, patients appreciate an honest answer and recognize that doctors do not always know the reason why something has happened. When a patient is told something which they subsequently find to be untrue they may question everything else they are told and the patient's doubt may extend to the whole health care experience. The importance of being open when things have not gone as planned should not be underestimated, with a clear and honest explanation of what has happened being provided. Patients are usually more interested in finding out what is being done to prevent the same thing happening to someone else than in seeking legal or disciplinary action. There is evidence that an apology and open disclosure will in fact reduce the likelihood of patients taking further action. An example is shown in Box 2.

• *Conflicting information*: If patients hear one proposed course of action from one professional which appears to be contradicted by another, then this causes confusion and anxiety. Patients are more inclined to believe the doctor in whom they have most confidence. It is very hard for a patient to hear what they perceive to be conflicting approaches to a medical problem and it gives them the impression that members of the health care team are making decisions in isolation. This poses the problem of how much information to give a patient. Should they be aware of discussions of various options or is this likely to cause further concern? They do need to know the options but the information needs to be delivered consistently, preferably by one designated person. It is important to explain to patients that a multidisciplinary team will be caring for them and this team will discuss various options for treatment and make a recommendation to the patient on which one seems

Box 2 Honesty

Regular check-ups showed that a patient who had had surgery ten years ago was doing well. However he was contacted two weeks later and told there was a shadow on his chest x-ray. Further investigation and an operation revealed that the tumour was inoperable. Three previous x-rays over an eighteen-month period had indicated the presence of cancer but no action was taken. The patient was told he had a life expectancy of 12 to 14 months. He was being treated at another hospital but felt that the dreadful situation was made worse by poor communication between the two hospitals. PALS was involved with the family and offered support in terms of organizing and sitting in on meetings together with assistance in making a formal complaint. At the meeting the trust acknowledged that it had failed to identify the cancer growth at an early stage and the family appreciated the straightforward way that the meeting was handled. They had expected to be dealing with people trying to avoid the truth.

most appropriate. It is vital to ensure that the patient is made to feel that they are involved in the decision and that they will be kept informed.

Staff can also receive conflicting information from various family members. Staff members must be aware of the rules on confidentiality and ensure that information is only released with the patient's permission. Where the patient lacks capacity then an individual with responsibility for the patient and his/her affairs should be identified. An area where problems often arise is in relation to 'do not resuscitate' decisions which should primarily be discussed with the patient although many family members often do not wish this to be the case. Clinical teams have to manage this situation but must remember that the primary duty of care is to the patient and where possible they should be asked if they wish their family to be involved in the discussion or informed of the outcome.

- *Making judgements*: Staff members are frequently ill-prepared for the behaviour of patients. Patients have a right to be treated compassionately and fairly and staff members have an obligation to provide care, taking the patient's views and beliefs into account and ensuring that they are not judged by their behaviour or attitudes. Any information recorded in the clinical notes about patients must be impartial and objective and no statements made which could be misinterpreted. It is wise to anticipate that anything written down could be read out in a court of law.

When treating patients who may have made a complaint, care must be taken so that there is no perception that the complainant is being discriminated against. Indeed there should be no record in the patient's notes that they have made a complaint. Where events have taken place which may have led to the relationship between a patient and a member of staff being damaged, every effort should be made to resolve these and PALS can be instrumental in facilitating this.

Key points in ensuring effective communication with patients:
- Have I understood? Reflect back what they have told you.
- Has the patient/family understood?
- Are you speaking to the right person?
- If they are angry, ask what you can do to help.
- What outcome do they want?
- Be honest.

Conclusion

PALS was intended as a way of making health care more accessible for patients. It has succeeded in this but has also had the effect of making the management of complaints less time consuming for staff. That having been said, it does not mean that patients' concerns are taken less seriously. The experience of PALS should be used to learn how to work in ways that will not only benefit patients and staff but will also reduce risk.

Further reading

Parliamentary and health service ombudsman's principles of: good administration, good complaint handling, remedy. Published February 2009 http://www.ombudsman.org.uk/improving_services/principles/index.html.

Chapter 37

Patient and public consultation

Jilla Bond and Tom Magill

Key points

Patient and Public Involvement in the planning and delivery of services provides significant added value for patient and clinician alike, as follows:

- different perspectives on the same issue,
- diversity of input resulting in better decision-making,
- patient empowerment leading to better health and well-being,
- improved services through a patient-led NHS, and
- better outcomes and greater job satisfaction through positive feedback.

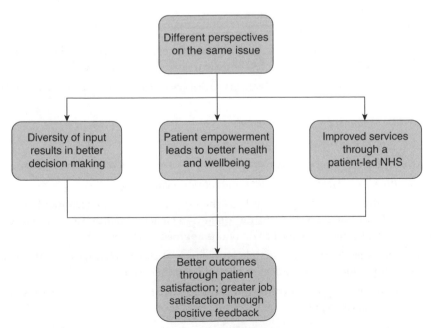

Fig. 37.1 Principles of patient and public involvement.

Introduction

NHS organizations are required to make arrangements to involve and consult patients and the public in:

◆ the planning of the provision of services,

◆ the development and consideration of proposals for changes in the way those services are provided, and

◆ decisions to be made by the NHS organization affecting the operation of services.

Patients have the right to participate in decision-making about their treatment as detailed in the NHS Constitution.

Different perspectives on the same issue

'Doctor knows best'....or does he?

◆ Does not the person receiving the treatment have an opinion on the effectiveness and success of the measures being taken on their behalf?

◆ What about also taking into account the accessibility and quality of the services and the observations of their family and carers?

It is upon these principles that Patient and Public Involvement is based.

The traditional view that doctors and nurses should never be challenged in their decisions has been slowly put into logical perspective. Of course clinicians are the experts in diagnosis and treatment but by encouraging input from the patient, clinician and patient become a team and, together, they enhance the healing process and experience for the benefit of all as:

◆ The doctor has the clinical expertise, and

◆ Patients know their own bodies and circumstances so their opinion about what is happening is critical to the success of their treatment and overall well-being.

Vincent and Coulter state that '*Patients have a key role to play in reaching an accurate diagnosis,*

◆ *deciding about appropriate treatment,*

◆ *choosing an experienced and safe provider,*

◆ *ensuring that treatment is appropriately administered, monitored and adhered to,*

◆ *identifying adverse events and taking appropriate action*'.

Shared decision-making strengthens the effectiveness of the treatment and is now enshrined in the NHS Constitution and in General Medical Council (GMC) Guidelines. Illustrations of the benefit of this approach include:

◆ an elderly gentleman with multiple problems who chose to have his incontinence as the top priority for treatment so he could continue fishing,

◆ a Muslim whose greatest concern was the osteoarthritis in his knees because he could not kneel to pray.

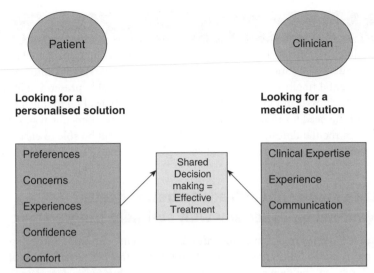

Fig. 37.2 Different perspectives in the clinician–patient partnership.

The involvement of the patient in prioritizing their treatment is critical to their overall well-being and the doctor making the right decision.

In addition, visitors to clinical environments notice things that those involved with the patient's clinical treatment may miss, such as:

◆ shortfalls in care: people not being fed, lack of respect,

◆ cleanliness issues and environmental changes that can be made, and

◆ access issues and creature comforts which can be improved.

All of these observations will greatly enhance the patient experience and well-being.

It is important to recognize the added value public involvement brings rather than treat it as a 'tick-box' exercise.

Diversity of input results in better decision-making

In the same way that family history and social circumstances are often taken into consideration when diagnosing the cause of a patient's ill health, lay opinions can contribute to better clinical results. When clinicians are busy in clinics or on the wards, it is easy to overlook the humanitarian view that is so vital. A successful medical procedure can be adversely affected by financial worries or visitors being unable to attend because of inadequate or costly parking or difficult travel. Including the public in the planning process allows this perspective to be addressed at the beginning. Involvement, however, needs to reflect the diversity of the local community and the users of the services. Older peoples' needs will differ from the needs of the young. Customs and attitudes will vary according to culture, religion, or gender.

Box 1 Patient involvement

Practicalities may dictate that people in crisis from mental ill health should present at an Accident and Emergency Department. Reality suggests that someone in a state of mental fragility or crisis will never feel comfortable presenting into the hurly burly of A&E and may therefore not present at all, leading to much greater crisis and the need for more extensive and expensive care. Someone who has suffered from mental illness, or a close friend or relative will be able to ensure that factors such as this are not overlooked when planning changes to such services.

Patient empowerment leads to better health and well-being; especially with self-help programmes

The Expert Patient Programme illustrates this well. Through this approach patients with long-term conditions are empowered to take control of their own case management, thereby taking ownership of their treatment. Those who complete the programme are encouraged to share their experience with others in similar situations, and even to train as a course tutor to deliver future courses. Extending this concept of patient involvement to the observations made by families, carers, and the general public will allow the medical profession to be better equipped to deliver the best and most appropriate services to their 'clients'.

Improved services through a Patient-led NHS; involving people in planning

Patient and Public Involvement and Engagement are fundamental to the concept of World Class Commissioning. Ideally PPI will be embedded at every level of an organization; from meaningful participation at Board level to Committees and focus groups which are researching, planning, or delivering services.

Key issues to consider are:

- The benefits need to be clear to all within each organization.
- Volunteers should be respected for the time and commitment they give and be engaged in a meaningful way – their views and opinions must make a real difference.
- Allocating clear roles, responsibilities, and accountabilities.
- Identifying adequate resources, practical support, and learning opportunities.
- Out-of-pocket expenses to be refunded.
- Feedback to participants on the results of their involvement.

PPI brings a balance to the decision-making process. It acts as a reality check. It is recognized that patients will more readily and honestly give their views and express their concerns to people who are not medical staff, making surveys or feedback collected by volunteers more effective. No successful business would contemplate operating without understanding the requirements and needs of its clients and health care needs to take the same view. Satisfied, contented patients will lead to a successful institution and greater job satisfaction for staff.

An example of a step in the right direction is the Choose and Book system. It empowers patients at the start of their treatment by giving choice according to expertise and locality.

- This gives the patient the opportunity to choose the practitioner and location for the care they will receive.

- The patient can prioritize whether it is more important to be treated nearer home or in a hospital further away in which he may have more confidence.

- By giving the patient control over these matters the patients have greater peace of mind; creating a better foundation for treatment.

Better outcomes through patient satisfaction; greater job satisfaction though positive feedback

Healing is a team effort and it is only right that the patient and their family be allowed to play a key role in this process. The medical profession may have been inclined to shy away from consulting and involving patients but there is much to learn from patients, those close to them, and the casual observer.

People's observations count. Anyone who drives or walks down the same street every day will know that significant changes can be made and passed by many times before they are observed, such as a tree being felled or a house painted a different colour. The same applies to the health care environment. A casual observer can spot changes that could be made for the benefit of patients, which those working there no longer see such as:

- Fire extinguishers fixed proud of the wall in a specialist department for the visually impaired,

- A shabby fitting room where patients are expected to try on prostheses, the trauma of having to face life with an artificial appendage being exacerbated by a dispiriting environment,

- Piles of rubbish outside the window where patients might be seeking inspiration or solace from trees and peaceful gardens,

- Poor attitudes, sharp voices.

Box 2 Patient feedback

The benefit of listening to patients has been exemplified by a system introduced in a Dutch hospital where a month after discharge, patients are invited back to comment on their care Everyone from the ward, cleaners to the consultants, is required to attend and listen without comment, while the patients discuss their experiences, good and bad. At the end of the session, the ward team is given the opportunity to ask questions about the comments they have heard. When this system was first introduced the wards were reluctant to participate but quickly they realized the benefits and positive learning that could be derived from such an honest exchange.

Small changes can make a huge difference to the experience of the person undergoing treatment.

How to involve patients and the public

Once the value of involving patients and the public is recognized, consideration must be given to the practicalities, challenges, and processes required in ensuring that all involvement work is meaningful and interconnected. Involvement can vary. Individuals and groups can participate in:

◆ Service change planning,

◆ Clinical Boards, Committee working or focus groups,

◆ Promotional health campaigns,

◆ Collaborative groups consisting of local people, employers, voluntary groups, and communities, and

◆ Readers groups for checking information is clear and consultations can be understood.

The methods used to converse with target audiences will vary in relation to:

◆ how representative of the population they are, and

◆ the capacity of participants to become involved.

Varied approaches to involvement should not be seen as differing in importance, but rather different tools which can be employed depending on the requirements.

Learning from complaints

'There is nothing either good or bad, but thinking makes it so'.

Hamlet, Act 2, Scene 2, Shakespeare

Some of the best sources of information from the public will be ICAS (Independent Complaints Advocacy Services), PALS (Patient Advocacy and Liaison Service), and Complaints. Information gleaned from analysing ICAS and PALS reports can give a valuable insight to service shortcomings. Likewise complaints should be seen as an opportunity to learn and possibly implement significant improvements in service delivery. In most cases, the focus of people's complaints is to try to ensure that what happened is not repeated, so it is vital to engage with the complainant promptly, understand their viewpoint, and learn from the incident.

The plurality of participation

Figure 37.3 lists the different stances that can be taken towards involvement and the methods or approach that can be used, ranging from providing information to supporting independent groups of local people. These require varying resources and levels of support.

Stances in summary

Level/stance	Information	Consultation	Deciding together	Acting together	Supporting
Typical process	Presentation and promotion	Communication and feedback	Consensus building	Partnership building	Community development
Typical methods	Leaflets Media Video	Surveys Meetings	Workshops Planning for Real Strategic Choice	Partnership bodies	Advice Support Funding
Initiator stance	'Here's what we are going to do'	'Here's out options – what do you think?'	'We want to develop options and decide actions together'	'We want to carry out joint decisions together'	'We can help you achieve what you want within these guidelines'
Initiator benefits	Apparently least effort	Improve chances of getting it right	New ideas and commitment from others	Brings in additional resources	Develops capacity in the community and may reduce call on services
Issues for initiator	Will people accept bo consultation?	Are the options realistic? Are there others?	Do we have similar ways of deciding? Do we know and trust each other?	Where will the balance of control lie? Can we work together?	Will our aims be met as well as those of other interests?
Needed to start ...	Clear vision Identified audience Common language	Realistic options Ability to deal with responses	Readiness to accept new ideas and follow them through	Willingness to learn new ways of working	Commitment to continue support

Fig. 37.3 Wilcox's Stances for Participation.
Reproduced from Wilcox, D., *The Guide to Effective Participation*, (1994), with permission.

When planning involvement projects, consideration should be given to any past, ongoing, or future involvement work which could inform or complement the proposed project. Patient and Public Involvement Teams and Voluntary Organizations can provide a wealth of knowledge, not only of their own activities, but also the work of other local bodies (such as voluntary organizations, the local Council, and other service providers). Coordinating efforts to inform, consult, and involve the local population can improve desired outcomes and ensure that other local activities are complemented rather than duplicated.

In the following section we will be looking at each stance in detail.

Information

In all communications, be it Public Health information or proposals for changes to services, it is crucial to ensure:

◆ the use of plain English,

◆ that the information is clear, and

◆ the text is concise and appropriate.

Consideration must always be given to the appropriate form of communication for the target audience. Is the information available in the relevant languages, format, on audio or pod cast, in large type, speech to text, or sign language? Involving everyone – staff, patients, and the public – in the production of communications (including leaflets, newsletters, posters, Open Days, and local press) is vital (see Chapter 39). There are many new and exciting methods of communication which have come into play in the last decade. People's opinions can now be gathered via:

◆ the internet (blogs, straw polls, YouTube),

◆ SMS/Text messaging, and

◆ traditional 'pen and paper' methods of letters, posters, and surveys.

Box 3 Time given to getting to understand the communities being served will be particularly informative

Arranging to meet with local Community leaders will facilitate better understanding of cultural differences. In one community of Asian males over 50 who spoke little English, it was well known that there was a high prevalence of coronary disease and diabetes and it was discovered that these patients believed that they would be cured simply by taking the pills prescribed by the doctors at the clinic. They had not understood the importance of also changing their lifestyle by increasing exercise, stopping smoking, and modifying diet. Through the Community leader, a meeting was facilitated for the highly respected clinicians to communicate to the group the importance of a change of lifestyle. This led to better health outcomes and gave a human face to the medical profession, increased mutual respect, and allowed the clinicians a valuable insight into the culture of these patients which informed future consultations.

Consultations

Consultation is based on developing a number of options and then seeking feedback on the choices. Cynicism has crept in because this leads to the feeling that public involvement is invited after critical decisions have been made making it seem an academic exercise. Consultations often fail because:

- Communication and explanations on the services and options proposed is inadequate.
- The documents appear slanted towards one outcome.
- There is no feedback on outcomes.
- No changes are made as a result of the consultation.

Priority should be accorded to giving feedback about how the information was considered and changes that were made as a consequence, or why no material changes could be made.

This can be done by including an option for respondents to subscribe to regular updates and other opportunities to get involved. This may also provide a contact list for other involvement and engagement activities. Effective and comprehensive consultation requires a budget, extensive planning, and professional expertise.

Deciding together

The benefits of joint decision-making have been explored extensively in the first section of this chapter. Respect is vital when engaging volunteers and seeking opinions. It is also important to outline clearly:

- the objectives,
- the time and commitment involved, and
- the outcomes anticipated as a result of their involvement.

Acting together

Patient Participation Groups (PPGs) have been established in many GP practices to give patients a voice in the development of services offered and to ensure the patient perspective is taken into account in decision-making. Similar groups can be established, and attached to specific services – these can act as 'focus groups', which will be able to act as a sounding board for any changes to services. The appointment of a new Out-of-Hours services contract was halted when members of the public raised such astute questions; it was decided to recommend the procedure involving the LINk from the beginning.

Supporting independent community initiatives

Community groups flourish when they are allowed to make their own decisions independently and decide the direction of their work. The relationships which independent community initiatives have with their local statutory bodies require careful management and hard work but can be an excellent source of well-informed volunteers and constructive engagement. By working in partnership with Local Authorities, voluntary bodies, and community groups, these groups can be highly motivated and focused with a large capacity for involvement. Local Involvement Networks (LINks) were introduced in the Local Government and Public Involvement in the Health Act (2007) and have been established to ensure that local people have a direct say in the commissioning of their services as well as feeding back local opinion on how health and social care services are actually being received on the ground. These too offer an excellent source of well-informed, willing, interested parties with a valuable contribution to make.

Summary

In recognition of the benefits of engagement there is now an obligation for Statutory Bodies and Service Providers to prove that the views of the patients and public have been sought and to demonstrate what actions were taken as a result. Even if recommendations could not be accommodated, it is now necessary to evidence the procedures that were followed in giving genuine consideration to the proposals made. Those who have embraced patient and public involvement have recognized the immense benefits it brings to the planning and delivery of health services and have found it to be an enriching experience for clinicians and patients alike. Openness and generosity to the views of patients, their families, carers, and the interested public will add colour and richness to the career of any clinician.

Further reading

Vincent, C., Coulter, A. (2002). Patient Safety: what about the patient? *Quality and Safety in Health Care* **11**, 76–80.

The expert patient: a new approach to chronic disease management for the 21st century (2001) Department of Health, http://www.dh.gov.uk/en/Publicationsandstatistics/Publications/PublicationsPolicyAndGuidance/DH_4006801.

For further reading on Mirror Meetings, *see*: Jonkers–Schuitema (2002), *Do Patient Groups Help Caregivers to Improve Research and Clinical Practice?* Academic Medical Centre: Amsterdam.

Additional information on Wilcox's stances can be found on http://www.partnerships.org.uk/guide/guide1.pdf.

The Engagement Cycle introduced in April 2009 and developed by IN Health Associates for the Department of Health.

Chapter 38

User feedback/surveys

Alison Wright

Key points

- Effective Clinical Governance requires the NHS to take patient feedback into account when planning care delivery.
- Patient surveys are an invaluable source of information that trusts have at their disposal for aiding improvement in the quality of care.
- Patient experience surveys and Patient Reported Outcome Measures (PROMs) create an information base that allows people to compare the performance of health care providers as reported by other patients.
- Patient experience and PROMS will form part of the Quality Accounts for each Trust and will contribute to assessment of performance by Commissioners and the Care Quality Commission.
- Other sources of feedback such as PALS, and compliments and complaints, should be used collectively to identify trends and build up a strong case for service improvement.

Introduction

In his *NHS Next Stage Review Final Report* 2008, Lord Darzi stated that *'High quality care should be as safe and effective as possible, with patients treated with compassion, dignity and respect. As well as clinical quality and safety, quality means care that is personal to each individual'* and *'If quality is to be at the heart of everything we do, it must be understood from the perspective of patients'*. Effective clinical governance recognizes the importance of the quality of patient care, determining this, at least in part using feedback from patients themselves. There are many methods to gather and receive patient feedback such as PALS and complaints, but the most rigorous and systematic is through surveys of patient experience.

Patients as consumers

Patient feedback and the associated assessment of the performance of health care professionals, has increased in prominence in recent years. This is attributed partly to concerns around patient safety and the resultant efforts to improve performance, but increasingly to a more consumerist approach to patient care that has emerged. In its publication *'Great*

Expectations' (2007), the NHS Confederation puts forward the argument that, in an age of rising expectations among service users, the focus on patients as consumers is critical.

The authors of *'Patient Insight: Harnessing the Power of Public Opinion'* suggest that *'Services should be designed with input from users, using the "wisdom of crowds" and drawing on delivery-end experiences to inform providers about the usefulness of the services they provide'*. Traditionally NHS trusts have not been dependent on patients for their income, but in recent years two key initiatives have begun to change this, they are:

* the introduction of greater choice and competition, and
* more focus on the incentivization of high quality care.

As patients are becoming more informed and being given more choices, health care organizations are becoming aware that dissatisfied patients can take their custom elsewhere. The national 'tariff' system means that the money to pay for patient care and treatment goes with them. Now, more than ever, the importance of acknowledging patient feedback in informing change is crucial.

Evolution of patient surveys

The content of patient surveys has moved on since the days of measuring patient 'satisfaction'. Satisfaction ratings do not inform providers what is right or wrong with a particular service, and therefore do not help guide which aspects of a service should be maintained or improved. In addition, most NHS patients are highly appreciative of the care they receive and, as a result, rate their care positively. 'Satisfaction' measures are subjective and are dependent on:

* culture,
* geography,
* patient expectations, and
* patient mood.

Well-designed patient experience surveys minimize much of the subjectivity associated with satisfaction surveys, by asking patients to report on exactly what happened with regards to various aspects of their health care episode (*'Did the doctor tell you the purpose of any new medications?'*), rather than their *evaluation* of what had occurred (*'How satisfied are you with…'* or *'How would you rate…the information given to you by the doctor about the purpose of any new medications?'*).

The National Patient Survey Programme (NPSP)

Since 2002, all NHS trusts in England have been mandated to:

* survey a sample of their patients each year, and
* report these findings to the health care regulator (the current incumbent being the Care Quality Commission).

During this time, the NPSP has used postal surveys to gather feedback from patients across a variety of health care settings:

* inpatients
* outpatients

+ emergency care
+ primary care
+ mental health
+ maternity services
+ paediatric care

Capturing patient feedback in this way via a central authority and using a standardized approach:

+ ensures comparability between trusts,
+ feeds into performance reviews by the regulator, and
+ facilitates change for the better.

Patient priorities

Attending hospital as an outpatient or inpatient can be a daunting experience and it is now widely recognized that communication and interpersonal skills are highly regarded in the partnership between the patient and the health care professional. Patients now rightfully expect clinicians and other health care staff to

+ listen to their concerns,
+ involve them in decisions about their care and treatment,
+ keep them fully informed, and
+ give them due respect.

Professional standards and guidance increasingly allude to these skills as key characteristics in the clinician's repertoire. Indeed, there is a worldwide evidence base that shows that patients who are actively involved in decisions surrounding their own healthcare

+ gain greater knowledge and confidence in managing their conditions,
+ adhere better to courses of treatment,
+ are more likely to participate in preventive schemes,
+ are more likely to receive treatment which is appropriate to them personally,
+ (in some cases) use fewer health service resources, and
+ achieve better health outcomes.

The importance of patient feedback in shaping improvements

In 'Patient Insight: Harnessing the Power of Public Opinion', a review was undertaken of 12 NHS organizations, examining board papers and minutes covering a six month period. A number of key findings emerged (see Table 38.1).

A common barrier in successfully engaging clinicians in utilizing patient feedback is the *perceived* lack of localized patient feedback results that are available. An organization that embraces patient feedback and truly appreciates its value is aware that it is not a one-step process of change but an ongoing, cyclical process (see Figure 38.1).

Table 38.1 Organizations' use of patient experience information

Data collection	General high awareness of mandated annual surveys but little use of other data such as clinical quality. Scant use of other data sources such as PALs
Analysis	Some trusts presented regular patient experience information at board meetings; others reviewed results on an ad hoc basis only.
Discussion	In the main, patient experience does not feature highly on board agendas
Follow-up	While some organizations used a systemic approach to following up patient experience based information, other trusts merely noted patient experience information but no follow-up was made. Conversely, complaints data tends to be regularly reviewed and followed up.

Optimizing use of patient feedback

Making the data from the National Survey Programme public is aimed at encouraging health care providers to

- review areas of need,
- inform quality improvement, and
- direct resources appropriately to the areas most in need of improvement as identified by patients.

The national survey programme provides a picture of an organization's health enabling comparisons against other trusts and providing a catalyst for quality improvements. The information provided by these survey contractors and by the health care regulator gives trusts the following outputs:

- External benchmarking:
  - access to the national picture, seeing how a trust performs against the average of all other trusts,
  - comparison against other similar trusts (e.g. all other trusts in the same SHA, versus other trusts of foundation status, versus all other specialist trusts etc),
  - an accurate picture of a trust's strengths and weaknesses and what is achievable.

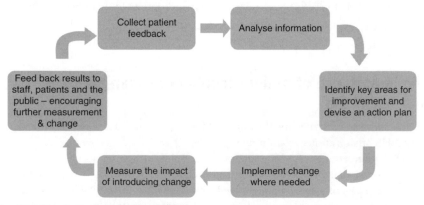

Fig. 38.1 The patient experience cycle.

- ◆ Internal benchmarking:
  - provides breakdowns of a trust's data by speciality, site, department etc,
  - facilitates sharing of good practice so that poorer performing teams can learn what constitutes a good patient experience,
  - helps engage staff in the improvement process since they can see how the results apply to them.
- ◆ Historical analysis:
  - allows trusts to see where improvements have been made when comparing performance against previous years, and
  - shows dips in performance.
- ◆ **Verbatim comments** – most patient surveys include a couple of questions at the end of the questionnaire, inviting patients to write free text comments in relation to the aspects of care they considered to be good and those aspects that could have been better. The information generated by these 'open' style questions is invaluable in supplementing the quantitative findings, as they
  - gives insight into why scores may be low on a certain measure (eg to explain why many patients state that their admission process was disorganised),
  - highlights any other areas of concern specific to that trust that are not covered elsewhere in the questionnaire – sometimes one comment can go far in clarifying why a service deficit may be apparent and what can be done to rectify the situation.

Formulating an action plan

A group needs to be formed consisting of staff (and ideally patients and the public) who have responsibility for disseminating the patient survey results and developing an action plan. The engagement of clinical staff and members of the Board is crucial; staff will be more supportive of change and view improvement initiatives as a positive step if they are involved throughout the process.

The group should:

- ◆ look at what other groups in the trust are doing already in terms of service improvements to compare data sources, combine resource and avoid duplicity of effort,
- ◆ prioritize actions – attempting to embark upon too many aspects at once will prove overwhelming,
- ◆ examine any aspects that are not so resource-hungry and could be improved using quick-fix solutions,
- ◆ set realistic targets and timelines and decide up front how 'success' will be measured.

Surveys outside of the National Programme

Any health care provider can undertake a survey of its patients at any time, without having to rely on the schedule of patient surveys as defined by the health care regulator. Many trusts implement ad hoc surveys to measure progress as a result of action planning, rather than waiting a year or more to re-evaluate success. However, the importance of good survey design must be recognized:

◆ as poor question design or a failure to test the questions rigorously may produce meaningless or misleading results, and

◆ localized questionnaires should employ a core set of tested and validated questions from within the national programme.

The majority of patient feedback programmes utilize quantitative methods since this is the approach needed to ensure that patient feedback is representative for an organization as a whole. However, sometimes, qualitative methods are used such as:

◆ focus groups,

◆ one-to-one in-depth interviews, and

◆ experience-based design.

These methods are used to explore ideas or experience in greater depth. The free-flowing conversational style of interviewing means that the content can be adapted to the individual patient depending on their own circumstances and experiences.

In late 2008, the Secretary of State for Health asserted that the patient must be '...*placed even closer to the centre of the NHS*'. His wish was for every hospital trust to engage in collecting immediate and ongoing feedback from patients in relation to their experiences of care. Many trusts are exploring ways to capture 'near real-time' or 'frequent' feedback using hand-held devices, kiosks, online surveys, SMS text messaging, or bedside TV surveys to collect information which can be quickly and regularly communicated back to staff and patients alike. The emphasis is on finding out what patients on particular wards or within different divisions have to say, with action planning tailored to these people, rather than a 'one size fits all' approach to quality improvement.

Patient Reported Outcome Measures (PROMs)

As of April 2009 the NHS became the first health system in the world routinely to collect Patient-Reported Outcome Measures (PROMs). Lord Darzi's 'Next Stage Review' emphasized the need for '...*understanding success rates from different treatments for different conditions. Assessing this will include clinical measures such as mortality or survival rates and measures of clinical improvement. Just as important is the effectiveness of care from the patient's own perspective which will be measured through patient-reported outcomes measures (PROMs) ...*'

As a result, NHS patients undergoing the following elective procedures will now be invited to complete a questionnaire:

◆ hip replacement

◆ knee replacement

◆ groin hernia surgery

◆ varicose vein surgery

Pre- and post-intervention, they will be asked about their health-related quality of life in terms of, e.g. mobility, psychological well-being, and pain to measure the effectiveness of the procedure.

The NHS Standard Contract now makes it a requirement that clinical quality performance reports include patient-reported outcome findings across these four areas. The inclusion of PROMs means that trusts and the NHS will be able to assess the treatments and interventions that are the most effective and gives the public detailed information on the performance of their local health care provider as reported by other patients.

Commissioning for Quality and Innovation (CQUIN)

Under this scheme in NHS England, the contracts between commissioners and health care providers will include conditions whereby a percentage of the final payment is withheld if the provider does not meet agreed standards on patient experience (see Chapter 42).

Patient feedback and measures of safety

Safety is at the core of quality in health care, the underlying principle being that patients should not be put at risk by the care they receive. To a large extent, the term 'patient safety' covers safety incidents, medical errors, and infections picked up while a patient is in the care system. Yet, it is just as important that patients are adequately told of the side effects of any new medications prescribed and told of any danger signals to watch for once they are discharged. Listening directly to patients who have experienced defects in their care or been subject to errors and mistakes can be a powerful tool for driving change. These 'patient stories' can be delivered in person to a clinical team or even a Trust board and can influence changes to services or systems which have failed and improve safety. Written stories which may be shaped as complaints or merely descriptive documents can also be included in performance or quality reports thus ensuring that the patient voice is heard at all levels within an organization. This approach can be extended to include families for instance in intensive care units so that staff can understand the perspectives and needs of those close to the patient.

There is some evidence to suggest that communicating effectively with patients and involving them in decisions can also go towards improving safety and as a consequence lead to a reduction in the number of complaints.

Summary

Patient experience must be addressed as part of the broader issue of clinical quality, with trust boards receiving regular feedback telling them about the experiences of patients under the care of their trust, and whether the experience of patients is improving. Patient experience surveys and effective use of the results will thus ensure that the patient experience is at the heart of quality.

Further reading

'Understanding what matters: a guide to using patient feedback to transform services' (2009). Department of Health.

'Using patient feedback' (2009). Picker Institute Europe. http://www.pickereurope.org/usingpatientfeedback.

Gerteis, M., Edgman-Levitan, S., Daley, J., Delbanco, T. L. (Editors) (1993). Through the Patient's Eyes: Understanding and promoting Patient Centred Care. San Francisco: Jossey-Bass Publishers. www.nhssurveys.org. A useful resource for those involved in the national surveys. Includes tools and resources to aid understanding of survey results.

Chapter 39

Patient choice

Ruth Robertson

Key points

- Giving patients a choice of elective care provider is part of a broader programme of system reform in the NHS.
- Patients should have been given the choice to be treated by any provider on a national list since April 2008.
- It is hoped patients' choices will lead to improvements in the quality of NHS service provision.
- Giving patients choice impacts on their experience of care, the GPs' process of referral and the organization of care within hospitals.
- Policies are developing which give patients more choice over *what* treatment they receive as well as *where* they receive it which has implications for the relationship between patients and clinicians.

Introduction

Patients in the NHS have always had some choice over how and where they receive treatment, but it is only recently that patient choices have been seen as a mechanism for improving the quality of NHS services. Since April 2008 NHS patients in England, referred by their GP for specialist care, have been able to choose to have elective treatment from any approved provider on a national list. This chapter provides the background on this policy and its impact to date, including:

- how patient choice and the broader programme of system reform was designed to work in theory,
- a brief policy history,
- how offering patients a choice has been implemented,
- the impact of patient choice on patients, GPs, and providers, and,
- other ways in which the government is seeking to empower patients and give them more control over their care.

Patient choice in theory

The theory behind the policy of giving patients a choice of provider is based on market principles outlined by Hirschman in his book *Exit, Choice and Loyalty*. He describes how when someone decides to 'exit' a poor service provider this sends a signal to that provider to either improve or leave the market. In health care, if patients choose to be treated by high quality providers, those performing less well should be motivated to improve to attract more business. For this quality improvement mechanism to work, four conditions must be met:

1. Patients must be given the opportunity to choose.
2. Information must be available to allow patients to select the provider that best meets their needs.
3. Alternative providers must exist from whom patients can choose.
4. Money must follow the patient.

The government has implemented policies to strengthen and extend patient choices as part of a broader programme of system reform. Figure 39.1 shows the four key elements of this programme which is intended to create a competitive market for NHS funded care. In addition to giving patients a choice of provider, the government has encouraged independent sector providers into the NHS market and NHS trusts to compete for patients' custom. A reimbursement system called payment by results (PBR) has been introduced, which pays providers per case treated with *'money following the patient'*. This means providers are financially penalized for losing patients, a change from the previous system of prospectively agreed block contracts. Independent regulation has been strengthened to ensure care provided meets agreed standards and provides value for money.

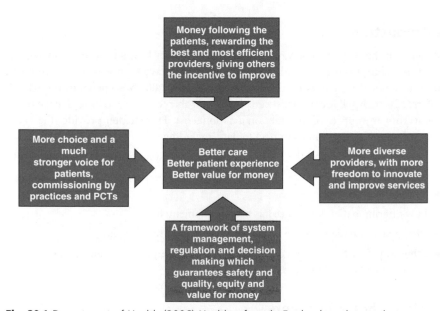

Fig. 39.1 Department of Health (2006) Health reform in England: update and commissioning framework.

Table 39.1 Patient choice policy: expected benefits and possible problems

Expected benefits	Possible problems
Improved efficiency of NHS provision	**Inefficient providers deteriorate further**
The PBR tariff is fixed per case treated to motivate hospitals to provide care below the tariff rate so they can retain any surplus to reinvest in patient care.	Poor performers may attract fewer patients and less money meaning the worst get worse as the good get better.
Improved quality of NHS provision and a more responsiveness service	**Quality of 'hotel services' and access improve only**
Hospitals will compete to provide a high quality service that attracts patients and the money that follows them. Hospitals will be motivated to improve their service in line with patients' preferences.	Lack of information and support mean choices may be based on areas on which information is easily available such as distance from home, waiting times, and available facilities.
Improved equity	**Reduced equity**
Some patients were able to 'work' the previous system and push for care from their hospital of choice or choose to pay privately. Requiring GPs to offer alternative providers to all should widen choice beyond this small assertive group.	Some may find it easier to exercise choice than others, meaning more educated or English speaking patients are able to access the best care while others are left with the poorer providers.
Better use of NHS capacity	**Difficulties for hospitals to meet waiting time targets**
The Choose and Book system lists options by waiting time allowing patients to easily choose the first available appointment.	Hospitals that attract a high number of patients may have difficulties meeting waiting time targets. They cannot reject referrals unless clinically inappropriate.
Empowered patients, improved convenience	**Implementation is critical**
Patients get more control over their care and are able to book appointments online at home or over the telephone.	Patients may not be offered a choice by their GP and buy in from GPs is critical to the policy's success.

The expected benefits as well as possible problems of giving patients a choice of provider are outlined in Table 39.1.

Policy history

The White Paper *Working for Patients* first included the aim of giving patients more choice over the services they received as part of its internal market reforms. In reality this programme actually gave more choice to GPs rather than patients. GPs could apply to become fund holders and hold a budget for parts of their patients' care. This gave them control over where to send patients for hospital care. The policy was designed to

♦ promote competition between hospitals trying to attract referrals, and

♦ allow GPs to negotiate higher standards with providers.

From 1997 the government moved away from the idea of using choice and competition to drive quality improvements within the NHS. However, this began to change and in 2002 when *Delivering the NHS Plan* announced a series of patient-choice pilots for patients who had been waiting at least six months for treatment. Selected patients were given the option of faster treatment from an alternative provider either within the NHS, independent sector, or in some cases overseas providers. Patients' choices at this time were intended to

* help make efficient use of capacity within the NHS, and

* decrease waiting times (a big concern at that time)

In 2004 the *NHS Improvement Plan* announced plans to give all patients a choice of provider at the point of referral. Patients would be offered at least four choices by their GP from January 2006 and by the end of 2008 would be able to choose any registered provider nationally (later to be delivered by April 2008). Offering patients a choice of provider was part of the government's plans to

* create a competitive market for NHS funded care, and

* improve the quality of services.

A patient's right to choose where they are treated has now been included in the NHS Constitution (2009), which places a duty on PCTs to facilitate those choices.

Patient choice in practice

When patients are referred by their GP for a first outpatient appointment, they should be offered a choice of providers from a national list that meet standards assessed by the Care Quality Commission and are willing to provide care at the NHS tariff price. This includes:

* NHS trusts,

* Foundation trusts,

* Independent sector treatment centres,

* NHS treatment centres, and

* Registered independent sector hospitals.

An electronic booking system called Choose and Book has been implemented to support patient choice. This can be accessed in a number of ways:

* GPs can access this system from their surgery and book an appointment for their patient at the provider of their choice.

* GPs may issue a booking request which gives the patient information on potential providers and a unique reference number. The patient can then either call a telephone booking line to book the appointment themselves, or do so online via their personal health space page.

* Some PCTs operate referral management centres locally which patients call to book their appointments.

There is still relatively little easily accessible information available to help patients choose between hospitals. The Choose and Book system gives information on waiting time and travel distance. Further information about facilities and performance in the Care Quality Commission's Annual Health Check assessment is available on the NHS Choices website. Results from the national programme of patient surveys can be found on the Care Quality Commission website, but awareness among the public of these information sources is low (For more information on patient surveys see Chapter 37). Patients should be given a 'Choosing Hospital' booklet by their GP which outlines local options, although most respondents in surveys say they did not receive a booklet.

Most comparative performance information is available only at organizational level, aside from cardiac mortality rates which are risk adjusted and published for each surgeon (http://heartsurgery.healthcarecommission.org.uk) and websites such as www.iwantgreatcare.org which allow patients to post opinions on particular clinicians.

Implementing patient choice

Despite national targets for acute trusts and PCTs and incentive payments for GPs, implementation of patient choice has been slow. Usage of the Choose and Book system, designed to provide electronic appointment booking, is still relatively low with less than half of first outpatient appointments booked using the system in 2007/08.

The Department of Health monitors implementation of patient choice with a bimonthly survey which shows under half of patients referred for elective care recalled being offered a choice of provider in July 2008. A similar number of patients were aware that choice was available before they visited their GP. There is still some way to go in raising awareness of the policy among patients and ensuring choice is offered. This survey along with figures on Choose and Book implementation previously fed into targets for PCTs and acute trusts that were monitored by the Healthcare Commission; however, these targets no longer exist and implementation is monitored locally. PCTs and acute trusts must also demonstrate compliance with a set of core standards developed by the DH and monitored by the regulator. One standard asks for evidence that patients are offered choice. It is not yet known how or whether implementation of patient choice policy will be monitored by the CQC.

The impact of patient choice on patients, GPs, and hospital providers

Giving patients a choice of provider has had some impact on the following:

+ patients' experience of care,
+ the process of GP referral, and
+ the way hospitals organize their clinics.

Impact on patients

Choice of hospital is popular with the public and the majority of respondents to the British Social Attitudes survey said they wanted a choice. However as discussed above, implementation has been slow and the number being offered a choice is still quite low. When asked which factors are important to them when choosing a hospital, patients in the Department of Health's monitoring survey most frequently mention the following:

1. cleanliness

2. low levels of infection

3. quality of care

4. waiting times

5. the friendliness of staff

6. the reputation of the hospital

7. location or transport considerations.

It is not yet clear whether patients are actively comparing hospitals on the factors listed above and selecting a provider based on their preferences. There is no evidence to suggest that patient choice is based on 'safety' considerations at present.

Impact on GPs

For GPs, patient choice has impacted on the way they refer patients into secondary care. There has been much resistance to the use of the Choose and Book system, in part because of technical difficulties accessing the system during consultations. Giving patients a choice of provider puts a responsibility on GPs to be the agents of choice. Some feel they do not have enough time in the consultation to go through the options with their patients and to book appointments. Some GPs are frustrated that referrals can no longer be made to a named consultant and some find it difficult to select the right clinic to refer a patient to on the system.

Impact on hospitals

The Choose and Book system has changed the way hospital clinics are organized. Hospitals have had to put new procedures in place for dealing with electronic referrals and concrete appointment slots which make it more difficult to overbook clinics to allow for patients not attending. Hospitals also now have to run paper based and electronic booking systems in parallel, using additional resources.

The fact that hospitals must accept any patient who chooses their care can bring challenges in terms of meeting waiting-time targets. As waiting lists reduce further in the future providers may be motivated to compete more for patients in their local health care market. There is no evidence as yet on whether patients' choices are leading hospitals to improve the quality of their services.

Giving patients a choice of provider is unlikely to be a major driver of improvements in patient safety. Cleanliness and hospital acquired infection rates are clearly a concern for patients and their choices might motivate hospitals to work harder to push down infection rates. However patients do not report using other safety indicators to choose between hospitals.

Other choices

Patients have many choices within the NHS, not just a choice of hospital for elective treatment, although this has been the main focus of policy in recent years. Patients are increasingly being asked to make choices not just over *where* they have treatment, but also over *what* treatment they receive. The broad aim of these policies is to

◆ empower patients,

◆ give patients more choice over their care options, and

◆ allow patients to personalize their care plan.

By the end of 2009, all women should have choice around where they give birth (at home, in a hospital, or in a midwife-led unit), the type of antenatal care they receive, and the location of their postnatal care. The final report of the *Next Stage Review* of the NHS published in 2008 announced plans to pilot the use of individual health care budgets for patients with *'fairly stable and predictable'* health care needs, such as those with long-term conditions. This scheme is similar to direct payments implemented in social care. Patients will be given a budget for care of their condition giving them more choice and control over which treatments and support they receive and who they receive them from. These policies are still in early stages of implementation and will require changes to the relationship between patients and clinicians.

Summary

The policy of giving patients a choice of provider aims to empower patients, increase competition between providers, and thus improve quality of care. It is not yet clear that many patients are actively comparing hospitals and the impact of their choices has not been extensively measured. Policies are also developing that give the patient more control over the type of services they receive and devolve some responsibility to patients for decisions about their treatment plan. Support for patients and clear information will be needed to make both choice of provider and treatment a reality.

Further reading

Department of Health (2008). Report on the National Patient Choice Survey - July 2007 England, London: Department of Health.

Fotaki, M., Boyd, A., Smith, L., McDonald, R., Roland, M., Sheaff, R., Edwards, A., Elwyn, G., (2005). *Access to Healthcare Patient Choice and the Organisation and Delivery of Health Services: Scoping review*. Manchester: National Co-ordinating Centre for NHS Service Delivery and Organisation, R&D (NCCSDO).

Le Grand, J. (2007). *The other invisible hand: Delivering public services through choice and competition*. Oxford: Princeton University Press.

Robertson, R., and Thorlby, R. (2008). *Briefing: patient choice. King's fund briefing*. London: King's Fund.

Chapter 40

Patient information

Claire Read

Key points

- Ensuring that patients receive appropriate information about their diagnosis and treatment is fundamental to the provision of safe and high-quality care.
- Good patient information is the result of input from a range of clinical and non-clinical professionals, as well from patients.
- Approaches to producing and providing information vary between organizations.
- There is national guidance on patient information.
- Many assessments of health care services – including those by The Care Quality Commission, NHS Litigation Authority (NHSLA), and Audit Commission – include standards on patient information

Introduction

With an emphasis on patient-centred care, the NHS Plan made patient information a key aspect of health care provision. The Plan made clear that providing appropriate information to service users was crucial to meeting an overriding goal – of enabling patients to become joint decision makers in their care. While different healthcare organizations have taken varied approaches to producing and providing this sort of information, there is a general acknowledgment that good information can be a significant aid to involving patients in their care and that, furthermore, it can improve safety. Creating such material is a challenge which can only be met through the contributions and expertise of a range of professionals.

The benefits of well-produced patient information

The aim of all patient information should be to help patients – and their friends, families, or carers – understand conditions, proposed treatments and investigations, and available services and support. While widespread internet usage and audio-visual equipment ownership now means this information could take the form of an interactive web application or a brief film on DVD as well as a traditional patient information leaflet, the overall aim remains unchanged.

When this aim is met, patient information can help create patients who:

- Protect and take responsibility for their health,
- Feel equipped to work with healthcare professionals to decide on the best course of treatment,

- Comply with treatments because they understand why they have been suggested, have played a role in deciding on them, and understand the consequences of non-compliance,
- Feel able to ask questions, allowing the speedy resolution of any concerns,
- Feel reassured and prepared,
- Are able to give informed consent, and,
- Feel able to share their opinion because they are confident it will be valued.

It is clear that this in turn creates significant benefits for health care professionals, for the organizations within which they work, and for the health service nationally. For example:

- A patient who is aware that regular INR checks are necessary when on warfarin is less likely to accept medication without first undergoing the tests she/he knows to be appropriate.
- A patient who understands the importance of hand hygiene in reducing the risk of health care associated infection is less likely to accept treatment from a professional who has not washed his/her hands.

Well-produced patient information can combat misinformation or misunderstandings. Consider the internet with its myriad of inaccuracies, or the problems of word of mouth, or the way in which the media may willfully portray stories to increase concerns and it is clear how valuable an opportunity this is and why every effort should be made to ensure it is not squandered.

The dangers of poorly produced patient information

If well-produced patient information can bring benefits to both patient and health care professional, including increased safety, then it follows that poorly produced information represents a risk. Just as poor verbal communication between professional and patient can confuse, worry or even alienate, so too can poorly produced patient information. The fact that such information is of a lasting nature should provoke additional concern. A leaflet which describes the risk of death in terms incomprehensible to the patient, for example, may be reviewed frequently over a lengthy period time, causing progressively greater anxiety. It may be passed on to family and friends, causing further worry, and potentially leading to pressure to not comply with suggested treatments or to make inappropriate decisions. Given that non-compliance can harm patients, it is not an exaggeration to say that poorly produced patient information is a risk to patient safety.

The challenge of creating patient information

It is vital, then, to create information for patients which engages and informs rather than concerns and alienates. This is undoubtedly a challenge, not least because health and health care are not simple topics. Individuals need to have information which:

- Makes complicated procedures understandable but remains clinically accurate,

+ Informs them about different treatment options, and
+ Helps them understand that risks attached to procedures are counterbalanced by benefits.

All this must be achieved while aiming at an incredibly diverse audience. Patients with chronic conditions may be very well-informed and need less detailed information than a newly diagnosed patient. Some patients have little knowledge and no desire to enhance it. Individuals with a 'traditional' understanding of the place of the patient in health care may not want to express or even form an opinion. In a multicultural society, the challenge of different perspectives on the patient–professional relationship and of patients for whom English is a second language – if it is spoken at all – must be addressed. Learning difficulties and sight impairments provide further accessibility challenges.

Meeting the challenge

Patient information is by its nature 'one size fits all'. The trick is finding the right size and different organizations take different approaches to meeting this challenge. Some place responsibility within the Patient Advice and Liaison Service (PALS) function. In others, the duty lies with what is generally described as 'communications', a department usually staffed by professional writers and editors who likely have a background in health communication but who are unlikely to have ever been clinical professionals. The team may have one or multiple individuals with sole responsibility for patient information or may have individuals for whom it is part of a wider remit, typically centred on publications.

While PALS can give a steer on the needs of patients, and communications support the production of a DVD or create a well-written leaflet, neither is likely to have the knowledge to create information that is fully robust from the clinical perspective. It is here that health care professionals have a crucial role to play. All health care professionals can expect to be asked to contribute to patient information since it is they who must provide details on clinical practice, explaining risks, benefits and alternatives, and the rationale behind treatment and diagnostic paths.

But health care professionals cannot create successful information alone. Doctors are not expert writers and editors – and nor should they be. They are further encumbered by the difficulties of communicating on a subject with which they are very familiar. It is all too easy to assume knowledge that the audience is unlikely to possess.

Forging collaborative relationships

If patient information cannot be successfully created by any one group then it is clear a variety of collaborative relationships is needed, such as:

+ The health care professional can give clinical information and advice on which information is needed at which point in the patient's care,
+ The communications professional can ensure information is clear and meets necessary guidelines. She/he can advise on which format is most suitable and on what information already exists locally and nationally.

- PALS representatives can help identify the subjects on which patients are most likely to require information – and in what depth. They can also assist in gaining feedback from patients, allowing for the continuing refinement of documents.
- External agencies such as charities and translation agencies can assist in making information accessible to all.

Adopting such an approach greatly increases the likelihood of success. And there is a real need to reach such an outcome, not least because many assessments of health care services contain requirements on patient information. The NHSLA's risk management standards include explicit requirements on archiving and updating leaflets but many more inspections contain general requirements – among them the Audit Commission's auditors' local evaluation (ALE) and the Care Quality Commission's annual health check. The latter particularly focuses on making information accessible to all.

Unfortunately, there is evidence that a great deal of written patient information is not connecting with its audience. A 1994 study of internet information on diabetes showed that a reading age of between 11 and 16.8 would be required to comprehend the sites – while finding that the average reading age of the UK population was around nine years. A recent study on schizophrenia drew similar conclusions.

The general principles

Advice on how to create successful patient information comes primarily from the NHS Brand Guidelines on patient information, produced by NHS Identity. These guidelines focus on written information, still by far the most common format used and thus the area on which the rest of this chapter also focuses. It is worth noting that many of these principles can be applied to other forms of information.

The NHS guidelines are detailed, offering advice on practicalities such as sourcing print suppliers. Many of these details are unlikely to be relevant to health care professionals working on literature, but it is worth being aware that there are requirements which whoever is responsible for layout and design will need to meet: the health care professional should not be surprised if the designed proof he or she receives back looks significantly different to the document submitted. That said, there is much within the guidelines which will be of help to any clinical professional charged with the creation of a patient information document.

In short, the guidelines consistently emphasize the need to consider the audience at which literature is aimed.

How to implement these principles

Everyone has an inherent understanding of considering audience – compare the way in which someone asks to borrow money from a stranger to how she/he asks a friend – but it is a principle which is all too often forgotten when preparing information for patients. A very simple way to keep audience in mind is to ask 'who, what, why, where, when':

- Who is this literature for?
- What are the needs of this audience? What is it hoped they will do after reading this information?

Box 1 Guidelines for drafting patient information literature

- Write from the patient's point of view
- Use 'patient-friendly' language
- Make sure the information given is relevant to the audience
- Explain all instructions
- Be concise: use short sentences and paragraphs; a question and answer format; and bulleted or numbered lists where appropriate
- Direct readers to further sources of useful information and make clear that information is available in different formats

- Why do readers need to know this information? Why is written literature is the best way in which to communicate this information? And, crucially, why should the reader care about what is being said and act upon it?
- Where and when will this information be given out? Will it be sent with admission letters? Will it be given in clinic? How does this affect what needs to be said?

If these questions are consistently considered while preparing a leaflet – and through the inevitable editing and revision stages – the likelihood is that the outcome will be a good one. Further work can then be undertaken as needed to make the document accessible to as many people as possible – perhaps by organizing translations, transcription into Braille, recording an audio version, or creating an 'Easy Read' version for those with learning difficulties.

How considering audience makes a difference

Consider a leaflet which tells a patient that she/he should not consume caffeine for six hours before a heart scan. Now consider a leaflet which states that caffeine should not be taken for six hours before the scan it describes, because caffeine increases the heart rate and so could make the results inaccurate, leading to the scan having to be repeated or to inappropriate treatment. It should be clear that it is the latter text which is more likely to achieve the desired outcome. The patient is likely to be just as keen as the health care professional to avoid inappropriate treatment and/or the need for another scan. But to decide not to take actions which could jeopardize clinical treatment, the patient needs to understand why such actions could have an effect.

Now consider the following sentences:

- Refrain from caffeine for six hours before the scan.
- We ask you to please avoid caffeine for six hours before your scan.

It should be clear that the second sentence is preferable. By asking rather than ordering, and by using personal pronouns such as 'you' and 'we', the instruction is much more likely to be obeyed. Note that 'refrain' is eliminated from the second sentence and replaced with 'avoid'. It is important to note that research has indicated as many as seven million people in England (roughly one in five adults) have difficulties with basic literacy and numeracy. Care should be taken to avoid words which are not in common usage among the majority of the population.

Finally consider the following:

◆ Before the procedure, an echo will be performed to monitor the pumping action of the heart.

◆ Before your operation, we will carry out an echocardiogram (you may hear this called an 'echo' for short). This painless ultrasound scan lets us see how well your heart is pumping blood around your body.

These examples highlight that writing effective patient information is not a case of eliminating all medical terminology. To do so would be of limited value since patients are likely to hear health care staff use such terms. The priority should be to explain all such terminology in clear terms which would be understandable to the majority of patients.

Summary

The task of creating successful patient information can seem overwhelming and is certainly not straightforward. It necessitates careful consideration of audience; a review of the rationale behind the information; and collaborations between many colleagues. However, it is a challenge worth meeting. Good information can help create patients who:

◆ Participate in decisions about their health

◆ Are aware of key safety issues

◆ Feel able to ask questions and share opinions

Such patients can form effective partnerships with clinical staff and health care organizations. However patient information, whether document, film, or audio, is by its very nature a 'one size fits all' solution. As such, it can never replace the face-to-face individually tailored communication between health care professional and patient (see Chapter 46). When done properly, though, it can serve as an invaluable aid to such communication.

Further reading

NHS Brand Guidelines on patient information. www.nhsidentity.nhs.uk/tools-and-resources/ patient-information.

Ollerenshaw, H. (2007). 'Patient information services: a strategic partnership approach'. *Health Expectations* **10**, (1): 92–100.

'Better information, better choices, better health'. Department of Health, 2004. http://www. dh.gov.uk/en/Publicationsandstatistics/Publications/PublicationsPolicyAndGuidance/ DH_4098576.

Patient Information Forum. An independent organization which promotes and supports the creation of high-quality information for patients, carers, and families http://www.pifonline. org.uk/.

Chapter 41

Self-management and the Expert Patient

Deborah Trenchard

Key points

- Recent policy in the NHS has focused on the importance of involving patients in the design and delivery of healthcare.
- The Expert Patient programme was developed to empower patients with chronic disease and enhance their control of their own health.
- Knowledgeable patients have improved life control and activity, often suffer fewer symptoms and are more resourceful.
- Healthcare staff have an important role to play, implicit and explicit, in encouraging self-management by patients
- Effective communication and respect are fundamental to the patient–doctor relationship and this must take into account culture, attitudes, and religious belief.

Introduction

The idea of self-management for those with long-term illnesses was the brainchild of Professor Kate Lorig, a researcher at Stanford University, California. During the 1960s and 1970s, she pioneered the idea of *'developing the confidence and motivation of the patient to use their own skills, information, and professional services to take effective control over living with chronic lifelong conditions'*. Lorig felt that educating patients and their carers would be an effective way of offering them more autonomy to manage their own illness.

In the United Kingdom, NHS policies have consistently emphasized the importance of the patient in design and delivery of services. There is also recognition that chronic disease, e.g. diabetes or arthritis, comprises the major part of the national burden of ill-health. *Saving Lives; Our Healthier Nation* (1999) announced the introduction of an Expert Patient programme and the NHS Plan (2000) set out the way this would be achieved. In 2001 the Expert Patients Taskforce published *The expert patient: A new approach to chronic disease management for the 20th century*, which recommended self-management programmes for patients. The first programmes were piloted in 2002 and an implementation, training, and support network established based on the Stanford model.

The underlying evidence indicates that empowered patients

◆ take their health seriously and are confident in managing it,

◆ communicate effectively with doctors and establish effective partnerships,

◆ ask appropriate questions, are realistic about their disease and its impact,

◆ seize opportunities to learn about their condition so they can lead rewarding lives, and

◆ are pro-active in managing their health.

The Expert Patient programme focuses on five core self-management skills (Fig. 41.1):

◆ Problem solving

◆ Decision making

◆ Resource utilisation

◆ Developing effective partnerships with healthcare providers

◆ Taking action

Today self-management is seen as a fundamental part of the way care is provided for those with chronic disease and it is as much about education as it is about motivation and confidence to manage their condition.

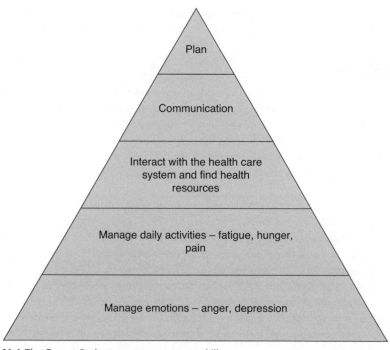

Fig. 41.1 The Expert Patient programme core skills.

The Darzi Review (2008) emphasized 'Increased control' for patients by '... *allowing people to exercise choice and be partners in decisions about their own care, shaping and directing it with high quality information and support. Empowering patients enables them to use their personal knowledge, time and energy for solving their own health problems'*.

Self-management: A case study

An expert patient with a chronic illness such as cystic fibrosis (CF) learns early on, to manage her daily routine of drugs and oxygen therapy. The CF patient knows the risks of her disease but also of the treatments; she accurately measures and administers medications, performs physiotherapy and knows what is and is not possible for her to achieve. She is scrupulous when questioning healthcare staff and wants to be fully informed about the side-effects of drugs she takes and if they are changed, how long it will take before the new drug starts to work and how this transition may affect her. The CF patient, and often her family, is well informed, and can accurately quote statistics about her condition and prognosis. She knows her physical limitations; and because of these boundaries, she is acutely aware of her life expectancy. She takes complete ownership of her condition and the eventual outcome. The example shown is a typical day in the life of a 30-year-old patient with cystic fibrosis, diagnosed at the age of five months. She manages her condition based on the advice and treatments prescribed by the medical team. She is highly compliant and has developed her daily routine around these interventions on the basis that this is the most effective way to stay healthy and prolong her life.

Box 41.1 Case study

- Before breakfast uses a DNASE nebulizer to loosen mucus and prepares her intravenous drugs.
- One hour later administers antibiotics through IV line followed by another nebuliser and breathing exercises lasting 45 minutes.
- This is followed by a second nebulizer, inhalers, and morning medicines.
- Breakfast and gets dressed.
- Before lunch administers another IV antibiotic.
- After lunch two hours of what she calls 'me time'!
- Another DNASE followed by a period of one hour before a further nebulizer is administered.
- This is followed by another 45 minutes of breathing exercises and percussion with the assistance of the physiotherapist.
- Dinner followed another IV antibiotic and maybe more physio depending on the condition of her chest.

Information leads to confidence and control

Patients need information and support to become empowered and take control over their condition and care. An informed patient is one in possession of appropriate and honest information who works in partnership with the healthcare team and is fully involved in their healthcare. They are prepared to take greater responsibility in order to manage their health effectively. Today, there are numerous Internet sites where people can find detailed medical information, but this cannot be a substitute for proper dialogue with the doctor and other members of the healthcare team rather it should be a way to initiate a dialogue with the physician. There is an expanding litera-ture written for and by patients but the following quote emphasizes the importance of the partnership between patient and medical experts and a discerning approach to information accessed through the Internet.

> ... mainstream medical websites can be a fabulous educational resource for medical infor-mation – and an educated patient is a good patient – but they also have the potential to be a big problem. Medical websites give you the ability to self-diagnose without the proper care and treatment of a medical doctor, at the risk of great harm and mental anguish. And as you've probably already heard, only fools have themselves for a doctor!

> *Medical Myths That Can Kill You* by Nancy L. Snyderman, M.D.

Patients can be frustrated by lack of information from medical teams as well as by confusing and conflicting information obtained elsewhere as the following anecdote illustrates. An educated middle-aged patient persistently questioned her hospital con-sultant and gained the impression he was convinced that it was not important for her questions to be answered to her satisfaction. Exasperated and emotionally charged, she took her illness in her own hands and trawled the Internet in search of acceptable answers. Before long, she realized that deciphering and understanding the informa-tion was immensely challenging and was not going to help her. This shows that many patients want to be fully informed but need structured and reliable information and failure of healthcare staff to respond appropriately and honestly can impair the partnership and render it ineffective.

Why patients may fail to become empowered

Whilst many patients do want answers, a significant proportion are reluctant to be inquisitive when it comes to their health or that of a family member. Typical reasons why patients feel unenthusiastic are as follows:

+ The unfamiliar environment of a consulting room or surgery
+ The time constraints of appointment systems
+ Lack of continuity with different staff meeting the patient and providing different or conflicting information
+ Lack of rapport with doctor and failure of communication particularly failure to listen to the patient's concerns

◆ Failure/reluctance of doctor to acknowledge patient strengths and respect their views and choices

◆ Patients arriving for the appointments ill-prepared without formulating their questions satisfactorily

◆ Deference to the assumed knowledge and authority of the doctor

◆ Failure to understand why it is important for them to engage with the healthcare team

Not surprisingly, a disproportionate number of people feel inadequate when it comes to getting involved with their health. Two things frighten them the most:

◆ Being told there is something wrong with them

◆ Meeting the consultant / specialist and not understanding what they are told

Being told there is something seriously wrong with very little explanation in language people can comprehend, or conversely, too much information, is overwhelming and distressing. A patient must be ready emotionally to hear and take in the information given by the doctor. This means it may be necessary to impart relevant facts and details about prognosis and treatment options in stages. If a patient is told that surgery is the only option, he or she may leave the hospital frightened and bewildered. Patients may feel intimidated, vulnerable, and disadvantaged when meeting a surgeon for example. This may be because they think they have a serious problem and it is usually a condition they know little about. The simple fact that the surgeon is addressed as 'Mr' may put him into a different and elevated category from a 'normal' doctor in the patient's eyes, which immediately results in a communication barrier. However, the surgeon is the very person the patient should be questioning extensively. Patients (elderly, disabled, those with language barriers) and their advocates benefit from knowing what their options are. Healthcare staff have a duty to ensure patents are informed, know what treatment strategies are available, and know where to go to get support or advice.

The doctor–patient partnership

Generally speaking, people are intimidated by words they are unfamiliar with and more so when they visit the hospital, or surgery, and words are used with no explanation of their meaning. Medical jargon, acronyms, and terminology are intimidating for patients and result in failures of communication, which impair the relationship. Whilst it is important to emphasize the doctor–patient partnership all too often, there is a doctor–patient barrier. According to Dr Nancy L. Snyderman, M.D.

> The doctor–patient relationship is a sensitive one, requiring respect and openness on both sides....To build a good relationship with our doctors, we must insist on clear, non-arrogant, and sensitive communication. Should you find that your doctor seems disinterested in you and doesn't seem to care about the details of your life, talks in language you can't decode, or is cold and insensitive, find another doctor. You deserve someone who is passionate about your care and whose answers and explanations make sense to you.

In her book *Big Pharma*, Jacky Law describes the need for the doctor–patient partnership to be one of equals moving from compliance to concordance.

> A doctor–patient relationship may be grossly imperfect in healthcare systems that neglect the time required to develop it, but it is arguably the most underrated resource there is for creating robust public health and reducing levels of anxiety....The idea of concordance between doctor and patient would seem as normal and natural a thing to aspire to as harmonious relations within a family. But it represents a radical departure for medicine, overturning centuries of practice where doctors have always known best and not taken kindly to challenges to their authority.

Patients across the spectrum (of age, education, class, or ethnicity) continue to fear medical authority. They fear that if they question then the doctor may take umbrage or be unkind and this may impact on the care they receive. In the patient's mind, doctors know best and consequently, the majority of patients find it difficult to question healthcare professionals even if they may have a burning desire to know something and from the other side patients who ask lots of questions are often seen as 'difficult'.

There are many doctors who are convivial, respectful, and keen to engage with their patients. They listen to, encourage them, communicate effectively, and are highly respected. This attitude, dialogue, and respect creates a plausible doctor–patient relationship and fashions confident and positive patients. However, a doctor can only be one channel through which the patient seeks information, advice, and therapy. Ultimately, a patient's decision and ability to challenge and conquer his/her own fears about his disease and become fully engaged in his/her own health goes beyond any doctor's remit.

Empowerment and culture

Respect for culture and beliefs is a vital part of patient empowerment. Understanding the traditions and practices of the diverse ethnic population for which the NHS provides care is fundamental. Beliefs in native rituals, the power of spirits, use of herbal

---

Box 41.2 A healthy doctor/patient relationship: Case study

A patient revealed her fear at the first meeting with her GP: her mother and sister had both died from ovarian cancer and she was concerned that she was at significant risk of developing the disease. The female doctor said that she too had lost her mother to the same disease at age 62. This common thread was used to build a constructive and healthy doctor–patient relationship. The patient continued to question and received appropriate answers. Two weeks later the results of some blood tests were received and the patient received a letter from her GP requesting a non-urgent appointment. The doctor spent some time explaining what the tests revealed about the patient's health and said that she had decided to call the patient in, instead of a discussion over the telephone, because she got the impression that the patient was the type of woman who preferred to see and discuss her results.

remedies, and the power of evil to cause illness can impact significantly on a patient's ability to understand their disease and willingness to manage it.

In some third world cultures, people still use traditional remedies to heal their bodies. They continue with rituals: belief that the rain and the wind, even the stars, and music of the sea will result in ill-health and that mother earth will provide a cure. Today, some 'new age' groups use yoga, meditation, and visualization to connect with their body, mind, and spirit. A plethora of remedies, vitamins, and herbal teas are available. People are turning to Chinese, ayurvedic, homeopathy, and other complementary approaches, including spinal manipulation and acupuncture. Advocates for these methods vouch for their efficacy in healing some diseases.

The chief reasons for seeking alternative approaches for health management appear to be the following:

- Remedies and alternative therapies are widely available with few apparent side effects.
- People think they can self-diagnose via the Internet.
- The 'customer' can chose the approach and the provider.
- The 'customer' is in control of the relationship – no hospital waiting rooms, no white coats; fear is at a minimum.

As an example, when a person arrives for an acupuncture appointment, the system is designed to set him at ease: a relaxed atmosphere, a holistic approach, total acceptance discussion. The patient is less apprehensive, since he feels he has been listened to and his questions have been answered. The treatment is carried out immediately and sensitively. He leaves feeling empowered; in charge of his mind and body. In spite of the fact that he has to pay, he returns for further appointments until he feels the problem is resolved to his satisfaction. Such individuals are interestingly often averse to the NHS prescription charge levied after a visit to the GP.

It is conceivable that a healthcare system that aims to promote health and heal people could, in some instances, perpetuate ill health. Anxiety, fear, and confusion are examples of how some patients feel after visiting their GP or a hospital and this disempowers them. Whereas the frequently more positive and constructive relationship with an alternative therapist produces a productive partnership.

Summary

The United Kingdom is a country made up of people from every part of the globe; the majority of whom have been conditioned to revere the medical establishment, not question it. This has inadvertently created what the Americans call 'the white coat syndrome'. Patients communicate more freely with a nurse and they're more likely to question their local pharmacist. Irrespective of their cultures and maladies, patients all have one thing in common: unlimited access to the NHS. In order for people to take full advantage of what the NHS has to offer they have to be empowered to participate more in their own health management. The Darzi report hopes to deliver on this and put patients firmly in the driving seat when it comes to healthcare but they need encouragement to take on this responsibility.

Further reading

Trenchard, D. (2008). *Raising Tiffany – Portrait of a Special Girl*, Foreword by Professor Michael A. Gatzoulis. Milton Keynes: Author HOUSE.

Kloss, J. (1939 (1st Edition), various updated editions available). *Back to Eden*. Lotus Press.

Holford, P. (2005). *The New Optimum Nutrition Bible*. Piatkus Publishing.

Roizen, M.F., and Oz, M.C. (2006). *YOU: The Smart Patient*. New York: Free Press.

Balch, P.A., and Balch, J.F. (2000). *Prescription for Nutritional Healing*. New York: Avery.

Section 7

Communication effectiveness

Effective communication is fundamental to safe health care. Traditionally we have relied on professional courtesy and common sense. However, some of the most dramatic failures in healthcare organisations have been the result of poor communication. This section illustrates the multiple facets of communication in healthcare, in what are often large organizations with many individuals and groups interacting, in complex way, with other people and organizations across the healthcare economy. Most Trusts have a professional communications department, which will interact with external organizations, the media, and the public (*Communicating with the public*) to deliver key messages around success, or attempt to limit the damage when there have been failures. Establishing effective relationships with stakeholders (*Communicating with commissioners*) or developing collaborative relationships (*Networks*) is a vital aspect of improving healthcare. Within healthcare organizations, communication at all levels must be planned appropriately. Both top-down (*Board structures, responsibilities, and communication*) and horizontal (*Communication with staff*) communication is needed to ensure the right messages are delivered and understood. Finally, and possibly most important of all, communication with patients can be challenging but is undoubtedly related to safety when dealing with issues of consent, confidentiality, and being open when things have gone wrong (*Communication with patients*).

Chapter 42

Communicating safety: With the public and the media

Murray Anderson-Wallace

Key points

- Developing an open, effective dialogue within and between the organization, its clinicians, managers, and local media is a critical aspect of developing safe, reliable care.
- Frontline NHS staff are, through the stories they tell about their work and organizations, highly influential in developing the climate of opinion.
- Significant differences exist between individual patient satisfaction and wider public perception of services.
- Communicating safety is fundamental to the everyday activity of all clinicians and managers and not solely the responsibility of the Trust Communications Department.

Introduction

It is widely accepted that developing an open and effective dialogue between clinicians and managers about issues that affect patient safety is critical to the development of safe, reliable care. Evidence suggests that open disclosure and honest conversations with patients who have suffered harm events is crucial. It is also known that healthcare systems, which have an active organizational discourse around patient safety, are more likely to develop strong safety cultures with associated positive impacts on staff and patient experience and outcomes.

However a strong safety culture cannot be developed solely through 'internal' discussion. Tackling some potentially difficult conversations within the public domain is a fundamental part of this process. NHS organizations have diffuse boundaries and healthcare workers are integral members of the communities they serve. They are often both providers and users of services and are central to both the production and consumption of the stories that shape opinion and perception about NHS services at a local level.

Patient safety is a difficult issue to address in the public domain. Airline passengers boarding a plane assume they will be transported safely, the crew being properly trained, briefed and operating within a broader system (engineers, air traffic controllers etc.), which takes safety seriously. Patients make similar assumptions about healthcare but evidence shows that the level of inadvertent harm caused by contact with services is high when compared to other safety-critical industries such as scheduled airlines. It is widely accepted that a significant proportion of this harm is avoidable.

Patient and public perceptions, and media influence

The media plays a very influential role in shaping public perceptions of safety in healthcare and most organizations struggle to proactively engage the media about patient safety issues. Most media coverage portrays the NHS as being in a permanent state of crisis. Newspaper headlines and TV documentaries regularly draw public attention to apparent failings of a system in meltdown. In this context, one might expect levels of individual patient satisfaction to be very low indeed, however, patient surveys repeatedly indicate high levels of satisfaction with NHS care.

Healthcare Commission Annual Surveys have shown successive increases in levels of patient satisfaction year on year. In 2007

- ◆ 77% of patients rated the hospital care they received as 'excellent' or 'very good'.
- ◆ 92% rated the way doctors and nurses worked together as 'good', 'very good', or 'excellent'.

A study by the Picker Institute reiterated this trend but showed that whilst individual patient satisfaction continues to rise, overall public satisfaction in the state of the NHS is much lower.

The NHS Confederation suggest that this divergence indicates that individual patients think they have simply been lucky in the care they receive and that their experience is not representative of the NHS as a whole. This gap in perception might also indicate that those not regularly in contact with NHS services probably rely on negative messaging from key 'opinion forming' sources when rating their satisfaction.

How are opinions formed?

The range of media sources used by the public to form opinions of the NHS is increasingly varied. The NHS Confederation has identified three of particular significance based on their consistently negative opinions, their reach, and degree of influence.

1. National Press and Broadcast Media (TV and Radio): In a highly competitive media environment, positive stories have limited newsworthiness and many national newspapers seem to have explicitly negative editorial policies regarding the NHS. In terms of credibility, the national press is often viewed with scepticism and is often regarded as sensationalist and inaccurate. Despite this, studies have clearly shown that press coverage continues to play an influential role in shaping climate of opinion around key healthcare-related issues. The broadcast media is considered to be a more reliable source being viewed by consumers as a more accurate 'reflection of reality' than the press.

2. Staff attitudes. Whilst generally supportive of the NHS and their own roles surveys suggest that staff tend to be more critical compared to other sectors, of the organizations within which they work. With over 1.3 million employees, a very significant

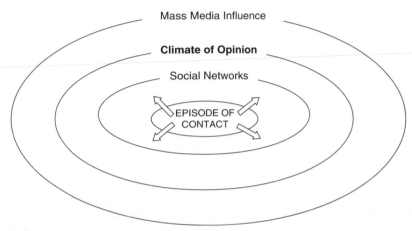

Fig. 42.1

percentage of people will know someone within their family or immediate social circle who works in the NHS. Stories told by doctors and nurses have significant reach and even though their views are often only representative of a tiny part of a huge system they are seen as highly reliable and credible. These stories have the potential to spread quickly within social networks and the media, thereby shaping public opinion. A study into public perception of HCAIs conducted by the NHS Institute for Innovation and Improvement found staff frequently cited cases where individual experiences and isolated incidents had received significant local press attention (Fig. 42.1).

3. Shaping the stories. NHS organizations can do much to enhance their reputation locally by improving their approach to engaging the media, but huge gains can be achieved through engagement with staff and via them, to local stakeholders.

The quality of the individual encounter with healthcare staff has a massive influence on patients' sense of the safety and quality of services. The way professionals behave, communicate, and respond both with and around patients and how the 'system of care' is organized are crucial elements in shaping perception. These encounters form the stories told by patients, and are quickly generalized and spread within family and social networks, both face-to-face and on-line.

A more proactive approach to directly involving frontline NHS staff in patient safety and quality improvement work combined with engaging the media around patient safety stories can significantly contribute to improved public perception and confidence in services. By actively involving staff in improving their working conditions and processes to create more effective and safer systems to work within is much more likely to lead to genuine stories of safety and reliability. The same conditions that create good morale amongst staff are also associated with

- encouraging a culture of safety,
- learning from error, and
- continuous improvement.

These in turn translate into

+ reduced mortality rates,
+ better patient experience, and
+ improved outcomes.

The changing face of the media

Newspapers and broadcasting are still hugely influential in shaping opinion, but the significant rise in the use of new media (from individualized mobile devices to screen media in public spaces) are revolutionizing the way the creation and the consumption of media is understood. The changing nature and status of the media in contemporary culture is also providing access to formerly privileged information and a level of insight into hitherto closed worlds of health and healthcare. Previously inaccessible minutes of Board meetings for example are now readily accessible. The power of 'word of mouth' and the influence of story-telling on behavioural change, especially in human systems such as healthcare, is amplified though new media channels. This influence can be seen in the number of health-related blogs often written by NHS staff, 'The NHS blog doctor' being a notable example.

New avenues of communication are inspiring new patterns of participation. The NHS is just beginning to be influenced by these developments. The growth of social media technologies such as GoogleHealth are showing how more accessible, personalized, and interactive information services will be central to new forms of engagement for patients and the public in the near future. It is clear that people no longer rely on a single source of information and increasingly make their own connections among dispersed media content. The ability to control the story "at large" through a single channel has gone.

Developing the public story

Excellent communications with patients and the public should be an integral part of the everyday activity of all clinicians and managers. Of course, Healthcare Communicators have a key role to play but it is only through skilful use of the clinical and managerial 'voice' that significant change can be achieved.

Four key strategies exist:

1. Recognition of the power of the story lived and told by staff.
2. Use of a broad range of communication approaches and strategies to create more targeted and focussed conversations with key audiences channelled in more creative and engaging ways.
3. Use of multiple media platforms to influence the climate of opinion and reframe the debate around safety.
4. Use of visible symbols within the care environment, i.e. how to use visible cues to influence confidence, behaviour, and action.

Engaging with the media

Research has shown that whilst trust in the news media is relatively low, their influence in terms of shaping attitudes and behaviour is high whereas trust in hospitals is actually relatively high but their influence is less. These two narratives need to be linked to create better outcomes.

Developing open and honest relationships with local media, newspaper and radio stations in particular, is worthy of consideration. The local media could be used for 'internal' communications work since staff groups may be more likely to learn about what is going on in their workplaces from the local paper or radio station than through internal newsletters.

A number of NHS Trusts have gained from senior managers and clinicians writing regular columns in local papers and using advertorial approaches to communicate to large groups of staff. Some specific steps have been found to be useful:

◆ Establishing regular briefings with the local media, covering both good and bad news in relation to the issues. Offering advanced briefings minimizes the need for staff to approach the press directly.

◆ Answering press inquiries promptly and where possible by the clinicians involved.

◆ Acknowledging a person's individual experience and where necessary apologizing directly for poor experience. Many studies have shown that an acknowledgement of the event and an apology is all people want when something has gone wrong.

◆ Pre-emptive explanations are beneficial since in the absence of a story people will 'backfill', which essentially means make it up!

Vital signs

Visual cues can play a major role in building or diminishing public confidence in the service. Often visible symbols in the healthcare environment do not communicate messages of confidence, proficiency, and professionalism. From unclear signage to contradictory messaging, visual symbols play a vital role in

◆ helping people know how to behave within a given environment,

◆ helping to set and manage boundaries, and

◆ inviting or discouraging certain sorts of behaviour in non-verbal ways.

The physical environment is also highly influential: a dirty toilet, apparently 'blood-stained' floors or 'discarded' clinical waste in a corridor is not easily forgotten. Whether any of these images have any real link with infection control or patient safety is irrelevant. What people remember, and act upon, is

◆ what they saw,

◆ what they experienced, and

◆ the meaning that they and others give to the experience.

Once again these are the stories that spread quickly in social and family networks and almost inevitably are what makes local news.

Cultural change and patient safety

Improving the safety of patients in healthcare organizations is about changing patterns of behaviour and systems of practice. Evidence on successful spread and adoption identifies observability (being able to see, feel, and hear about a change) and contestability (the process of dialogue, debate, and reframing) as key to the process of adoption. Put simply, enough people need to engage in the 'narrative of change' to make it happen and to sustain it. Few relatively isolated conversations amongst committed individuals may create pockets of excellent practice in some areas but will not create the critical mass of conversations needed to sustain a real change in culture and practice at all levels. To create large numbers of conversations about patient safety, a creative approach to 'internal' and 'external' communication across multiple media platforms is required. Successful approaches to spread and adoption are

◆ targeted,

◆ engaging, and

◆ interactive.

Simply trying to 'sell' an idea through persuasion is less effective and ultimately not sustainable (Table 42.1).

Summary

Communicating with the media and the public about quality and safety in healthcare is a new concept. The complexity of the messages, risk of creating anxiety amongst

Table 42.1

What you can do...	How you can contribute...
Start with your own practice	Ask yourself how you personally communicate safety and clearly define what you do that visibly demonstrates to your patients that you are putting their safety first.
Actively communicate about safety issues in the teams within which you work	Simply asking 'what can we do today to make patients safer?' is a good start.
Become a 'clinical champion'	Make it known within your organization and/or your professional body that you are willing to collaborate with the communications team to speak to the external media on clinical safety issues and ask for some media training.
Take responsibility for your own 'stories'	Be aware of how the stories you tell spread within your professional and social networks and in turn help to shape the climate of opinion. Be honest but take responsibility for the impact that your words will have.
Don't be naïve about the motivations of the external media	Be aware that if you speak to the external media that you will not have any control over how your comments are framed or interpreted. Always try to work within the local procedures for external press engagement.

those for whom care is provided, and fast moving and often hostile media environment makes for a challenging task. The reciprocal relationships between NHS staff, the communities they serve, and external media sources can be powerful tools to support change but need to be managed effectively.

Clinicians and managers have to decide if it is satisfactory for the climate of confidence and opinion of the NHS to be set by a media that knows little of the day-to-day struggles and successes of caring for patients. It is time to harness the significant shaping power of our interactions with each other and our patients to create different realities that can be confidently related and spread across our networks of influence.

Further reading

Edwards, N. (2006). *Lost in Translation: Why Patients Are More Satisfied with the NHS than the Public*. NHS Confederation, www.nhsconfed.org.

Engaging Patients in Quality and Safety Improvement. The Picker Institute, www.pickereurope.org.

Farr, M. (2006). *Segmenting NHS Staff: Towards a Strategy for HCAI Intervention*. NHS Institute for Innovation & Improvement / Dr Foster Intelligence, http://www.institute.nhs.uk/safer_care/mrsa/our_product_tools_and_resources.html.

Anderson-Wallace, M. **and Blantern, C.** (2005). Working with Culture, in *Organisational Development on Healthcare*, Ed: Peck, E. Oxford: Radcliffe.

Chapter 43

Relationships and communication with NHS Commissioners

Nicholas Hunt

Key points

♦ The NHS is divided into a purchasing arm, which commissions, monitors, and pays for care, and a provider arm, which delivers care in hospitals and the community.

♦ Establishing sound processes for relationship management and communications between these two is crucial for efficient NHS organization and care delivery.

♦ The relationship between providers and commissioners is structured through a series of timetabled meetings throughout the year.

♦ Commissioning for Quality is now central to the relationship between purchasers and providers with financial incentives to provide high-quality, safe care through Commissioning for Quality and Innovation (CQUIN).

♦ Safe care is cost-effective and there are strong strategic and financial reasons for this to be a fundamental driver in the NHS.

Introduction

Under the overarching governance of the 10 Strategic Health Authorities (SHAs), which run the National Health Service (NHS) in England, the NHS is divided into two organizational arms – purchasers and providers. In general
  • *providers* are those who deliver direct patient care in hospitals or the community
  • *purchasers* are those who commission, monitor and pay for care
Establishing sound processes for relationship management and communication between these two is crucial to efficient care delivery.

Each SHA is subdivided into Primary Care Trusts (PCTs), of which there are 152 across the country, which purchase and commission patient care. NHS general acute, teaching, and specialist hospitals need to form and maintain a good relationship with their host PCT but, dependent on location, type, and range of services, also have to establish relations with other PCTs or commissioning bodies such as SHA-wide Specialised Commissioning Groups (SCGs) or the National Specialist Commissioning Group (NSCG), established in April 2007. The relationship between service provider and service commissioner is typically organized through a series of timetabled meetings throughout the year supplemented and complemented by email exchange, formal

letters (e.g. contract and contract variations) and through forming cordial relationships so that differences and disagreements between purchaser and provider can be handled through a sensible and mature relationship between officers of what still is a single NHS. Possible areas of disagreement could include;
- identification and funding of local priorities,
- arrangements for 'prior approval' of certain low-volume high-cost treatments,
- overall affordability of proposed annual activity plan, and
- issues around access to care.

The so called purchaser–provider split of the NHS is now an embedded organizational reality of the NHS in England (NB: arrangements for organizing and delivering care in Wales, Scotland, and Northern Ireland are markedly different), and it has resulted in a dynamic, complex set of relationships between the two arms, driven not least by the almost continuous organizational change which the commissioning side of the NHS has been through in recent years.

The structure of the NHS (see Fig. 43.1)

The current organizational arrangement for the NHS wherein the country is divided into 10 Strategic Health Authorities, each containing a number of PCTs and acute trusts, is the latest of a series of organizational changes that have taken place and which have seen the number of PCTs shrink from nearly 400 to under 200 and the emergence of Specialised Commissioning Groups (SCGs), GP Practice Based Commissioning (PBC), and a variety of lead or sub-contract arrangements including contracting out the commissioning function to the private sector.

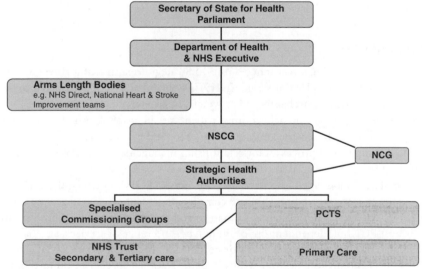

Fig. 43.1 The structure of the NHS in England.
NB: This is a highly simplified structure to show the separation of provider and commissioner bodies.

There are ten Specialised Commissioning Groups (SCGs), one per SHA, each acting on behalf of a population of about 5 million. Services commissioned at SCG level include blood and marrow transplantation and haemophilia services. The National Commissioning Group (NCG) commissions services on a national basis for a specific group of extremely rare conditions or very unusual treatments, mostly where the national caseload is less than 400 per year, e.g. heart and lung transplantation. Ministers make final decisions on the designation (and de-designation) of nationally commissioned specialized services, based on recommendations from the NCG and confirmed by the National Specialised Commissioning Group (NSCG), which is an advisory body overseeing the national commissioning function and facilitates collaborative working at a pan-SCG level. The NCG is a standing committee of the NSCG.

For the purpose of this book, the establishing and management of relationships with commissioners is best understood from the perspective of the provider as a large local teaching trust providing some areas of specialist patient care on a regional, national, and local basis. From the perspective of this type of hospital trust, the following key areas are crucial:

- How relationships are established and maintained with commissioners

- Who/what those commissioners are

- How commissioners are organized

- How their organizational arrangements impact on the relationship with the hospital

The difference between an NHS Trust and NHS Foundation Trust in relation to communications and relationships and the burgeoning world of marketing in the NHS influencing patient choice and maximizing income are both increasingly important.

NHS Foundation Trusts (FTs) are a new type of NHS organization, established as independent, not-for-profit public benefit corporations with accountability to their local communities rather than central government. FTs have greater freedoms and flexibilities than NHS Trusts in managing their affairs. FT status provides a means through which local people can officially become involved in the democratic process of influencing the provision of their health services. A comparison of non-Foundation and Foundation Trusts is shown in Table 43.1.

Types of commissioners and how they work

- Most commissioning or purchasing of NHS care is undertaken by PCTs.

- Some highly specialized services of high-cost and low-volume (e.g. heart and lung transplant) are purchased on a national basis by a National Specialist Commissioning Group.

- The commissioning of specialist services not commissioned by the NSCG have increasingly been handled by Specialist Commissioning Groups, which purchase care on a consortia basis on behalf of all the PCTs in that SHA, e.g. haemophilia services. The benefit for the management of specialized services with the emergence of SCGs is the single point of contact in each SHA rather than multiple contacts spread around PCTs.

◆ At local level, there has been relatively limited growth in services purchased by GP practices known as Practice Based Commissioning (PBC). The introduction of PBC enables GPs to purchase, for example, rehabilitation or diagnostic services from multiple providers not just their local hospital.

Table 43.1 Comparison of Foundation and non-Foundation NHS Trusts

NHS Foundation Trust	NHS Trust
Not directed by Government so has greater freedom to decide own strategy and the way services are run.	Directly responsible to the Government through the Department of Health and the Secretary of State.
Governed by a Board of Governors comprising people elected from and by the membership base drawn from patients, the public, and staff. The Board is more responsive to the needs and wishes of the local community.	Headed by a Board consisting of executive and non-executive directors, and chaired by a non-executive director. Non-executive directors are recruited by open advertisement.
Both are part of the NHS and exist to provide and develop healthcare services for NHS patients according to core NHS principles – free care, based on need and not ability to pay.	
Authorized, regulated, and overseen by Monitor, an independent regulator.	Authorized, regulated, and overseen by the Government, Department of Health, and the SHA.
Greater financial freedom to support the delivery and development of services. Freedom to retain financial surpluses and to borrow to invest in new and improved services for patients and service users. Freedom to access capital on the basis of affordability instead of centrally controlled allocations.	Limited financial freedom. Financial surpluses may not be retained for investment by the Trust. Capital investment is based on a system of centrally controlled allocations.
Accountable to the local community, Commissioners, Monitor, and Parliament. Freedom from Whitehall control and performance management by SHAs.	Accountable to SHAs, Central Government, and Parliament. Regular performance management by SHAs.
No requirement to agree and review an annual activity and performance plan.	Required to agree an annual (and quarterly reviewed) activity and performance plan with the SHA.
Both are inspected by the Care Quality Commission for compliance with healthcare standards and targets.	
Local flexibility to tailor new governance arrangements to individual circumstances.	Strict governance as laid out in the NHS statutory framework.
Clinical activity for private patients is strictly limited.	No limit on clinical activity for private patients, but provision of services should not prejudice the interests of NHS patients or disrupt NHS services.

National Service Frameworks (NSFs) and Care Networks (CNs)

The principal instruments through which commissioners are guided in what to commission from where are the National Service Frameworks, Care Networks, and a set of recently emergent service specification standards covering most, but not all, services.

- NSFs are directories of best practice and standards to be achieved by providers in delineated fields of service. NSFs do not exist for every type of health service but are directed by public health policy. Thus, there are NSFs for
  - children's services,
  - coronary heart disease, and
  - cancer;

  but not for, say, COPD.

  Commissioners require providers to adhere to and/or move towards the best practice as established in a NSF or service standard and to monitor and report regularly to them on a set of measures to demonstrate adherence to best practice, e.g. age-sex standardized admission rates for heart failure by PCT and SHA. Hospital Trusts are also subject to inspection and audit from external organizations nationally and locally, e.g.
  - a local coronary heart disease network will review activity and accessibility of rapid access chest pain clinics;
  - specialized cancer services networks are subject to national peer review process;
- Care Networks facilitate the progress of a patient's journey, providing a means of communication and collaboration between various agencies involved in their care management. This includes the NHS (primary, secondary, tertiary, and home care), social services, and local government. The aim is to provide a high quality of service to patients and carers by integrating service planning and delivery. Effective communication between the organizations involved is essential to ensure that policy and practice work together.

Service standards documents (e.g. September 2009 Paediatric Cardiac Surgery Services) are much more detailed than NSFs in detailing best practice.

The Annual Operating Framework and National Guidance

The industry of monitoring, reporting, and exchanging information between NHS sectors is augmented each year by the publication of an Annual Operating Framework outlining broad and detailed expectations of the NHS (e.g. every organization will have a pandemic flu emergency plan and will be set a detailed target on reducing hospital acquired infection). The contracts between purchasers and providers expect full adherence to national guidance in areas such as

- MRSA screening for elective admissions,
- reducing the numbers of mixed sex wards,
- achieving maximum wait time targets in A&E, and
- child protection.

Formal contract and negotiations

There is a current National Standard NHS Contract applicable to NHS Trusts and NHS Foundation Trusts. They are typically of three years length with each year's activity being negotiated in January and February. The negotiations are only partly about activity projections, income, and expenditure; an increasing amount of negotiations focus on performance reporting and targets relating to patient safety and the quality of care.

In *High Quality Care for All*, Lord Darzi, recent Minister for Health, defined quality of care as 'clinically effective, personal and safe' and concluded that publishing quality performance would help patients make informed choices about health care and allow clinical teams to benchmark their performance. The report is expected to inform the developing regulatory system for healthcare and as a result the Department of Health (DH) has introduced legislation, which requires NHS providers to publish annual Quality Accounts (QAs) to inform the public on the quality of care provided. QAs will improve public accountability and engage boards in understanding and improving quality.

Since 1 April 2009, a proportion (0.5%) of a provider organization's total NHS income is directly linked to an agreed set of performance targets for patient safety and quality. This proportion is heralded to increase over the years as part of a policy drive to link income to quality of care as much as volume of care. *High Quality Care for All* included a commitment to make a proportion of provider income conditional on quality and innovation, through the Commissioning for Quality and Innovation (CQUIN) payment framework. For local agreement, CQUIN schemes must cover

- safety,
- effectiveness (including clinical outcomes and patient reported outcomes),
- user experience (including timeliness of provision), and
- schemes for innovation and improvement as well as those indicators covering the DH's national priorities.

CQUIN is a welcome development in introducing a dialogue between purchaser and providers about the quality of care they provide rather than just the cost. Indeed, it is widely recognized that safe, high-quality care is less expensive.

Representatives of the hospital/provider will meet monthly with their host and other PCTs, under the terms of the contract to review

- activity, e.g. numbers of patients treated,
- expenditure, e.g. cost of treatment, cost of drugs excluded from the contract, and
- performance as measured by, e.g. achievement of waiting list targets.

That review may result in the hospital being required to draw up an action plan in response to failure to meet targets or achieve a required standard, e.g. patients not being seen within 4 hours in an accident and emergency department.

Each NHS Trust is also required to agree an annual activity and performance plan with its SHA, which is reviewed on a quarterly basis. The parties to the agreement have a mutual responsibility to respond to the health needs of their populations.

The annual activity and performance plan must ensure that activity, finance and workforce plans are consistent. The plan should include the following:

+ national priorities will be met,
+ local priorities are identified and met, and
+ plans are consistent with the agreed contract.

The parties work together to ensure that the Activity Plan is constructed, monitored, and reviewed to reflect changes in the distribution profile of activity and casemix, and the capacity requirements of national and local targets and standards. Within the Plan, demand management is shared (Commissioner manages external demand, Provider internal demand) so as to achieve the performance standards identified in the Commissioners' Commissioning Intentions. The Provider is required to review capacity and demand and ensure that all Services are provided to patients within the timeframe set out in the SLA.

For NHS Foundation Trusts, there is no requirement to agree such a plan with the SHA but instead has to with Monitor, the FT regulatory body, which issues a licence to operate. NHS Foundation Trusts can keep any financial surplus created unlike NHS Trusts, which have to return annual surpluses to their SHA.

Both Trusts and FTs are required to report various breaches or failures directly to the SHA within set timescales, e.g. Serious Untoward Incidents (SUIs) are required to be reported to both the SHA and PCT within 24 hours.

Service developments and new business

The emergence of NHS Foundation Trusts, coupled with Government policy on encouraging patient choice and a plurality of providers, has resulted in the growth of marketing in the NHS where organizations can now vie for custom and introduce new services to attract business providers, and are learning to advertise their services and also to deploy marketing skills in support of new services or delivery strategies such as the development of a primary angioplasty service (more popularly known as heart attack centres), or transfer of a clinic from a secondary to a primary care setting.

Providers must increasingly offer patients and referring clinicians more information about their services, thus facilitating informed decisions about care and treatment. Promotional activity providing information supplementary to existing national sources of intelligence (e.g. the NHS Choices website) is also a growth area with some health services using radio and public transport for advertising. Marketing may be seen as a misuse of resources intended for patient care but could be a way of realizing greater value from existing resources.

The DH understands the new need for self-promotion, but has also pointed out the risks. *The Code of Practice for the Promotion of NHS-Funded Services* (2008) highlights the importance of safeguards to protect referring clinicians, patients, and the public:

+ information patients receive must be accurate and not misleading, or damaging to the reputation of others,
+ the reputation of the NHS must be protected, and
+ expenditure on marketing must not be excessive.

It suggests a framework for self-regulation, aligning recommendations to the Advertising Codes administered by the Advertising Standards Authority (ASA).

Referral data from companies such as Dr Foster enables high-risk patients to be identified and targeted in a cost-effective way that makes them more likely to respond. For example, a campaign in Slough identified patients at high risk of diabetes (7% of the local population). Through direct targeting, the PCT saw a 164% increase in the early detection of diabetes in the first 3 months.

Metrics to evaluate the success of marketing and show the value of promotion to the wider NHS must be sought in the same way the commercial sector uses hard metrics (revenue, profit), soft qualitative metrics (loyalty, satisfaction), and value or perception metrics (brand awareness).

New service funding

The formal contract and national guidance allows for the introduction of new services but obtaining funding for them is not equally straightforward. Different PCTs across the country have very different views on what they will pay for. Similarly, PCTs may withhold payment for a drug or device if it has not received National Institute for Health and Clinical Excellence (NICE) approval. Commissioners and providers need to ensure that drugs or device usage is compliant with relevant NICE guidelines. However, 'pass through payments' exist to allow PCTs flexibility to make additional payments for care not yet approved but proven to be better than the equivalent funded through the national tariff, which may have longer term efficiency benefits, e.g. reducing the likelihood of repeating a procedure.

All PCTs have Exceptional Treatment Panels which can be applied to for special funding for a service (usually drug or device based) not routinely expected or funded.

Disagreements, disputes, and data queries

Alongside an almost endless stream of data flowing across the NHS has emerged a workforce of data analysts to query the veracity of such data and much of the communication traffic between providers and PCTs relates to this. Most data queries are dealt with quickly and easily but some result in disputes for which there are rules of arbitration but unless the stakes are significant, i.e. hundreds of thousands of pounds, most organizations will sort it out amicably. The need for resolution of such disputes is one of the main reasons to always maintain cordial relations between purchasers and providers.

Summary

The commissioning process promotes safe, high-quality care, a top priority of *High Quality Care for All*. Effective communication between purchasers and providers is absolutely vital to ensuring efficient and safe care delivery. Across the NHS over the last decade, capacity and investment have increased, service, and systems reform has been achieved through wide-ranging initiatives (e.g. 18-week maximum wait, patient choice). The next step will be to capitalize on the results of this reform and use the additional capacity to transform services to deliver high-quality care for patients in hospitals of their choice whilst demonstrating real value for money.

Further reading

Code of Conduct for Payment by Results, Department of Health, April, 2009.

National Service Framework for Long Term Conditions, Department of Health.

Marketing for Health Services: A Framework for Communication, Evaluation, and Rod Sheaff; *Total Quality Management.*

Leo Tolstoy. *War and Peace,* 1869.

World Class Commissioning – An Introduction, Department of Health, October, 2009.

Chapter 44

Healthcare networks

Angela Walsh

Key points

- Networks are a form of partnership arrangement that can support clinical staff working collaboratively across organizations.
- There are many types of networks, which may be based on client group, disease, specialty, or function.
- Clinical staff can be attracted to and engage with networks to gain experience in leadership and multi-disciplinary working as well as the delivery of projects across organizational boundaries.
- Communication in networks relies on having the right relationships with the right people and organizations. Networks support the 'let's fix it' approach.
- Networks are aimed at improving the quality, safety, and reliability of care.

Introduction

The NHS National Workforce Project programme describes clinical networks as 'linked groups of health professionals and organizations from primary, secondary and tertiary care, working in a co-ordinated manner, unconstrained by existing professional (and organizational) boundaries to ensure equitable provision of high-quality and clinically-effective services. They are "whole systems", partnership-based virtual organizations'.

Networks are based on the premise that working collaboratively with others can be more effective than working alone. Clinicians are attracted to networks because of their focus on specific clinical issues, many of which have been raised by clinicians themselves. Networks create a form of partnership, a way of linking up individuals, groups of professionals, and organizations to underpin working across and beyond traditional organizational and professional boundaries. Working as a strategic or collaborative alliance, networks can support delivery of common aims, projects, or work streams between or through organizations, which may even be in competition with each other. Good networks tend to be thin on tiers of management or hierarchy and have a degree of flexibility with the work they undertake. Being agile, they can respond quickly. This adds to the appeal for clinical staff.

Types of networks

Networks (Fig. 44.1) can be categorized in various ways, including by

- patient or client group,
- disease,
- service speciality, and
- function.

In a health care setting, networks might work across

- a clinical speciality such as cancer, diabetes, cardiac or critical care,
- primary, secondary, and tertiary care following particular patient care pathways,
- health, social, and voluntary services in a geographical locality, and
- a geographical region like an SHA or series of SHA regions.

Goodwin (2003) described a continuum of network forms:

- Informational networks
- Co-ordinated networks
- Managed networks.

The variation arises from the core roles the network undertakes, as well as the resource and infrastructure arrangement.

Informational networks

Informational networks have been described as the most common form of network with this model providing best practice guidance, policy, and strategy development.

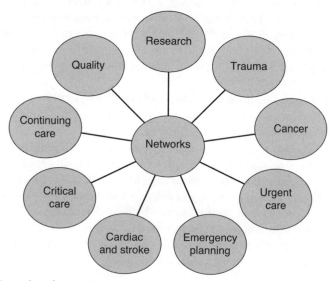

Fig. 44.1 Examples of networks.

Coordinated networks

Coordinated networks have developed greater integration between organizations though clinical and financial responsibilities have remained separated.

Managed clinical networks

Managed clinical networks have the most developed roles. These may include

+ managing demand for a service,

+ strategic and operational planning,

+ setting quality and safety standards,

+ monitoring the quality of a delivered service, and

+ performance management and audit.

Many networks have improving patient safety and clinical governance across the service as primary goals.

Networks: A case study

Critical care (intensive care and high dependency care) is a highly resource-intensive service, which is essential to underpin and enable a wide range of acute emergency and elective hospital services. It poses a commissioning challenge because

+ it is complex,

+ it is clinically far removed from primary care, and

+ its costs and benefits may be poorly understood by those outside the immediate field.

In response to well-publicized failures of service due to under-capacity, the DH commissioned a national review of critical care services. In addition, mounting evidence demonstrated that patients on acute wards frequently suffered preventable mortality and morbidity due to sub-optimal care. The main recommendation from these and subsequent assessments was that critical care services must be planned and delivered systematically across the whole health system.

To facilitate this, the establishment of clinical networks was proposed, which would

+ involve groups of Trusts,

+ work to common standards and protocols, and

+ take responsibility for all the critically ill in all specialties within a geographical area.

The North West London Critical Care Network is the only funded critical care network in London and covers both the NHS and independent sector including 17 Trusts and 8 independent hospitals plus the London Ambulance Service.

The network harnesses and channels tremendous goodwill, inspiration (as well as criticism of some existing service pathways) from clinical staff keen to collaborate across organizations and in partnership with commissioners to deliver critical care to appropriate patients more effectively.

Membership is via an annual membership fee and covers both PCTs and NHS/Independent Providers for which a range of functions and services are facilitated or provided. These include, for example

- An inter-organizational critical care transfer governance process and clinical review for all critical care patients arising in network organizations, which demonstrated a 50% reduction in clinical risk over 2 years. This is now being sought by Trusts in other parts of London and both North Central London and South West London sector commissioning agencies are considering the roll out.
- Supporting modelling/introduction of benchmark prices and organ supported currency for critical care using the DH pilot project to benchmark.
- Delivery of standardized guidance across the sector.
- Core expertise and clinical advice on all issues and guidance/best practice relating to critical care with rapid access to independent high level clinical expertise.
- Critical care specification for front-line ambulances being commissioned for delivery of anticipated increase in primary and secondary critical care patient transfers under service change initiatives.
- Development of quality standards and audit for critical care services.

The critical care network board has clinical/management representation from organizations within the network and is chaired by an acute Trust Chief Executive. There are two medical leads, a nurse lead, and an allied healthcare professional lead as well as established clinical groups including a medical forum, nurse practice development forum, physio forum, short-term task groups, and quarterly multi-disciplinary events, which bring acute commissioners and clinical staff together agreeing approaches to services and issues. A Network Director and project staff support the delivery of these initiatives.

Engagement in clinical networks

Networks provide many opportunities for clinical staff (including medical, nursing, therapists, and technicians) wanting to

- meet with peers, share emerging practice, develop guidelines, or negotiate a common approach to improving care,
- develop skills in delivering collaborative projects and in multi-disciplinary working,
- take a leadership role working in a broader environment than a single directorate or trust/organization, and
- develop strategic responses to local clinical service problems.

The right relationships and good communication

For networks to operate successfully, they are dependent on having the right relationships in place. These may be between

- individuals,
- groups of clinical staff,

- managers,
- patient/patient groups,
- health and non-health organizations,
- other networks, and
- any combination of these.

The relationships required depend upon the type and function of the network and may vary by work stream, project, or task. As in life generally, network relationships require good communication to be effective. Good communication within a network is dependent on the ease of access to the network for individuals, groups, or organizations. Having some central infrastructure as well as clarity about role and function supports this. For example, access may be via

- physical or virtual methods,
- engagement in network boards,
- steering groups,
- collaborative events,
- task groups,
- email groups,
- web sites, and
- using web or telephone based video links.

With little formal managerial authority networks also have to be transparent about who their constituents are, their relationship with them, and who they are trying to influence in any situation. 'We've taken that on board' is a common statement in management situations, but networks do not just want something taken on board, they want the super tanker to change direction. Communication of clinician-driven initiatives is a cornerstone in achieving this.

The approach that many clinical staff take when trying to communicate an idea or proposal for sharing or for action is to produce a document using a style of writing best suited for getting a research or a scientific paper published. These styles do not work generically, particularly where people have limited knowledge of the subject and are pressed for time. Things really do get lost in translation even when one might (not unreasonably) assume everyone speaks the same 'health' language.

Communicating effectively within and across a network can be easy so long as 'who, what, where, when, how and so what' are kept in mind.

The audience must be clearly identified:

- Who are they?
- What do they need to know?
- What do they need to understand?
- What will be their perspective (what is in it for them)?
- What is required from them in terms of action?
- Where are they located?

- When will they be targeted most successfully?
- How will they engage with the project in question?

The 'so what?' is needed to test whether the implications from the audience's perspective have been spelt out adequately. It is essential to highlight what is in it for them and make it clear. Short, well-signposted communication targeting existing mechanisms is essential and it may be necessary to meet people on their own territory to really engage them. A mixture of communication approaches need to be employed but it is important to observe a few fundamental principles:

- Written documents should use headings, numbered paragraphs, and clearly labelled figures/graphs/exhibits particularly when a paper or proposal is being discussed in meetings or groups.
- Setting out a map with points of reference to consider is helpful for complex issues.
- Specific decisions or actions being sought as well as key findings should be at the start of the paper together with its purpose and a short summary of the issues. Background and evidence or more findings can be provided later.

Effective communication within a network includes

- differently angled communications for different audiences about the same thing – one size may not fit all,
- feeding back progress, difficulties, and success,
- using data to demonstrate points,
- using different staff/contacts for different issues,
- ease of sharing/promotion,
- details of project, deliverables, service model, and pathways first, and
- leaving discussions about resources until after the principles have been agreed.

Clinical governance and improving patient safety across a network

Goodwin stated that 'Exercising management across (a network of) organisations brings special challenges because a manager cannot readily exercise direct authority ... success in managing networks requires that:

- effective collaboration is secured,
- the right assembly of resources is achieved,
- shared sense making is created amongst the people involved'.

A project delivered by the North West London Critical Care Network (NWLCCN) illustrates this. NWLCCN was set up to benchmark and enhance the quality and safety of critical care delivery across health organizations in the North West London area.

Example: 50% risk reduction in 12 months using a networked approach to critical care transfers

This particular project was initiated to quantify and tackle perceptions from clinical staff within the network hospitals that

◆ significant numbers of critically ill patients were undergoing critical care transfer for organizational reasons (no bed available, no staff available),

◆ escorting staff were inadequately trained in undertaking such transfers, and

◆ avoidable patient safety incidents were occurring.

Commissioning organizations were unaware of these perceptions or concerns.

The network core task group established for the project comprised three doctors from different Trusts, a nurse and the Network Director, though many others contributed views, information, and advice. A simple quality improvement method, 'PDSA' approach of plan, do, study, act was adopted and to this was added a clear overall aim: to reduce potential risk of harm to patients from critical care transfers (see Chapter 51). It was also agreed that measurement was required to demonstrate benefit or change.

Clinical context

The context for the work was that the transfer of critically ill patients is associated with patient safety incidents, increased morbidity, and mortality. Such risks may be tolerable when moving patients for specialist treatment, but a reduction of transfers for organizational (no bed, no staff) reasons would result in reduced risk exposure and reduce harm for patients and distress for their relatives.

Assessment of the problem and analysis of its causes

There was no record of transfer for these patients, so a transfer document to capture clinical and organizational data was developed by clinical staff and implemented across network organizations in a rollout programme. Critical care transfers across all 19 organizations were captured and audited using this documentation. Dynamic review of this data highlighted:

◆ Two-thirds of all transfers were found to be for *organizational* reasons rather than for clinical reasons.

◆ Escorting staff were inadequately educated on issues surrounding critical care transfers.

◆ There was poor transfer preparation of patients and staff.

◆ There was inconsistent involvement of *senior* clinicians in decisions to transfer patients and inadequate escalation of problems encountered to senior management.

Strategy for change

The network task group proposed a multifaceted solution with implementation initially planned over a 2-year period. This included

- scripts presenting data *and* solution proposals developed for various audiences,
- the profile of critical care transfers was raised by targeting presentations and reports to existing local management and clinical meetings within hospitals, with healthcare funding organizations – PCTs and with the strategic health authority,
- collation of hospital-specific transfer data, reported quarterly and annually, then every month with data summary targeted at junior and senior clinical and managerial staff, including capture and reporting of safety incidents during transfers,
- development of a transfer training faculty using staff from all Network hospitals with a designated network transfer lead in each hospital,
- adaptation and implementation of a critical care transfer training course developed by a Practice Development Officer from the military services,
- local, national and international presentations, lectures, and publications.

Measurement of improvement

Dynamic analysis of data from the transfer documentation was performed and all staff attending the new training course were issued with questionnaires.

Effects of changes

As a result of implementation and subsequent refinements,

- the number of transfers between hospitals for organizational (lack of bed, staff) rather than clinical reasons *decreased* by 50% (see Table 44.1),
- 100% of the 164 responding staff attending the initial training courses felt it would improve the standard of subsequent transfers in which they were involved,
- analysis of delays arising during transfers, physiological changes, escorting staff experience, and developing trends was now possible,
- all documented critical care transfers are now subjected to senior clinical review and subjective experience suggests that the standard of transfers has increased, and
- two other London sectors have now adopted the same critical care documentation and audit.

Table 44.1 Numbers of transfers between hospitals for organizational reasons in North West London

Critical care transfers	Year 1 No. of transfers	Year 2 No. of transfers	%age change between years
Total non-clinical (no bed, no staff, or no kit)	274	138	–50%

Lessons learnt

◆ The project quantified perceived 'sub-standard' practice and provided the evidence to challenge the status quo.

◆ The network developed and implemented the strategy collaboratively across all network hospitals to improve practice using *clinical* and management mechanisms and data at junior *and* senior level.

◆ Changing behaviours required high-quality data and feedback reporting.

◆ Change arose from empowering individuals (with information, data, and network wide messages) to challenge local assumptions and behaviours.

◆ Economy of scale was achieved in terms of collaborative effort, standardization of approach, audit, and response.

◆ Subsequent change is also being audited and acquired information utilized to influence future strategy.

◆ Improved patient safety within a specified clinical area.

◆ Created a benchmark model that could be applied to a diversity of 'patient-risk' situations.

The project worked because it mattered to all those involved and especially patients. The aim was to improve patient safety and reduce risk of harm. The concerns identified were clinical, and clinicians developed the response. It was easy to get engagement because those who understood and experienced the problems derived and implemented the response. Response alone by one organization would have been much more difficult; the project gave a critical mass to the work. An economy of scale and effort was achieved and other benefits arose as a consequence.

Summary

Key principles for clinical networks are summarized below:

◆ MCNs must be managed with clear structures and lines of responsibility. A clinician or a clinical manager should take a lead role with clear responsibilities for core team members.

◆ The purpose of the networks is to improve patient care in terms of quality, access, convenience, and co-ordination.

◆ Work undertaken must be evidence-based. Networks support research and continuous professional development.

◆ Outcomes must be measured and audit is an integral part of network activity.

◆ A quality assurance programme is necessary for all clinical networks.

◆ Each network should produce a written annual report that is made available to the public.

◆ Networks must be multi-disciplinary and multi-professional. A properly functioning network needs appropriately trained clinicians with adequate facilities, working in partnership. Training and continuing professional development (CPD) should be an integral part of the networks.

◆ Patients must be involved in the network and each network must have a policy on disseminating information.

Further reading

Fraser, S.W. (2008). *Undressing the Elephant, Why Good Practice Doesn't Spread In Healthcare.* Sarah Fraser/Lulu Publishing.

Sun Tzu. *The Art of War.* 6th century Chinese military treatise.

Howarth, A. ed. (2005). *Networks Briefing: Key Lessons for Network Management in Healthcare.* NHS Service Development Organisation Programme.

Chapter 45

Trust Boards structure, responsibilities, and communication

Nick Coleman

Key points

- Boards have overall responsibility for Trust activities with a focus on future direction, operational boundaries, values, and outcomes.
- Boards function by establishing committees to deal with pieces of work, each with specific tasks and delegated powers. The main committees are: audit; remuneration and terms of service; clinical governance; risk management; and (for PCTs) the Professional Executive Committee.
- Boards lead the Trust. To be effective, they rely on excellent communication: the directors need to understand what is going on in the Trust; and their directions and decisions need to be understood by all in the Trust.
- The worst failings in Trusts invariably include failures in Board communications and operation. If Boards and their committees do not work properly then patient safety is compromised.

Introduction

NHS Trusts were established in the 1990s with governance frameworks modelled on private sector organizations. This included each Trust having a Board with overall responsibility for future direction, the boundaries within which the Trust operates, its values, and its results. How Boards themselves operate, including roles of directors and committee structures, were also modelled on the private sector. For example, all Trust Boards have a non-executive chair and equal numbers of executive and non-executive directors (NEDs), giving an overall majority of non-executives. There is no distinction between the Board duties of executive and non-executive directors: they have shared accountability for the direction and control of the Trust and are equal in law.

As with the private sector, there is a fundamental distinction between the Board and the Executive. For a Board to do its job and add value to a Trust, it must

- be disciplined in sticking to the highest-level issues it is accountable for,

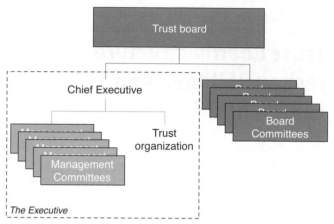

Fig. 45.1 NHS Trust Board Structure.

- deal with them efficiently,
- not do the Executive's job, and
- not become an excessive burden on the Executive.

    The distinction also applies to the directors:

- The executive directors are accountable for Trust operations (so having inherent conflict of roles).
- The non-executive directors (NEDs) are independent (not part-time members of the executive team).

    The distinction also applies to committees: Boards may delegate tasks and powers to board committees, which are different from committees in the executive structure. For example, the Remuneration and Terms of Service board committee is composed entirely of non-executive directors because it sets the employment terms and salaries of the top executives.

The role of NHS Boards

The duty of an NHS Board is to add value to the organization, enabling it to deliver healthcare and health improvement within the law without causing patient harm. It does this by providing a framework of effective governance within which the organization can thrive and grow.

    Within this overall duty, NHS Boards are expected to focus on the following:

- *Direction*: setting the Trust's strategic objectives and ensuring human and financial resources are available for delivery,
- *Values*: setting and maintaining the organization's values or '*how we do things here*',
- *Boundaries*: setting the boundaries within which the Trust should operate. This is achieved via a framework of controls that enable Trust activities to be delivered

effectively and in compliance with external requirements while risks are assessed and managed. In other words, *'how the organisation is wired'*. Controls can be

a. 'hard', such as policy, rules, standards, and prescribed processes,

b. 'soft', which include organizational culture, ethics, commitment, and leadership of the Board, effective communication, appropriate incentives, and adequate training,

♦ *Results*: reviewing management performance

a. Is the Trust achieving its objectives in both non-financial and financial terms?

b. Are the required values and standards working?

c. Are the controls operating as intended?

If Trust Boards are to deliver on these areas, there must be clear and direct communication channels – both upward from the frontline of the Trust to the Board, and downwards from the Board to the frontline staff.

Committee structures

To assist in discharging their duties, Boards delegate tasks and powers to committees and sub-committees, and hire advisers. They can set up as many committees and sub-committees as they wish, but best practice is to have the minimum number of permanent committees. The essential areas these must cover are:

♦ Audit

♦ Remuneration and Terms of Service

♦ Clinical governance

♦ Risk management

♦ (for PCTs) The Professional Executive Committee

If the Board has particular issues to deal with, it may establish temporary committees to focus on, for example, investment during a major capital project.

♦ *Audit*: Every NHS organization must have an Audit Committee reporting to the Board with responsibility for ensuring effective internal control, i.e. making sure the internal controls and processes are working as intended to minimize risk. A tension often exists in Trusts:

• The most important matters are clinical and patient safety processes and controls; but

• audit is traditionally a field of financial systems, financial information, and compliance with the law.

Therefore it is important to maintain a proper balance between non-financial and financial audit. The Audit Committee needs to ensure that these responsibilities are either addressed directly, or through a carefully designed sub committee structure. Through its scrutiny and reports, the Audit Committee enables the Board to have confidence in control systems. Membership of the Audit Committee is restricted to NEDs – executive directors being conflicted.

♦ *Remuneration and Terms of Service*: Every NHS organization must have a Remuneration and Terms of Service Committee reporting to the Board. Its task is to advise the Board about appropriate remuneration and terms of service for the Chief Executive and other senior executive staff. Membership of the Remuneration Committee is restricted to NEDs – executive directors being conflicted.

- *Clinical governance*: All Trusts must have a Clinical Governance Committee, usually a committee of the Board (though for PCTs, it is a Committee of the PEC, reporting to the Board through the PEC). Its task is to focus on the systems in place to ensure, monitor, and improve the quality and safety of healthcare provided for patients. Membership of the Clinical Governance Committee does not have to include a NED, but often does because this is such an important area of activity, which impacts on the work of the Audit Committee.

- *Risk management*: All NHS organizations must manage risks to the organization's activities. A risk is an event that, should it occur, would result in material damage, e.g. by harming patients, or by threatening the Trust's ability to provide healthcare in future as a result of reputation damage. Risks lie in all areas:
  - Clinical
  - Quality of care
  - Financial
  - Staff related.

The Risk Management Committee must ensure that the Trust manages risks effectively by

    (a) constantly tracking and responding to emerging risks,

    (b) maintaining a clear action plan to reduce the likelihood of risk events occurring,

    (c) ensuring mitigation plans are present to minimize the impact should a risk event occur.

Various ways to organize the Board's risk management activities exist.

It can be included in the Audit Committee's business or it can be incorporated into a joint clinical governance and risk management committee. The key output is the report of the top 10 or 20 most significant risks to the Board to assist in understanding the key threats to the organization and the controls and contingencies in place to manage them. The Risk Management Committee does not have to include a NED, but often does because this is such an important activity which impacts on the work of the Audit Committee.

- *Professional Executive Committee (PEC)*: All PCTs have a Professional Executive Committee (PEC) as a Board sub-committee. The PEC focuses on:
  - clinical change,
  - clinical engagement,
  - interfacing with acute sector clinician partners,
  - ensuring the PCT has a whole-systems approach to care,
  - delivery of the clinical agenda,
  - health improvement.

The PEC brings together clinical and managerial perspectives and takes a leading role in these functions on behalf of the PCT. The PEC is also responsible to the Board for the Clinical Governance and Risk Management systems of the PCT. Particularly important to PCT Boards and PECs are communication and reporting arrangements necessary to fulfil its governance and accountability obligations.

Foundation Trusts will also have a Nominations Committee, and may need to establish a dedicated Investment Committee.

Effective board communications

All Boards need systematic reporting and monitoring, which keep them informed

- of progress towards their objectives (non-financial and financial),
- on whether the required values are effectively in place,
- on whether controls are operating as intended,
- on whether threats to the Trust's achievement of objectives (i.e. 'risks') are being recognized, assessed, and managed by the executive.

Boards only meet occasionally (usually monthly), and all NEDs are part-time. So to achieve all this and be effective, Boards and their committees depend on having intelligently prepared information, which needs to be focused on the right issues, in the right level of detail, and presented clearly.

Directors need a sound understanding of how the Trust operates and what its activities are. For NEDs, this is difficult since most come from non-clinical backgrounds. Therefore, information feeds to the Board need to include general briefings and immersions to build the NEDs' understanding, as well as sharply focused Board papers.

Finally, communication with Boards and their committees is two-way. As well as putting directors in a position to be effective and make full use of their expertise, the best Trusts have a clear and uncluttered flow of information on Board decisions back into the organization, so that their directions and decisions are understood by staff and it operates as a coherent unit.

Board papers

It is easier to prepare a long Board paper, which includes everything than to produce a short one intelligently distilled into essential points. The latter is a test of the author's real understanding of the matter.

Strategic information for the Board should

- be structured in the context of specific strategic goals,
- provide objective context such as performance trends in clinical and safety indicators, clinical quality, patient experience, finance, and business development,
- set out relevant forecasts and anticipate future performance issues, and
- encourage an external focus – looking at the Trust from the outside.

Operational performance information should

- provide an accurate, balanced picture of current and recent performance including clinical, financial, regulatory, and patient perspectives,

- Focus on the most important measures of performance highlighting exceptions and variance analysis,
- Be appropriately standardized to take account for factors which affect outcomes, e.g. the age and deprivation profile of patients,
- Compare the Trust with peer organizations' performance – benchmarking.

All information should

- be clearly and simply presented, including graphs and narrative,
- be up to date,
- direct Board attention to key issues – significant risks, issues and exceptions; and
- provide the right detail for the Board to understand the issue.

  It also helps to distinguish between

- issues which need to be reported routinely at a certain level of detail,
- issues which need to be reported only if there is a demonstrable problem, e.g. where performance significantly deviates from peer Trusts, and
- issues which change slowly and only require review on a quarterly or six-monthly basis.

  And it can help to distinguish between

- items which are for information only,
- items which are for decision, and
- items which are for discussion.

When it goes wrong

Common problems with communications to Boards and their committees include

- poor agendas,
- long unfocused papers,
- too many committees,
- committees debating issues outside their remit,
- too many people present, and
- the executive spending too much time servicing the committees.

  At a more substantive level, there can be governance problems such as

- unclear, overlapping accountabilities,
- conflicts of interest,
- lack of clarity on which directors are independent, and
- cultural and behavioural factors interfering with effective Board operations.

  The most severe Board failures can best be illustrated by looking at some major Trust breakdowns. Whenever there is a major safety incident in the NHS, the subsequent inquiry's report invariably includes a section on where the communications with the Board contributed to the incident.

Maidstone and Tunbridge Wells NHS Trust

The Healthcare Commission's report[1] concluded that, relating to the Trust's Board and infection control:

- 'Prior to the outbreak [the Board] only monitored the MRSA rate, as that was a priority to which a target for performance was attached.
- The Board considered the annual report on control of infection as a retrospective document rather than a prospective planning framework,
- Although a specific case of *C. difficile* was brought to ... the Board ... and a review promised, there was no follow up when this did not happen,
- The chief executive controlled the information that went to the Board,
- The second outbreak was declared on 12 April 2006 but it was not discussed by the Board in public until 25 July 2006,
- Following the declaration of the outbreak .... an immediate action plan to tackle issues was not taken to the Board,
- The Board had considered ... infection control from time to time ... but did not have a presentation from the infection control team, even during the second outbreak,
- For an organisation claiming to focus on the safety of patients ... the Board did not receive a paper on the mandatory hygiene code in the autumn of 2006, nor the gap analysis and action plan for compliance with the code until March 2007, when the code had been introduced in October 2006,
- When three new non-executive directors took up post in mid-2006 ... no basic induction on infection control and their role in its assurance, was organised. ... an expectation that the individuals would pick it up ... . two had no experience of health services,
- The information presented to the Board on the outbreak of C. difficile and infection control was often incomplete or inaccurate, leaving non-executives at a disadvantage'.

Stoke Mandeville Hospital, Buckinghamshire Hospitals NHS Trust

The Healthcare Commission report[2] concluded that, relating to the Trust's management of clinical risk and decisions by the Board:

- 'The structure established to bring clinical risk to the Board obstructed the flow of appropriate information to the Board,
- Although many issues required consideration and resolution at a strategic level, they were not discussed at the governance committee or by the Board,

---

[1] © 2007 Commission for Healthcare Audit and Inspection
[2] © 2006 Commission for Healthcare Audit and Inspection

- The main purpose of the reporting of incidents had been missed, as weaknesses in the underlying systems and broader strategic issues were not identified and resolved at the highest levels of the Trust. This was a significant failing,
- The Trust did not act as though a key part of its responsibility was the management of risk,
- In the context of the first and second outbreaks of *C. difficile*, the Trust did not appear to act on the principle that risks should be identified and appropriate changes implemented to protect the interests of patients,
- ... the members of the Board, sitting as the finance performance and information committee, heard about the pressures that the hospital was under, but decided to continue to pursue the Government's target for a maximum wait of four hours in A&E,
- There was no evidence of any discussion of the outbreaks by the Board in public until after the outbreaks had been reported in the national press.'

Summary

Trust Boards are responsible for future direction, the boundaries within which the Trust operates, its values, and its results. Under all of these ensuring patient safety within the organization must be the focus. Boards need to ensure that they receive all relevant information on performance, quality, and safety and that their decisions are transparent and clearly communicated to Trust staff. Setting a clear direction for the organization as well as establishing sound values and aims will ensure that an appropriate culture is developed which puts patients first.

Further reading

Governing the NHS: A guide for NHS Boards. DH NHS Appointments Commission, June 2003.

The Intelligent Board. Dr Foster, February 2006.

Healthcare Commission: Investigation into outbreaks of *Clostridium difficile* at Maidstone and Tunbridge Wells NHS Trust, October 2007.

Healthcare Commission: Investigation into outbreaks of *Clostridium difficile* at Stoke Mandeville Hospital, Buckinghamshire Hospitals NHS Trust, July 2006.

Chapter 46

Communication with staff

Robert Craig

Key points

- Typically hospitals are large organizations with thousands of staff: effective communication is a challenge.
- Poor communication has been identified as the cause for many organizational failures, particularly in relation to patient safety.
- Effective communication is vital to ensure that key messages are delivered to the relevant audience whether this is 'routine' organizational information or specific messages related to particular issues.
- Communication can be through formal structures such as committees or through informal routes, which reflect the organization's culture.
- The keys to effective communication are consistency, reinforcement, and multiple approaches: person-to-person, 'grapevine', electronic, formal letters, memos or minutes and through posters, alerts, and presentations.
- Training in communication can be effective for various professional groups including use of tools such as SBAR for both managerial and clinical staff.

Introduction

How do you recognize a good safety culture? What does it look like and what are its characteristics? Most commentators agree that an 'open' culture in an organization lies at the heart of a strong focus on and a good track record in patient safety; openness, for example, in

- incident reporting and investigation,
- willingness to challenge and be challenged about current and best practice, and
- good communication between and within staff groups and across the boundaries between clinical and managerial staff.

If good communication is an important piece of the patient safety jigsaw, how do organizations improve and maintain their communication? How do they identify communication problems and solve them? Isn't good communication just common sense and professional courtesy?

Walk into any hospital on any day and one could hear a phrase like 'I never hear anything: communication is terrible here' several times over. Why? Are all hospitals just equally dreadful at keeping staff informed and fostering good communication, or is it very hard to do so consistently well at the level that modern healthcare organizations require? While walking round that same hospital, one might also overhear a conversation between senior staff (whether managers or clinicians) bemoaning the fact that news of who did what to whom at the last Christmas party spreads like wildfire, yet Mr Bloggs' severe penicillin allergy seems to remain a closely guarded secret kept from many of those who need to know.

It's a cliché, but like most clichés, it's true: hospitals are large, complex organizations. In fact, most NHS Trusts would be large enough to be quoted in the FTSE 250 and it's worth remembering that such scale in hospitals is generally concentrated on one or two big sites, not (like most FTSE 250 companies) spread through multiple branches and locations across the country, or even overseas. What's more, hospitals are very 'people-driven' enterprises. Typically (and not only in the United Kingdom) a hospital's salary bill accounts for around 70% of its operating costs, significantly higher than large organizations in other sectors. Not only then are hospitals large institutions, but they employ large numbers of people for their size, and it's not hard to see why: they're open 24 hours per day, 7 days per week, every week of every year. Typically, that means three staffing shifts per day or, in some departments, 'in-hours' staff backed up by skeleton staffing or 'on-call' arrangements out-of-hours. Just to maintain its continuous services, hospitals employ thousands of people, a local general hospital might have 5,000 or more staff on its books: a small town in its own right, with all the internal communities, loyalties, and rivalries that implies.

And if they never close, there is no opportunity to take stock (or even draw breath, it seems), no annual shut-down, no two-week break when everything is closed, when staff and managers can take time to address problems and ensure solutions are worked though, tested, and refined before being implemented. Instead, every change and development has to be built into or grafted onto a working organization, with all the inherent risks that suggests. The lack of 'down-time' and continuous activity means that communication must be effective at every level all the time, whether the message is about an organizational issue (e.g. introduction of a new clinical service, the results of an external assessment, implementation of a policy) or a specific message pertaining to patient safety (such as how chest drains are to be inserted or how to ensure correct patient identification). Communication takes a variety of forms, from formal processes of committees and reports, to informal social interactions within professional groups and amongst colleagues.

Formal communication

Hospitals are complex organizations with a life and character of their own, and communication will not work well if left to chance, common sense, and professional courtesy. Ensuring that everyone who needs to know information does so, that they get it when they need it and that they know whom they need to pass it to or how to respond, takes time, commitment, and resources. Public sector organizations are often criticized for a 'meetings' culture, where nothing can be done without first calling a meeting (or several), setting up a working party and reporting to a higher authority for permission to proceed or to ask for resources. Hospitals are not immune from such charges, but in an environment reliant on so many different people of every discipline, skill, and background, meetings are an essential, if unlovely, part of working life if, and only if, they are managed well. Formal meetings can be categorized in four types:

- Team-based
  - Communicating with closest working colleagues
- Project-based
  - Coordinating service changes and developments
- Topic-based
  - e.g. patient safety
- 'Cascade'
  - News and updates on organizational initiatives
  - Reports/directives and presentations

Team- (or department-) based meetings (e.g. for theatre staff or a heart failure service) need to be regular and sufficiently frequent (no less than monthly) to promote and maintain cohesion and a sense of teamwork. They should be led by the team leader or manager, and include information internal to the team – changes in personnel and working arrangements being obvious examples – as well as news from the rest of the organization, particularly from services with which the team works closely.

Project-based meetings (e.g. for the development of a new service) will be led by the project manager and depend on the nature and progress of the project itself. In its early phases, frequency will be greater as the purpose, objectives, and resources of the project are established, debated, and refined, as members of the project team are introduced and as tasks are assigned. Once the project plan is in place, a regular pattern of meetings is important to maintain focus and monitor progress. As the project nears completion, more frequent meetings will be needed to ensure no 'loose-ends' remain and to ensure implementation, including communication of the project's implications, runs to plan.

Topic-based meetings (e.g. review of NICE guidance) will typically bring colleagues from across the organization together on an established, regular pattern to review, e.g. Medicines Management, Patient Safety, or Financial Performance. Members usually either bring relevant expertise to the group, or represent a group of colleagues, or both. Topic-based groups will often formulate or inform policy and advise senior managers of the organization's performance in that regard, recommending action and deployment of resources.

'Cascade' meetings are a means by which corporate messages can be passed into the organization and (in theory) feedback received. A regular brief (e.g. from the Chief Executive's office or the Board) will be passed out to senior managers and included in every team-based meeting, cascading down through the organization; at the same sessions, feedback received on the previous briefing can be gathered and passed back 'up the line'. Their effectiveness depends on good coordination of team meetings, so that

messages pass through an organization quickly; and on evidence that the 'feedback loop' works, and that reactions to the 'corporate' message are heard and understood. Feedback is important to demonstrate the extent to which communication channels are open and working, e.g. to show the impact of a top-down drive to reduce the numbers of operations cancelled after a patient's admission, mandating changes in process in order to improve patient's experience of their treatment.

Of course, every meeting takes time away from front-line services, multiplied according to the number of people involved in each one. What's more, there will, and should, be overlap between them: Team meetings will pass on not only the 'cascade' messages, but also the deliberations of topic-based groups and the work of project groups. Whether they know it or not, hospitals commit vast resources to communication of this sort, the key to its success is how well that time is used. Effective 'cascade' meetings need to

- be regular and reliable – same time, same place,
- be well-attended – wide-appeal information staff won't want to miss,
- be punchy – concise, well-crafted news items, and
- encourage feedback and pass it on.

Increasingly external organizations and regulators look for evidence that both internal and external communication is or has been effective, e.g. reporting serious untoward incidents to Commissioners, ensuring alerts, e.g. from the NPSA have been circulated to identified individuals. Systematic approaches to communication of this type must be developed, implemented, and monitored.

Communication does not have to be face-to-face but it helps: research at the National Training Laboratories in the United States shows that of what we learn, we retain approximately:

10% of what we read; but
50% of what we see and hear

However, electronic communication is quicker and cheaper. Internal e-mail and intranet systems provide the perfect platform for many forms of information for example

- alerts which require rapid dissemination (such as drug recalls),
- advice on when to go and get flu vaccinations, and
- information about educational opportunities or guest speakers, which need to reach a wide audience.

Computers, whether desktop, laptop, or hand-held, can be useful notice boards via screen savers or start-up messages (but they need to change frequently in order to maintain users' attention). Clearly e-mail only works if staff access their accounts regularly; whilst administrative staff and managers may spend much of their time at a desk, clinicians rarely do, and so it is important to understand how e-mail users function, e.g. it may be better to e-mail or send a copy to a consultant's secretary asking him or her to draw the relevant individual's attention to the information. However, if a laboratory wants to highlight abnormal test results then direct person-to-person communication via telephone is more likely to be effective, particularly if prompt action is required, e.g. to recall a patient. In addition, there is a tendency for staff to ignore or delete emails, which are sent to large groups (e.g. "all users") on the basis that if the information is important and specific to them, they will be notified by other means. At times a formal letter is the only way to ensure that a particular individual receives a key piece of information. The challenge in the twenty-first century is how to ensure, among the deluge of electronic information washing over us every day, that the right information is received and understood at the right time.

Informal communication

The relative speed with which the news from the Christmas party and the news of Mr Bloggs' allergy spread throughout a hospital show that to rely solely on formal communication methods is likely to be only part of a successful story. Informal methods, particularly those which reinforce the formal messages and methods, are an essential part of the armoury.

Experience suggests that identifying and working the 'informal channels' is at least as important as the formal messages themselves. Every organization has its opinion-formers and leaders who play no part in the formal management structure, but who are enormously influential in shaping organizational culture, leading staff reactions to developments, and assessing the impact of new or proposed initiatives. Those leading projects, or seeking to implement change, will always be well-advised to find these informal leaders, gauge their views, and engage their support for the cause. At the very least, talking ideas through with one of their number will avoid outright opposition when it meets the light of day; at best, it will get active support from a key ally at the right time. How to identify those people? There's only one way: getting to know the place and keeping your ear to the ground.

Techniques for ensuring effective communication

Whilst much communication will be of the informal type it is important to consider how to optimize transmission of the key message and this can be done in a planned way with more formal communication methods. Clearly any message must be framed to suit the group(s) to whom it is directed at in terms of language and presentation but also a well-structured message is more likely to succeed whether the communication occurs in a meeting or a part of an 'all users' e-mail. The key steps are outlined in Box 1.

Taking time to frame the message correctly and focusing on the issue in hand will help to ensure that it is clear to recipients what they need to do with the information received. Often key messages are lost in a sea of extraneous information, which detracts from or obscures what is required. It is vital to decide if the message is

- providing information or
- an instruction to which a response is required.

Furthermore, the way the message is communicated can affect its impact – thoughtful use of a wide range of communication methods (verbal, written, and pictorial) significantly contributes to the success or failure of a particular message. Some messages benefit from being delivered more than once in a variety of ways, e.g. a combination of e-mail, posters, and use of a screen saver to promote good hand hygiene practice.

Box 1 Key steps in structuring an effective message

- **Prepare**
  - What is relevant to the message to be delivered?
- **Précis**
  - Distil – reduce word count to the minimum necessary to provide the key information
- **Prioritize**
  - Put the most important elements first
- **Big Hits**
  - Ensure that critical information is highlighted
- **Big Picture**
  - Set the context and boundaries for the message
- **Relevant Detail**
  - Only include information which is pertinent to the issue being communicated

---

Some specific communication tools are being introduced into the health service having been successful in other industries. The SBAR tool (Situation, Background, Assessment, Recommendation) was developed in the US nuclear submarine industry to ensure that communication was focused on getting key information across and an appropriate response obtained. It is being promoted to facilitate communication between clinical staff about patients but increasingly is being used by managers to provide updates to senior staff on particular projects or initiatives. Whilst many believe that good communication is the result of common sense and professional courtesy, experience shows that many patient safety incidents and organizational failures result

Managerial problem	Clinical problem
Situation Patients waiting too long for admission **Background** Breaching national standards; worsening performance **Assessment** Poor use of capacity and scheduling **Recommendation** Review scheduling arrangements and capacity utilization	**Situation** Patient is breathless with increasing work of respiration **Background** Previous history of spontaneous pneumothorax in an otherwise well person **Assessment** Saturations are 85% in air, pulse rate 110 sinus rhythm CXR shows a left pneumothorax **Recommendation** Requires review and chest drain insertion in the next 15 minutes

from poor communication. Timing and content is fundamental to ensuring that staff get the right message at the right time and know how to respond.

Small is beautiful

All of this suggests that large hospitals will always struggle to ensure effective communications. There is no doubt that smaller hospitals should perform better in this regard than larger ones. On a human level, we will always respond better to 'John in Haematology', someone we acknowledge in the corridor, than the anonymous on-call Biomedical Scientist whom we're never likely to speak to again. Evidence from the United States suggests an optimum size of hospital for patient safety purposes as between 250 and 450 beds, large enough to support resources dedicated to patient safety, but not so large that there are too many layers in the management structure, too many 'links' in the chain of command for effective action to follow whenever a lever is pulled at the top of the organization. This last point is a direct consequence of the communications challenge: with the best – and clearest – will in the world, a long chain of command will inevitably allow messages to become diluted and other priorities to cloud the original objective. Smaller hospitals enjoy the benefit of decisions being made much closer to where they need to have an effect and should be able to use this to everyone's benefit: patients and staff.

Summary

Hospitals offer a multitude of challenges for effective communication, but good communication is possible when it is recognized that the challenge needs time, commitment, and resources; when formal processes and structures exist and are used effectively; and, particularly, when the importance of informal communication channels is recognized and exploited.

Further reading

Leonard, M., Bonacum, D., Taggart, B. (2006). *Using SBAR to Improve Communication Between Caregivers.* Institute for Healthcare Improvement.

Leonard, M. (2006). The SBAR technique: Improving verbal communication and teamwork in clinical care. *PONL Bulletin,* **2**(1).

Leonard, M., Graham, S., Bonacum, D. (2004). The human factor: The critical importance of teamwork and communication in providing self care. *Qual Saf Heath Care 2004,* **13**: i85–i90.

Maison, D. (2006). The interdisciplinary team perspective. Effective communications are more important than ever, a physician's perspective. *Home Healthcare Nurse,* **24**(3).

Chapter 47

Communication between patients and healthcare staff

Elizabeth Haxby

Key points

◆ Effective communication is fundamental to the provision of good healthcare and to ensure a true partnership between patients and healthcare staff.

◆ Communication of complex information requires time and skill, and failures of communication between patients and healthcare staff are a common cause for complaints.

◆ All patients have a right to receive information in a way that they can understand in order to make decisions about their health and treatment.

◆ Good communication is particularly important when seeking consent for interventional procedures and when 'Being open' if something has gone wrong during the care process.

◆ Effective communication includes the duty of confidentiality to protect information imparted during a consultation.

Introduction

Effective communication is fundamental to the provision of healthcare and ensures that patients are equal partners in making decisions about their health and treatment. The definition of communication includes both imparting information as well as receiving it. In the past there has been much emphasis on training healthcare staff to impart information and very little on ensuring that they assess how much the patient has received or understood. The paternalistic approach in which the healthcare professional decides how much information he or she is going to disclose regardless of patient needs or desire for information is now changing in recognition of the fact that it is the patient who should decide how much information they would like in order to make an informed decision. There are three key areas that need to be covered in this chapter:

◆ Informed consent

◆ 'Being open' when things have gone wrong

◆ Confidentiality.

The latter is included because it is very important that healthcare staff recognize their duty of confidentiality and know what information may or may not be disclosed or communicated to a third party without the patient's permission.

Consent

Consent is a patient's agreement for a healthcare professional to provide care and it is fundamental in any interaction between healthcare providers and patients. The need for patient consent stems from two considerations;

- *Ethical*: Every adult of sound mind has a right to determine what shall be done to his own body (Kant).
- *Legal*: Under the Law of Tort touching a person without their consent constitutes a trespass and doing anything to them might be construed as a battery.

A number of documents and publications are available from the General Medical Council, British Medical Association, and the Department of Health, which set out the legal and ethical frameworks in more detail and emphasize the importance of communication in the consent process. In particular the GMC document 'Consent; patients and doctors making decisions together' states '... *you should see getting their consent as an important part of the process of discussion and decision-making...*'.

There are three elements to consent, which must be fulfilled for the consent to be valid:

- The patient must have capacity to give consent.
- The patient must make a voluntary decision.
- The consent must be informed.

This chapter on communication will focus on the subject of informed consent. However, for the sake of completeness the other important principles relating to consent are set out in Box 47.2. It is important to emphasize that consent is required for any interaction between patient and healthcare professional:

- This may be implicit in relation to the provision of routine healthcare, e.g. blood pressure measurement.
- For interventional procedures that carry significant risk, express consent is required.

The communication aspects of seeking consent lie in relation to

- the description of the procedure,
- the disclosure of intended benefits and any potential risks,
- the availability of alternative therapies, and
- the impact of not having the treatment.

Clearly the discussion should take place in an appropriate environment, which is private and quiet although this may not be possible in an emergency. The patient may require support in terms of a relative or someone from the PALS team may be suitable. It is important that the information is given in a way that the patient can understand including the use of interpreters, translations, pictures, audio tapes, and written material as required. The aim of the discussion is to assist the patient in coming to a decision and therefore needs to focus on providing answers to their questions and giving them time to think things through. Patients will be variably informed about their illness and the treatment options with some having detailed knowledge gleaned from the internet and various types of literature and others having no knowledge at all beyond the most basic understanding. Communication must be tailored in each case to ensure the patient has the information they need to make their own decision.

Disclosure

In terms of deciding what information should be disclosed, there has been a historical debate between providing minimal information and telling the patient about every minor and remote risk. In the 2008 publication, the GMC advises that *'in deciding how much information to share with patients you should take account of their wishes. The information you share should be in proportion to the nature of their condition, the complexity of the proposed investigation or treatment and the seriousness of any potential side effects, complications or other risks'*.

The GMC advises that basic information should be included as set out in Box 47.1. As a general rule patients should be informed

- of any significant risk which is likely to occur with a 1% incidence or greater, e.g. wound infections, failure of the procedure, etc.,
- of the risk of death or neurological injury however remote, e.g. neurological complications of epidural analgesia. Whilst it would be fairly easy to construe that any intervention might possibly result in death, it is important to remember that the disclosure must be 'proportionate' to the risk, however it is the patient who decides

---

Box 47.1

- Diagnosis and prognosis
- Any uncertainties about the diagnosis or prognosis including options for further investigation or not to treat
- Purpose of proposed investigation or treatment
- Whether a treatment is part of a research project or an innovative treatment programme
- Who will be involved in/responsible for the provision of care
- The right to seek a second opinion
- Any bills the patient may have to pay
- Any conflicts of interest the practitioner or organization may have
- Any treatments that may be available elsewhere which may be of greater potential benefit than those which can be provided in your organization

if he/she wants to run that risk not the doctor. Historically, much of what is disclosed has been based on the 'reasonable patient test', i.e. what would a reasonable person in these circumstances wish to know? Research has shown that this is not a very useful approach since all patients are individuals and their needs, attitudes, and values will vary. This reiterates the need to communicate effectively with each individual patient and come to a joint decision,

♦ of the healthcare professionals' own outcomes for a particular procedure, e.g. deaths after CABG or revisions of hip replacements where available,

♦ of unit and national figures, which may also be useful but it is important to balance the risk of confusing the patient with lots of figures against providing them with comprehensive information,

♦ of the scope of what the patient is being asked to consent to; is it a clearly defined procedure or is the diagnosis uncertain and an exploratory procedure is to be undertaken which may have a number of different outcomes?

Risk must be explained using unambiguous terms. Clear and consistent language must be used and efforts made to ensure the patient has understood.

♦ Terms such as 'high risk', 'low risk', 'rare', and 'possible' do not have clear definitions and caution should be exercised when using them.

♦ Verbal descriptions may also be interpreted differently; 'likely' may mean 60% to some and 90% to others.

♦ Numbers are appealing since they are supposedly easily understood and compared although a certain level of numeracy is required.

Both doctors and patients have difficulty understanding statistical information and so often a combination of qualitative and quantitative information is most helpful. Healthcare professionals must not make assumptions about a patient's understanding or the importance they attach to certain outcomes.

The final part of the consent process is to check the patient has understood the information they have been given and to what they have consented. This can be done in a number of ways using open ended questions such as 'can you tell me what the key points of our discussion are?' rather than 'have you understood everything ?' to which a patient will almost invariably say 'yes' since they do not wish to appear foolish. A period of time between the consultation and the procedure is beneficial since it allows the patient to go away and think about what they have been told and pose further questions if clarification is needed. Claims may arise on the basis of 'failure to warn' so it is vital that the healthcare professional ensures that any important information relating to risks of complications has been fully understood.

Occasionally patients indicate that they do not wish to receive information concerning risks of a procedure particularly relating to mortality or major complications. This is mostly due to fear and anxiety and it is important to explore this with the patient. It is always important to explain that the patient is being asked to make a decision based on the balance of risks, i.e. the short-term risk of the intervention versus the long-term risk of the disease or impairment. Finally, research indicates that patients retain approximately 7% of the content of a consultation and so the benefits of providing

Box 47.2 Principles of consent

- The individual who is intending to carry out a particular procedure on a patient is responsible for ensuring that informed consent has been obtained although the seeking of consent may be delegated to another individual provided they have been trained and are subject to audit.
- Under the Mental Capacity Act 2005, all adults are assumed to have capacity to give consent unless otherwise demonstrated.
- Written consent is not a legal requirement but is advisable for any procedure which involves significant risk (DoH).
- There are particular requirements for consent in relation to research, screening, children, and testing for serious communicable diseases.
- There is no time limitation on consent, which is enduring unless the patient's condition or the nature of the procedure have changed to the extent that the potential risks and benefits have also changed.
- In an emergency interventions necessary to save life may be carried out without consent.

written information to support what was discussed cannot be overemphasized. This is covered in more detail in the chapter on patient information (Chapter 40).

'Being open'

There is extensive research to support the fact that approximately 10% of patients suffer some sort of harm as a direct result of their healthcare and in roughly 50% of cases this is preventable. When things go wrong, it is very important for healthcare staff to be open and honest with the patient and/or their family about what has happened. These are often very difficult conversations and staff need to know how to manage them effectively and sympathetically. Professional bodies (Box 47.3) are quite clear that staff have a duty of candour to disclose information about the event including

- describing what has gone wrong,
- offering an explanation, and
- expressing regret at the outcome.

Box 47.3 General Medical Council guide to good medical practice

'If a patient under your care has suffered serious harm, through misadventure or for any other reason, you should act immediately to put matters right, if that is possible. You should explain fully to the patient what has happened and the likely long and short-term effects. When appropriate, you should offer an apology.'

Box 47.4 The NHS litigation authority guidance 2002

'It seems to us that it is both natural and desirable for those involved in treatment which produces an adverse result, for whatever reason, to sympathize with the patient or the patient's relatives and to express sorrow or regret at the outcome. Such expressions of regret would not normally constitute an admission of liability, either in part or in full, and it is not our policy to prohibit them, nor to dispute any payment, under any scheme, solely on the grounds of such an expression of regret.'

In the past, healthcare staff and organizations failed to recognize the needs of patients and their families in these circumstances and often explanations were inadequate. Frustration at this type of response led to complaints and litigation. Surveys of patients' views on this reveal that they wish to receive an apology and an explanation and this is in preference to the desire to punish those involved or receive financial compensation. In addition, staff are anxious about giving an apology lest that be interpreted as an admission of liability (Box 47.4).

The NPSA in its 'Being open' Publication in 2006 established the principles that healthcare staff should observe when dealing with the aftermath of a patient safety incident;

1. Acknowledge that something has gone wrong
2. Provide truthful, timely, and clear communication with the patient/family
3. Offer an apology about what has happened
4. Recognize patient and/or carer expectations
5. Provide professional support for staff
6. Engage with risk management processes to ensure systems improvement
7. Recognize that there is multidisciplinary responsibility and avoid blaming individuals
8. Maintain the confidentiality of all those involved
9. Establish how future care or remedy will be provided

Effective and timely communication is key. The initial conversation may occur shortly after a safety incident has occurred when all the facts are not yet available and the full extent of harm unknown. It is vital to plan the communication with the patient/relatives in a systematic way and ensure that it is clear who will be able to provide information and when. One way of planning and structuring the communication is set out in Box 47.5.

Confidentiality

Doctors are under a duty to respect patient confidentiality for two reasons:
- Information about a person's health is a private matter.
- If there is no assurance information will be kept confidential patients may not disclose information which is significant in relation to diagnosis and treatment.

Box 47.5 The 'Being open' process

Initiating the 'Being open' process

- Establish the facts with the clinical team
- Agree who will meet with the patient/family
- *Plan what you will say*

The initial discussion

- Meet with the patient/family
- Be honest and give them the facts – do not speculate
- Apologize/express regret
- Answer their questions truthfully
- Outline what will happen next
- Agree the time/trigger for further meetings if necessary

Documentation

- Ensure all discussions are documented in the notes
- Record the date and time, who was present, what was said and agreed
- Ensure other staff are informed on a 'need to know basis'

The Data Protection Act 1998 sets out how personal data must be stored and processed sensitively and usually release of any health-related information pertaining to a particular individual requires the consent of that individual. The DH Confidentiality Code of Practice sets out the requirements of healthcare organizations in relation to management of confidential information and the BMA and GMC set out the relevant ethical issues. The duty of confidentiality is not absolute and there are clearly defined circumstances when the public interest in information disclosure outweighs that of protecting an individual's confidentiality, for example, the reporting of notifiable diseases, prevention of terrorism, detection of crime, or as directed by a court.

The principles of good medical practice in relation to confidentiality as set out by the GMC are shown in Box 47.6. In 1997 a review of the use of patient-identifiable information (PID) in the NHS was chaired by Dame Fiona Caldicott and published by the DH. This review laid out 6 principles as follows:

1. Justify the purpose for which information is required.

2. Do not use PID unless absolutely necessary.

3. Use the minimum necessary PID.

4. Access to PID should be on a 'need to know basis'.

5. Everyone with access to PID should be aware of their responsibilities.

6. Understand and comply with the law.

Box 47.6 Confidentiality

If a doctor is asked to provide information about a patient to a third party he must

- inform the patient about the disclosure or ensure they have already received information about it,
- anonymize data where unidentifiable data will serve the purpose,
- be satisfied that patients know about disclosure necessary to provide their care, e.g. clinical audit and that they know they can object, and
- seek patients express consent for disclosure where identifiable data is required for any purpose other than healthcare except as directed by the law.

The incompetent, children, and the deceased

Incompetent adults are also owed a duty of confidentiality but due to the need for others to be involved in their care treatment, information will have to be disclosed in certain circumstances when 'essential' to their medical interests. Children are entitled to confidentiality in respect of certain areas of information such as medical records. For young children clearly providing appropriate information to the parents is appropriate but for children who are competent to understand the nature of the information and do not wish it to be disclosed then this must be respected. The ethical duty of confidentiality also continues after a patients' death and any request to keep certain information confidential by a patient before their death must be respected. In the absence of such a direction before releasing information the following should be considered:

- Whether the information would cause distress or benefit to family members
- Whether disclosure would in effect disclose information about the family or other third party
- Whether the information is already in the public domain or could be anonymized
- The purpose of the disclosure.

Summary

Effective communication with patients is fundamental to good healthcare. Key areas include the consent process, being open when things have gone wrong, and respecting patient confidentiality. Failures in communication are common causes of complaints and claims. Healthcare staff must ensure that they are familiar with legislation and national guidance on management of patient identifiable information and ensure that disclosures can be justified and consent obtained wherever possible.

Further reading

Department of Health (2003). Confidentiality: NHS Code of Practice. http://www.dh.gov.uk/en/Publicationsandstatistics/Publications/PublicationsPolicyAndGuidance/DH_4069253.

General Medical Council (2006). Good Medical Practice. http://www.gmc-uk.org/guidance/good_medical_practice/index.asp.

National Patient Safety Agency (2006). 'Being open': communicating patient safety incidents with patients and their carers. http://www.npsa.nhs.uk/nrls/improvingpatientsafety/patient-safety-tools-and-guidance/beingopen/.

Section 8

Fundamental principles

Doctors no longer work in isolation, but as part of a healthcare team delivering increasingly complex integrated care. This section examines the responsibilities that doctors have, both individually and in teams (*Accountability, safety, and professionalism*). The functioning of healthcare teams is examined (*Team working*), and the nature of team leadership explained (*Leadership*). Finally, how the many teams within a healthcare structure function together, and form the identity of the hospital or healthcare delivery system, are explained (*Safety, systems, complexity and resilience*).

Dr Kieran Sweeney sadly died from mesothelioma on Christmas Eve 2009. Whilst writing the chapter on complex systems in this section Kieran had known that it was likely to be published posthumously. An obituary detailing his extensive work, and effect upon others, was published in the *BMJ* on February 8th 2010.

Chapter 48

Accountability, safety, and professionalism

Edwin Borman

Key points

♦ Accountability confirms that doctors provide safe care for patients. Openness regarding quality of care contributes to the trust in, and status of, the medical profession.

♦ Accountability is structured in layers. Doctors are accountable to their patients, their colleagues, their employers, and to regulatory authorities for the safety and quality of their practice.

♦ Accountability is an evolving concept. It varies according to the expectations of patients and of society, and according to the development of professional standards and regulatory methodologies.

♦ Accountability need not always hurt but, on some occasions, it may have to. For most doctors accountability systems confirm the good quality of their practice; however, such systems also should identify doctors who are having problems with their performance.

♦ Accountability is a key component of the regulation of the medical profession. Accountability in doctors' working lives fulfills a necessary condition for the recognition of their professionalism.

Introduction

The 1990s in the United Kingdom saw a series of high-profile medical 'scandals' following which the medical profession's ability to regulate itself has been challenged repeatedly. In order to maintain trust in the profession, society increasingly requires doctors not only to practise in a professional manner, but also to demonstrate the quality and safety of their clinical performance.

Accountability is one component of the complex systems now required for the regulation of the medical profession. Regulation determines how doctors fulfil their responsibilities to patients, society, and to their profession. Regulatory bodies set the standards that are expected of doctors, and the mechanisms to attain them. Accountability provides a means by which doctors can confirm that they are achieving these standards.

This accountability is essential to maintain the considerable trust that is invested in doctors. As events have demonstrated, trust is not a static phenomenon, nor is accountability. As society changes, so expectations of the profession change. Accordingly, professional responsibilities must evolve, in order to demonstrate that individual doctors, and the medical profession as a whole, recognize the privilege of medical practice and continue to justify that trust.

While some doctors may feel that the status of the medical profession has fallen, most recognize that it is a considerable privilege to practise as a doctor. Even following the 'scandals' of the 1990s, individual patients, and society as a whole, readily entrust doctors with their lives, and repeatedly confirm that doctors fulfil that trust. As a result of this – whether measured financially, in status, or in power – from an objective perspective, the medical profession still enjoys considerable privileges.

The first safety net: Individual accountability

Everyone has a personal ethos that determines their interaction with society. In the case of doctors, this ethos significantly determines how they practise their profession.

To a large extent, people regulate themselves, and tend only to be consciously aware of this in unusual circumstances; most of the time it is implicit. Given the demanding nature of modern medicine, the fact that doctors are only rarely conscious of accessing their personal ethos demonstrates how ingrained and effective it is.

This 'conscience' develops through a variety of means: in families, at school, and at university. Given this variety, it is remarkable that, for doctors, there is so much convergence between their personal professional ethos and the collective professional ethos. While that convergence can be considered to be a measure of the success of the ethical education process, it is likely that most doctors rely on a combination of learning methods: from implicit learning, by watching role models, to attending formal didactic lectures, to reading documents on the standards and ethics of practice.

All doctors have a duty to develop their personal ethos and, further, to ensure that it continues to develop. Not all of what is considered appropriate now to the medical profession will be in 50 years time.

Until recently the dominant model for stating the standards and ethics of practice followed the 'Thou shalt not' model; defining what a doctor must not do. That has shifted to a more positive statement of professional duties, that set out more clearly what doctors should be doing, as well as what they must not.

'The Duties of a Doctor', the opening section of 'Good Medical Practice', the key guidance document provided by the General Medical Council (GMC), emphasizes these responsibilities. Doctors must not act in an unprofessional manner *and* they must practise in accordance with high standards.

This change in emphasis recognizes the change in expectations of doctors by society. No longer is it acceptable simply not to be a bad doctor, it also is expected that a doctor should be a good doctor. As every doctor is required to follow this guidance, with time, a more rounded form of personal professional ethos should develop.

For most doctors, who practise safe, good quality medicine, individual accountability should be little more than showing that they are practising in accordance with expected standards. However, for a relatively small number, individual accountability will mean the recognition that they should improve, or will be required to.

What happens if a doctor transgresses the 'thou shalt not' parts of their professional standards? In most cases, their own sense of personal or professional conscience will fulfil the necessary act of 'self-policing'. However, should that not occur, it will be necessary for other parts of the 'accountability layers' to intervene.

Ideally, problems should be identified early, limiting the potential consequences for patients and for the doctor, and permitting the greatest opportunity for remediation. Occasionally however, more serious problems, or failure to respond to justified concerns, will necessitate regulatory intervention.

As an example, consider a doctor who has alcoholism. This is likely to affect clinical performance, either through the acute effects of inebriation, or through the longer term effects on the doctor's health. There certainly is sufficient societal and professional consensus that it is unacceptable for a doctor to practise under such circumstances. Most doctors understand this, and would limit their alcohol intake to socially acceptable amounts that would not affect their ability to practise.

Only a small proportion will not adhere to these standards. Of these, a number, through some form of prompting, will recognize that they have a problem and will alter their behaviour, or seek help from one of a range of support groups. Both are examples of remediation through individual regulation. However, a small number may not be able to alter their behaviour and will fall through this first safety net of individual accountability.

The second safety net: Accountability in teams

Modern medical practice is reliant upon doctors and other healthcare professionals working in teams to deliver care. Within teams, doctors can perform more complex interventions, provide more comprehensive treatment, and achieve better outcomes.

Clearly, this benefits patients, but it also benefits doctors. Doctors no longer practice in isolation. All doctors know, or certainly should, that they work alongside colleagues who contribute skills and abilities that support and complement their own.

Doctors are also being encouraged to work more effectively with other healthcare team members, with particular focus on patient safety and good communication. Good team-working is particularly important in healthcare, as the teams within which doctors work change frequently.

One example is the World Health Organization's 'Safe Surgery Saves Lives' campaign, in which all members of the theatre team take responsibility for ensuring that specific safety checks are made. This has the added benefit of binding the team more closely together.

Another example is in Emergency Medicine where, using the principles of Team Resource Management, each team member is designated a specific task, and is required to confirm out loud when this has been completed.

These examples also provide the opportunity to consider those doctors who do not want to be good 'team players'. While it is unusual for a doctor to be deficient in only one aspect of their performance, some may even be 'excellent clinicians' who reject the benefits of working co-operatively with colleagues. As healthcare becomes more complex and more reliant on multi-disciplinary interaction, dysfunction of an individual within a team will become ever more evident.

Increasingly, there are national initiatives that define standards required of the team, not just of the individual practitioner. Medical Royal Colleges provide templates for team audit projects, and Trust Clinical Governance departments expect these to be applied, and the results acted on. All doctors already are, or soon will be, familiar with their clinical performance being commented on by colleagues, as part of the annual assessment of their practice, through multi-disciplinary 360° appraisal.

Every doctor has a duty, when working within a team, to ensure that their own clinical performance, and that of other members of the team, is of an appropriately high standard, and to work together towards the best possible result for each patient.

To date, this team ethos has received relatively little attention, but recent developments are changing this. The GMC now requires doctors to address concerns they may have with the performance of another team member. Thus, when doctors work in teams, not only do they have a duty to *not* to 'look the other way', they are required to act on a concern that may impair the quality of patient care.

In the example of the doctor who has alcoholism, each team member who works with this doctor should act by raising their concerns with a more senior colleague, or by themselves discussing this problem with the individual. While this may lead to initial discomfort, such action is more likely to result in early remediation, addressing a potential problem before it becomes a significant one.

On some occasions, however, regulation through this second safety net – of accountability as a member of a team – may fail, and more significant intervention may be required.

The third safety net: Accountability within the workplace

Most doctors in the United Kingdom are employed, or have quasi-employed status. However, unlike most employees, doctors make decisions that, to a significant extent, determine the nature, quality, safety, and cost of the services they provide.

Doctors justify this unusual position by referring to their level of qualification, and to their professionalism, which necessitates putting their patients' needs first. However, doctors also have a duty to recognize the consequences of their decisions, not only for their own patients, but also for the organization within which they work, and for the NHS as a whole.

The introduction in the NHS, during the 1980s, of clinical management, was a major step by employers to developing some level of financial control in a service that, until then, had been relatively unaccountable for its expenditure of public money. This initiative also provided the opportunity for hospital managers to exercise greater scrutiny of their most qualified and high-spending employees.

Since then, more and more methods of reviewing clinical practice, and of ensuring accountability, have been introduced within the workplace. The implementation of many of these has been resisted by the medical profession, as it perceives these changes as an erosion of its power, and their imposition as an unnecessary, and unwanted, distraction from the 'real business' of patient care.

These arguments increasingly have been refuted by evidence collected by doctors themselves, of the incidence of clinical adverse events, the improvements that can be achieved by the adherence to and more rapid implementation of guidelines for best practice, and also differences between units, even when justifiable statistical corrections are made, in patient care, outcomes, and costs.

In short, it is doctors themselves who are showing that patient care can be improved by more rigorous clinical management. Most recognize this, and support the implementation of clinical governance systems incorporating audit and adverse events monitoring.

However, more work needs to be done to persuade all doctors of the additional benefits of an annual appraisal. Perhaps it is because appraisal is a contractual responsibility that doctors feel this way; a requirement, together with a senior colleague, to review their practice.

What many consider an unnecessary burden, and some perceive as a threat, in reality can be an opportunity. Appraisal provides a format openly to demonstrate the high quality of a doctor's work and continuing professional development, and also to promote the services they provide for their patients.

The clinical governance systems that progressively have been introduced in the medical workplace may also help to identify, perhaps at an earlier stage than otherwise would have been the case, the small number of doctors who have problems with their practice.

This may apply in the case of the fictitious doctor with alcoholism who, at appraisal, may request help, or who might have difficulties with clinical performance sufficiently serious to require specific review. Should the problem reach this stage, it is important that the Medical Director (or equivalent) is involved. Whilst intoxication on duty contractually is a disciplinary offence, in most cases employers recognize the medical needs of a doctor who has alcoholism, and will balance their actions by encouraging, or requiring remedial interventions. Should this doctor pose a risk to patients, or not respond to remedial support, the Medical Director would be required to ensure further referral, to the National Clinical Assessment Service (NCAS) or the GMC.

The fourth safety net: Regulatory accountability

National Regulatory Bodies, such as the GMC, are responsible for

- confirming that doctors are registered to practice,
- ensuring appropriate standards for medical education,
- determining the standards and ethics for medical practice, and
- acting when a doctor's fitness to practice may be impaired.

In the case of the GMC, all of these powers are provided by statutory authority that permits interventions ranging from simple advice to the withdrawal of a doctor's practice privileges.

While problems of fitness to practice attract much media attention, the number of cases requiring a GMC hearing is relatively small, approximately 360 per year, given that there are approximately 226,000 registered doctors. This bias in media attention means that other aspects of the GMC's work largely go unnoticed.

In 1999 the GMC determined that 'every doctor, on a regular basis, should be able to demonstrate their continuing fitness to practice'. This decision committed the GMC to implementing a system of revalidation, and all doctors engaged in active clinical practice to comply with this new requirement.

After more than a decade, repeated interventions from Government, and many changes to the GMC's proposals, it is likely that revalidation will be introduced by 2011. It is intended that, rather than a 'one-off' assessment, revalidation will be a continuous process. This increased accountability and openness will be a major demonstration of a new form of medical professionalism.

In order to maintain the support of doctors, who do not want to be overburdened with conflicting requirements or an excessive bureaucracy, it is essential that revalidation is informed by evidence that can easily be collected in the workplace. Quite reasonably, doctors do not want to have to jump through meaningless hoops, or have to comply with assessment tools that have not been validated.

The GMC plans that a more rigorous form of appraisal will provide the essential information for revalidation. Additional evidence will probably be required, most likely from multi-source feedback, in which patients, colleagues, and managers will be invited to comment on a doctor's performance (360° appraisal).

The primary intention of revalidation is to confirm that doctors are practising to suitably high standards. It is also hoped that the more regular scrutiny of all doctors should help to identify, at an earlier stage, the small number who have problems.

Rapid communication has made medicine international, a necessary development given that rapid transport has globalized the spread of illness. However, it also requires regulation to become more international.

Through the revalidation process, or following a formal referral to the GMC, the fictitious doctor with an alcohol problem may find his fitness to practice under scrutiny. In such cases, the GMC has an approach that can be described as support with firmness. The doctor is required to have a psychological assessment, to make commitments to abstain from alcohol, and to comply with treatment. Should the doctor not adhere to these requirements, the GMC will restrict or withdraw the doctor's practice privileges.

Were the GMC to restrict the registration of this fictitious doctor, mechanisms should exist to ensure that, if the doctor were registered to practice in other countries, those Regulatory Bodies would be alerted.

Summary

Doctors, like most people, understandably have concerns when invited to demonstrate greater openness and accountability regarding their performance at work. In the United Kingdom it is clear that society increasingly expects greater accountability from those who serve the public, whether they are Members of Parliament or doctors working in the NHS.

Rather than being perceived as threatening, greater openness and accountability will allow most doctors to demonstrate the good quality of the work they do, and to confirm their continuing fitness to practice. Improved mechanisms of accountability will, in the small minority of doctors who have problems, permit earlier identification, thereby increasing patient safety. In addition, through earlier referral, this should improve the opportunities for remediation, which would be of benefit for doctors.

Further reading

'Good Medical Practice' (2007). General Medical Council. www.gmc-uk.org.

'Budapest Declaration on Ensuring the Quality of Medical Care' (2006). UEMS, www.uems.net.

'Portugal Agreement' (2007). Healthcare Professionals Crossing Borders, www.hpcb.eu.

'Safe Surgery Saves Lives' (2009). World Health Organization, www.who.int/patientsafety/safesurgery/en.

Chapter 49

Team working

Allan Goldman and Guy Hirst

Key points

- Effective teams have been shown to improve safety and outcomes for patients and staff.
- The fundamental requirement of a team is that all members share a common goal.
- The dynamics and function of a team are very different from those of a group.
- Team Resource Management involves accepting that individuals will make errors, and organizing the group to avoid, trap, and mitigate the consequences of those errors.
- Non-technical skills (NOTECHS) are increasingly recognized as being vital in healthcare teams.

Introduction

Historically in healthcare the concept of teamwork has not been high on the agenda. The acquisition of the skills required to be a team member or a team leader have not been considered as important as the technical skills required by healthcare professionals. As in other safety-critical industries, awareness of understanding human interaction is now accepted as being instrumental in developing a safe culture. Team working is at the core of developing such a culture. The fundamental of a team is that all members share the same common goal, and in healthcare that common goal must be delivering the best outcomes for patients.

Evidence suggests that the following benefits to patients are achieved by effective team work:

- Reduced patient mortality (hospitals with 60% of staff in functional teams reduced mortality by 5%)
- Reduced errors contributing to improved performance
- Reduced patient time in hospital (demonstrably saving more money than the cost of running the teams)
- Reduced sickness rates for doctors
- Improved service provision through streamlining services
- Improved patient satisfaction

◆ Improved decision-making
◆ Improved staff motivation and well-being:
  • 35% of staff in no teams reported above threshold stress levels
  • 30% of staff in loose teams or groups reported above threshold stress levels
  • 21% of staff in real teams reported above threshold stress levels
Effective teams have improved patient outcomes, reduced hospital stay and cost, with the added benefit of staff having a good day at the office!

The history of teamworking

The emergence of the team approach can be traced back to the classic Hawthorne Studies conducted in the 1920s and early 1930s. These involved a series of research activities to examine what happened to a group of workers under various conditions. Analysis suggested that the most significant factor was the building of a sense of group identity, a feeling of social support and cohesion that came with increased worker interaction. Elton Mayo, one of the original researchers, identified certain critical conditions for developing an effective work team:

◆ The manager had a personal interest in each person's achievements.
◆ He took pride in the record of the group.
◆ He helped the group work together to set its own conditions of work.
◆ He faithfully posted the feedback on performance.
◆ The group took pride in its own achievement and had the satisfaction of outsiders showing interest in what they did.
◆ The group did not feel they were being pressured to change.
◆ Before changes were made, the group was consulted.
◆ The group developed a sense of confidence and candor.

These conditions could still be used to judge the effectiveness of a team today.

Teams and groups

It is almost impossible to differentiate leadership from team working. It takes a leader to galvanize a group of people into a team with a focus. However, team working should be distinguished from group working.

Healthcare workers often think that they work in teams, but analysis by team inventory reveals that they actually work in groups (Table 49.1).

The difference can be summarized as follows:

◆ *Group working* involves individuals coming together to perform a task or achieve a target.
◆ *Team working* involves a broader vision requiring a leader able to develop that vision with the team and to use all the talents of the team to achieve the objective.

Table 49.1 Differences between a team and a group

Team	Group
Decision by consensus	Decisions often not made
Disagreements discussed and resolved	Unresolved disagreements
Objectives well understood and agreed by members	Objectives often not agreed
All members contribute ideas	Personal feelings often hidden
Frequent team self examination	Discussions avoided regarding group functioning
Members understand their roles	Individuals protect their roles
Share leadership on as-needed basis	Leadership appointed

Especially, team working depends upon the ability of all members of the team to put the team's needs above their own individual interests. Members must also fill in for others in the team who lack skills or need help, and work flexibly between skill domains to achieve the agreed objective. Conflicting opinions are to be expected and the process of resolution enhances the strength of the team. Openness and honesty are also essential.

Team leaders

It is difficult to define what qualities make an effective leader. Dick Vermeil, one of the most successful American Football coaches in history, made the following points about good team leaders. They:

◆ provide clear vision for the team,

◆ hire the right people,

◆ build relationships,

◆ bring energy to the team, not suck energy,

◆ delegate and define responsibility,

◆ engender honesty and integrity,

◆ lead by example showing that hard work never loses its value, and

◆ create an atmosphere where people enjoy working and are proud of their results and being part of that team.

The NHS is acknowledged to be the third largest employer in the world. The sheer size and complexity of the organization means that team working in healthcare in the UK is inherently problematic. The somewhat amorphous structure means that team structures and interfaces are often indistinct and constantly changing. As we have evolved to more supra-specialized care, and with the implementation of the European Working Time Directive, the number of teams, and interfaces between teams, has mushroomed (Fig. 49.1). On many occasions, the Chief Medical Officer has commented

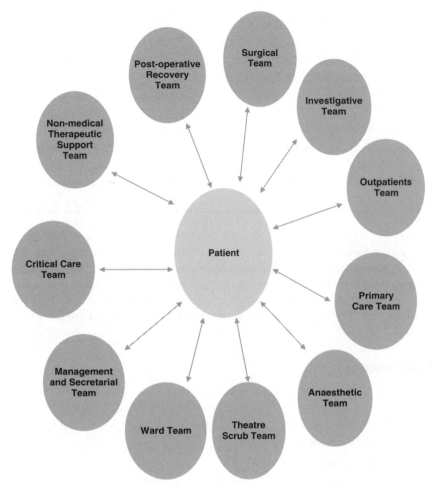

Fig. 49.1 Multiple teams in NHS.
Reproduced from *The Leadership and Management of Surgical Teams*, The Royal College of Surgeons of England 2007, with permission.

that healthcare must learn from other safety critical industries, in particular in the areas of team working and leadership.

Team resource management

As a result of some spectacular accidents (e.g. the 737 at Kegworth and Space Shuttle Columbia), and heroic recoveries (e.g. the Hero of the Hudson US1549) in other high risk industries, it is now understood that there is no substitute for effective and practical teamwork training. In aviation, this training has been developed over the last 30 years and is now into its fifth generation. The original focus was on error *avoidance*, which is a worthy goal but also an impossible one. Subsequently, academics concluded that the overarching justification for such training should be error *management*. Following Professor James Reason's groundbreaking work on human error in the 1990s, the latest training is based upon the premise that human error is ubiquitous and inevitable, but is also a valuable source of information. Given that error is inevitable, teamwork training principles can be seen as a set of error countermeasures with three lines of defence.

Defence No 1: AVOID
Defence No 2: TRAP THE ERROR
Defence No 3: MITIGATE THE CONSEQUENCES

The ideal team understands these principles, develops appropriate strategies, and trains for them. It is crucial that in large organizations, such as teaching hospitals, consistency of training in ever-changing teams ocurrs. In similarly large commercial aviation companies the flight crews seldom fly together, but by developing training protocols, routines and Standard Operating Procedures (SOPs), these obstacles have been overcome.

Many 'safety critical industries' have introduced a variety of resource management training programmes. Although medicine is probably more complex, and patients more idiosyncratic than aircraft, ships, or power stations, they do share a critical similarity in that they all rely on effective multi-professional teamwork, and effective communication in highly stressful and fluctuating environments.

Medical practice is also particularly challenging as critical decision-making is often made on the basis of incomplete evidence. Nonetheless, other safety critical industries have learned the 'hard way' about the introduction of human factors training and the development of the skills needed to cope with these challenges during the last 25 years. By learning from their experience, there may be an opportunity to shorten that journey in healthcare.

Senior airline crews put up considerable opposition to the introduction of resource management training in aviation. They felt it called into question their technical ability, and the way they had always conducted themselves, and managed their on-board team. However, this training developed in spite of such opposition, and these new 'softer skills' are now accepted as being as important as the technical skills, and as such should be taught from recruitment to retirement to all personnel who are part of the operational division of an airline. This realization is now gaining traction in healthcare.

A teamworking framework

In order for resource management training to be mandated in the airline industry, the teaching and the vocabulary had to be formalized. Objective frameworks to measure the effectiveness of human interaction were developed. The essential skills were divided into two domains, cognitive and social. The initial research developed for use in aviation was called the NOTECHS (Non-technical skills) system. The EC Directorate General of Energy and Transport, and the Civil Aviation Authorities of France, Netherlands, Germany, and the United Kingdom sponsored the NOTECHS project, which ran from March 1997 to March 1998. The central goal of the project was to provide a feasible and efficient method of assessing an individual pilot's non-technical skills in a multi-crew environment.

The NOTECHS behavioural marker system describes human interaction in four main categories:

1. Situational awareness

2. Decision making

3. Leadership

4. Teamworking

The first two skills are cognitive, whereas the second two are social.

The raw NOTECHS system has now been extrapolated for use in various research studies within medicine:

- Non-technical skills for surgeons (NOTSS)

- Anaesthetists' Non-Technical Skills (ANTS)

- The Oxford Notechs

- Team Self Review (TSR)

Team awareness

Statistics from the Joint Commission on Accreditation of Healthcare Organizations (JCAHO), and other research, indicate that in over 75% of events resulting in death or serious physical, or psychological, injury not related to the patient's illness, communication failure is one of the root causes of these incidents, and in over three-quarters of the cases resulted in the death of a patient. Communication lies at the heart of teamwork.

It is clear that multi-disciplinary medical teams must improve the way they deal with events and situations that occur as a result of the complex environment and interactions in which they operate in order to improve patient safety. One way to do this that is routinely employed in many safety critical industries, is to set aside a few moments at the start of the day where the team can meet, and prepare themselves for the day ahead. This is known as a *Team Briefing*.

Briefing is a skill and needs to be developed. It is much more than a mere exchange of information and includes subtle values such as the lowering of the authority or power/distance gradients. Breaking these hierarchical gradients empowers more junior team members to speak up with concerns, or ask questions to clarify uncertainties.

Although a pre-shift briefing should be encouraged in all clinical settings, the same skills are required to conduct mini briefs during the working day to alert all team members of alterations to plans or changes of situations. It is only by this form of communication that all team members can have the same mental model of their environment and challenges. It is recommended that these briefings, or updates, should be encouraged in periods of lower workload when the team have greater cognitive capacity.

Humans often fail to recognize that others with whom they interact have a totally different perception of the world around them. These differences are based on experience, role, background, and personality types amongst numerous other factors. Every time there is a perception mismatch, so is there the opportunity for misunderstanding and potential for error to occur.

In addition to briefing prior to a work period, an effective team will also debrief after the event. Effective debriefings are an opportunity to learn from the events of the day. They are also pivotal in understanding why things went well. Finally they are an opportunity for the team members to thank each other.

Two case studies

The two following case studies demonstrate how a series of individual human errors can combine to cause a catastrophic situation. In each case, there were many opportunities for other people present to question the actions of the team leaders before the event became a disaster.

Case study 1: Wrong site surgery

A patient was admitted for right nephrectomy. Due to a clerical error, the admission slip stated 'left'. The operating list was transcribed from the admission slips. The patient was not woken from sleep to check the correct side on the pre-operative ward round. The side was not checked from the notes or consent form.

The side was questioned by the consultant surgeon on the patient's arrival in theatre but was not confirmed either way. The consultant instructed the surgical trainee (SpR) to carry out the operation. The consultant mistakenly put the correctly labelled x-rays on the viewing box back to front. The consultant supervised the positioning. The SpR did not check the side and was not alerted to this being the wrong side by noticing the normal pulsation in the renal artery of the kidney he was removing.

A medical student observing the operation suggested to the SpR that he was removing the incorrect kidney but was told by the SpR that she was wrong.

The following factors contributed to the incorrect response of the surgical team:

1. A series of communication errors allowed the incorrect transcription to remain unnoticed.

2. A lack of team situation awareness was evident because no team briefing was conducted.

3. An open communication atmosphere was not evident as the medical student felt unable to assert herself in an effective way (steep authority gradient).

The mistake was not discovered until two hours after operation. The patient tragically died.

Case study 2: Wrong engine shutdown, Kegworth, January 1989

The operating crew shut down the No. 2 engine after a fan blade had fractured in the No. 1 engine. The faulty number 1 engine subsequently suffered a major thrust loss due to secondary fan damage after the power had been increased during the final approach to land.

The following factors contributed to the incorrect response of the flight crew:

1. The combination of heavy engine vibration, noise, shuddering, and an associated smell of fire were outside their training and experience.

2. They reacted to the initial engine problem prematurely and in a way that was contrary to their training.

3. They did not assimilate the indications on the engine instrument display before they throttled back the normal No. 2 engine.

4. As the No. 2 engine was throttled back, the noise and shuddering associated with the surging of the No. 1 engine ceased, persuading them that they had correctly identified the defective engine.

5. They were not informed of the flames, which had emanated from the No.1 engine and which had been observed by many on board, including 3 cabin attendants in the aircraft cabin.

The aircraft was destroyed in the accident and 47 passengers tragically died.

The two case studies above show that human beings are very vulnerable to making errors. An effective team assumes that errors will be made and creates an environment where those errors can be trapped, or mitigated, by team members. Such a team carries out briefings to ensure that all team members share the same awareness, and create an atmosphere such that any member of the team can raise concerns over safety issues without fear of retribution.

Summary

There is now good evidence that effective teamwork leads to improved patient outcomes, reduced costs, and improved staff morale. Key elements of the human factors programme developed in aviation over the past 25 years can be extrapolated to medical teams, provided key differences in medicine are recognized. It only seems sensible to learn from other industries where appropriate, and adapt the successes from their programmes to assist in making our patients even safer.

In healthcare, human factors, and thus teamwork training, should be considered to be as important as technical training. The goal should be to introduce such training from the first day at medical school until the last day of a career. Indeed, healthcare is so much more complex than any other industry that there is a strong argument that understanding of human factors and teamwork in healthcare is more imperative than anywhere else.

This is now beginning to be recognized and non-technical skills increasingly included in healthcare teaching and training curricula.

Further reading

Reason, J.T. (1997). *Managing Risks of Organisational Accidents*, Aldershot: Ashgate.

Flin, R.H., O'Connor, P., and Crichton, M. (2008). *Safety at the Sharp End*, Aldershot: Ashgate.

Cox, J. *et al.*, (2006). *Understanding Doctors' Performance*, Oxford: Radcliffe.

Catchpole, K., Giddings, A., Wilkinson, M., Hirst, G., Dale, T., De Leval, M. (2007). Improving patient safety by identifying latent failures in successful operations. *Surgery* **142**(1), 102–110.

Sexton, J. B., Thomas, E. J., and Helmreich, R. L. (2000). Error, stress and teamwork in medicine and aviation: cross sectional surveys. *British Medical Journal* **320**, 745–749.

Chapter 50

Leadership

Nelson Phillips

Key points

- While there are many definitions of leadership, at its most fundamental leadership is about influencing people and situations towards ends desired by a leader.

- Every leader must have at least one follower. Followership and leadership are therefore inseparable and leadership success depends on the commitment and capabilities of followers as well as the leader's ability to understand the needs of followers.

- Effective leadership in a clinical setting has been found to be associated with better health outcomes, lower levels of stress, higher levels of innovation, and an enhanced ability to embrace change.

- Leadership is a significant challenge for many clinicians often called upon to provide it, despite little preparation or enthusiasm for the role, especially as physicians have been described as a group that is particularly 'challenging' to lead.

- There are numerous theories and frameworks available for understanding leadership. Transformational leadership and emotional intelligence are two of the most useful approaches to leadership, and leadership development in healthcare.

Introduction

The study of leaders and leadership has been a central focus of attention in management research for over 100 years. During that time, thousands of articles and books have been published describing great leaders and effective leadership. But, while there are almost as many approaches to leadership as there are books and papers on the topic, some general themes are clear:

- The most general definition of leadership is that a leader is someone who is able to influence people and situations in order to achieve ends that he or she values.

- Leaders have identifiable traits, skills, or behaviours that make them successful as leaders, but that these vary depending on the context in which the leader wishes to lead and, in particular, vary with the followers he or she is attempting to influence.

- Leaders can be developed. That is, the effectiveness of leaders can be improved through various combinations of assessment, experiential learning, and reflection.

In healthcare, leadership among clinicians is an important concern. Effective leadership in a clinical setting is associated with a range of positive outcomes including better patient outcomes, fewer errors, more innovation, and lower stress among team members. The importance of the topic is reflected in the large and growing number of papers and books on the subject, the many conferences and workshops on leadership in healthcare, and the growing number of degrees and diplomas focusing on leadership in health. Yet, there is still a general perception that much needs to be done to develop leaders in healthcare that are up to the many challenges the sector faces. In particular, clinicians face challenges when taking up leadership roles due to a general lack of enthusiasm for the task, a lack of training and support, and the problems of leading peers who are notoriously bad followers.

History

The study of leadership dates back to at least the time of the ancient Greeks. Leadership studies in these early times focused on the study of 'Great Men', with the idea that by reading about successful leaders and reflecting on their lives a reader could improve his or her approach to leadership. This approach continued up until the early 1900s when it began to be supplanted by more systematic research looking at the traits of successful leaders.

Trait theories of leadership began to be developed by social scientists in the 1930s and 1940s. Much of this work was funded by the American military as it sought to define leadership in a military context, and to develop more effective ways to choose individuals with leadership potential. The assumptions of this approach are threefold:

1. People are born with inherited traits.

2. Some traits are particularly suited to leadership.

3. People are good leaders when they have the right combination of these traits.

From this perspective, leadership is an inherited ability not something that can be learned. The challenge, therefore, is to choose people with the right traits for particular leadership positions.

As the limitations of trait theories of leadership became clearer, researchers began to focus more on behavioural theories of leadership. This view of leadership argues that it is not the traits of the leader which determine success but, rather, the behaviours they enact in their leadership role. Researchers working from this perspective began an extensive research programme to understand what behaviours are associated with effective leadership. This view focused attention away from selecting leaders based on their traits, and instead focused attention on developing leader competencies so that they were able to enact the correct behaviours to inspire and motivate followers. Much of modern leadership development, and a preponderance of work on leadership in health care, is based on ideas from this stream of research, with emotional intelligence and transformational leadership being two of the central frameworks developed in this area.

Building on behavioural theories of leadership, researchers also began to explore the complex relationship between leader behaviours and factors like the context and the characteristics of followers. The situational leadership model developed by Blanchard is the most widely used example of this line of research focusing directly on the nature of the followers, and highlighting how leadership behaviours must change depending on the experience and motivation of followers.

Models of leadership that underpin current understandings of leadership success and development draw on various aspects of this complex body of work. They combine an acceptance that there are some traits that are important to leadership in any organization, although they may differ from one organization to another, but that leadership behaviours, and a sensitivity to the context and the characteristics of followers, are also key to successful leadership. Defining and clarifying this model – often called a 'leadership competency model' – is a key part of the leadership development activities of any organization. It is also a critical part of the leadership development of any individual leader.

Transformational leadership

In his highly influential work, Bass developed the notion of transformational leadership and differentiated it from transactional leadership. A transactional leader leads through exchange. He or she leads by exchanging one thing for another as in 'if you do A, I will see that you get promotion B'. This sort of leadership is the sort of leadership exemplified by management by objectives and other sorts of management frameworks based on forms contingent rewards.

Transformational leadership, on the other hand, is about inspiring and stimulating followers to achieve extraordinary outcomes. Transformational leaders help followers to grow, and develop themselves into leaders by empowering them, and helping them to see what is possible. Transformational leaders work by aligning the objectives and goals of the individual with those of the group and the wider organization. This combination of inspiring, developing, and aligning is the core of transformational leadership and the source of its impact on outcomes.

How does a leader do this? According to Bass, there are four elements that make up transformational leadership:

1. The leader must be charismatic so that followers seek to emulate him or her.
2. The leader inspires followers through challenge and persuasion.
3. The transformational leader is intellectually stimulating, expanding followers abilities and skills.
4. The leader is individually considerate, providing the follower with necessary mentoring and coaching.

Combined, this approach leads to high levels of performance across multiple dimensions and effective programmes of change. In healthcare, a transformational approach to leadership has been linked to improved health outcomes, increased patient satisfaction, and more effective innovation. The focus of transformational leadership on the needs, opinions, and feelings of followers has been shown to be particularly important in the context of clinical teams.

Emotional intelligence

The concept of emotional intelligence, or EQ, was developed by Goleman in the 1990s and is based on data on leadership characteristics, and corresponding leadership success, collected from almost 200 companies. His work forms the basis of many leadership development programmes and various leadership capability instruments. Emotional intelligence is a type of social intelligence that involves the ability to be aware of one's own, and others' feelings and emotions, and to use this information to act appropriately. The focus of Goleman's work was very much on the behaviours and skills that underlie successful leadership.

Ideas of emotional intelligence begin with the observation that highly intelligent people are often not the most effective leaders. In fact, everyone seems to know a story about someone who is very intelligent but a failure as a leader. What is often missing in these anecdotes is an ability to understand and manage people. This ability to manage social relationships is rooted, according to Goleman, in emotional intelligence. In healthcare organizations, emotional intelligence has been linked to staff satisfaction, staff retention, and patient satisfaction.

Goleman identified five components that make up emotional intelligence and that are fundamental to effective leadership. The components are as follows:

1. Self-awareness

Self-awareness refers to the ability to recognize and understand one's emotions, moods, and reactions. The hallmarks of people with self-awareness include the ability to realistically assess oneself, self-confidence from knowing one's strengths, and a self-deprecating sense of humour.

2. Self-regulation

Self regulation consists of two elements. First, the ability to control one's reactions and moods, and redirect impulses that would be disruptive or counterproductive. Second, it involves the ability to suspend judgement and to think carefully before acting. Individuals who are able to self-regulate are able to act with integrity and trustworthiness and are more able to deal with change.

3. Motivation

Leaders must be highly motivated and must therefore understand the sorts of situations that motivate them. While leaders generally have a strong need to achieve (a trait), understanding and managing situations to keep personal motivation high is a common behaviour of highly effective leaders. This ability allows individuals to pursue goals with energy and persistence in the face of difficulties and remain optimistic even in the face of failure.

4. Social awareness

Just as self-awareness refers to being sensitive to one's own emotions and drives, social awareness refers to being sensitive to the emotions and drives of others. It requires the recognition that every individual is different, and having to pay attention to the emotions and drives of others not assuming that they are 'just like us'. Individuals with this ability are good at building and retaining talent, and tend to be sensitive to cross-cultural differences.

5. **Social skills**

This refers to the ability to manage relationships and build networks. Building on social awareness, it involves knowing what the correct action is to get the desired result in a social situation. Individuals who are skilled in this area are good at inspiring others and leading change. They are also adept at building teams and are often very persuasive.

Of particular importance is Goleman's finding that emotional intelligence, unlike IQ, can be learned. Therefore, it is not a matter of choosing people with high emotional intelligence but developing it. Furthermore, while IQ declines with age, emotional intelligence increases. In general, people become more emotionally intelligent as they gain experience with people.

Leadership development in healthcare organizations

Leadership development is a complex process through which the quality of leaders in an organization is enhanced. The term can be used to denote activity carried about by an individual to enhance his or her leadership effectiveness, or carried out by an organization and focused on the entire leadership cohort.

While the term 'leadership development' is most often used for structured programmes in larger organizations, leadership development is not limited to formal programmes. In fact, successful leaders are ones who take control of their own development, seek out feedback on their leadership activities wherever they can, and create opportunities for personal growth such as:

- seeking informal feedback from colleagues,
- seeking more rigorous feedback with the help of human relations professionals,
- finding a successful clinical leader who will act as a mentor, and
- seeking out reading material and attending short leadership courses to inspire and challenge.

Self-development is the cornerstone of great leadership, and an awareness and acknowledgement of personal strengths and weaknesses, and efforts to build on strengths and bolster weaknesses, are the first steps to truly great leadership.

But, leadership development is not just an individual activity. Many large organizations have formal leadership development programmes focused on developing the current and future leadership of the organization. While this is generally less of a focus in clinical settings than in the corporate world, there is increasing evidence that this is an incredibly important area of development for public sector health organizations.

Leadership development involves a number of interrelated processes that, when combined, ensure that the leadership of an organization has the capacity to move the organization forward. The elements of a comprehensive organizational leadership development programme include the following:

1. **The evaluation of current strengths and weaknesses**

Once appropriate individuals are identified for inclusion in the programme, the first step is to determine their current leadership capabilities relative to the leadership capabilities that the organization has defined as important (usually in what is referred to as the organization's 'leadership competency model'). This can involve a number of different evaluation techniques including the use of internally developed 360° evaluations (that is, evaluations that include people above and below in the organization, as well as patients and others), the use of externally available instruments for evaluating leadership capabilities, and the engagement of external consultants who provide leadership evaluation.

2. **The creation of individual development plans**

Central to any leadership development programme is the development of a personalized development plan. Beginning with the personal goals of the leader in question and the results of the evaluation of their current strengths and weaknesses, a structured plan is developed to accelerate their development. This plan might include coaching, attending formal leadership development programmes, and plans for personal skill development when required (for example, a course in giving effective feedback, or being more assertive).

3. **The provision of experiential learning opportunities**

Learning to lead is not something that can just be read about and reflected on. Real change and development requires increased self-knowledge and experiences, which push leaders out of their comfort zone. A range of learning experiences are available to challenge leaders ranging from outward bound experiences (for example, winter camping expeditions), to role playing and rapid decision-making simulations. By carefully combining these sorts of activities with input from experts, and time to reflect and share with peers, programmes that challenge and develop leaders can be constructed that rapidly develop the sorts of leadership capabilities required by the organization.

4. **Individual coaching**

Coaching is the practice of providing one on one support and feedback to individuals or small groups in order to help them improve the effectiveness of their leadership activities. Coaches are usually external consultants who are brought in to provide an objective and confidential perspective for key leaders in an organization. Coaching has become a centrepiece of leadership development activities in many organizations and most executives near the top of large organizations will have had a coach. It is important to differentiate between coaches and mentors. While coaches are external people who are generally paid to help leaders develop their leadership skills, mentors are generally unpaid people who are more senior in the organization, and who volunteer to provide advice and networking opportunities to more junior people in order to advance their careers.

Summary

Effective leadership has been shown to have important effects on a range of health outcomes, on healthcare teams, and on the ability of teams to change and innovate.

At the same time, leading in a clinical setting is a challenge for many clinicians due to a lack of time, preparation, and enthusiasm. In addition, physicians are notoriously difficult to lead and are therefore challenging followers. However, there are good frameworks available for thinking about leadership in healthcare, and individuals can have a significant effect on their own leadership practice by recognizing the importance of leadership in clinical settings, by honestly evaluating their own leadership effectiveness, and by beginning to focus on their leadership practice as well as their clinical practice.

Further reading

Firth-Cozens, J. and Mowbray, D. (2001). Leadership and the quality of care, *Quality in Health Care* **10,** ii3–ii7.

Hersey, P. (1985). *The Situational Leader.* New York: Warner Books.

Goffee, R. and Jones, G. (2001). Followership: it's personal, too, *Harvard Business Review* **79**(11), 148.

Goleman, D. (2000). Leadership that gets results, *Harvard Business Review* **78**(2), 78–90.

Robbins, B. (2007). Transformational leadership in health care today, *The Health Care Manager* **26**(3), 234–239.

Chapter 51

Safety, systems, complexity, and resilience: What makes organizations safe?

Kieran Sweeney and Mike D Williams

Key points

- Healthcare organizations are complex adaptive systems consisting of inter-related sub-systems of micro-communities of individuals.
- Emergent properties of healthcare systems can be explained by complexity theory.
- Individuals make errors but good teams can reduce their number and impact.
- Resilience refers to an organization's ability to maintain its systems whilst adapting to external pressures.

Introduction

In this chapter it is proposed that when viewing the activities of a hospital, it is helpful to see that organization as a complex adaptive system (CAS). Complex organizations are constructed of inter-relating subunits (like departments), and those subunits, in turn, consist of micro-communities of individuals (like doctors and nurses). The reciprocal interaction of these micro-communities co-creates the culture of these subunits and, by scaling up, the culture of the organization itself. In this chapter, healthcare organizations are viewed as complex adaptive systems, requiring the application of systems thinking, and safety is seen as an emergent property of the inter-relationship of subunits and the individuals within them.

Safety, governance, and emergent properties

Safety is part of clinical governance, which was rather opaquely defined by Scally and Donaldson in 1998 as:

> 'a framework through which NHS organizations are accountable for continuously improving the quality of their services, and safeguarding high standards of care, by creating an environment in which excellence in clinical care will flourish.'

Seven pillars of clinical governance were identified – clinical effectiveness, risk management, patient experience, communication effectiveness, resource effectiveness, strategic, and learning effectiveness. Once established however, these domains tended to spawn silos of enthusiastic people scurrying about doing their best to spread the word. NHS organizations became governance aware, acutely so in some cases, when visited by the Health Commission, but not much excellence was flourishing. It became apparent that it was the inter-relationship between these domains that could lead to a culture more conducive to excellence, but to achieve this, leadership, teamwork, good, clear communication, and above all systems awareness were needed.

It became apparent that the pillars should not be seen as separate domains at all – this was like thinking about the weather, and considering temperature, pressure, humidity, and local geography separately, whereas each of these parameters, although measurable independently, is inter-dependent on all the others.

For healthcare, it is crucial to see safety as an emergent property of the interaction of all the seven domains of clinical governance, co-creating a quality environment. To grasp this idea theoretically, an understanding of systems, and their complexity and adaptability is required.

Healthcare organizations as complex adaptive systems

Early management approaches to strategy in the NHS regarded organizations as machines operated from the centre and, more importantly, predictable in their responses and outputs. The introduction of systems thinking into NHS management in the 1990s changed this. In systems theory, one accepts that a system (here, an organization like a hospital) consists of a collection of subunits, which interact with one another to produce an output that is greater (and more complex) than the outputs of the individual subunits. Theoretically, there are four features of systems that help us consider how they operate. These are shown in Table 51.1.

While these four features are not mutually exclusive, it is easy to see that hospitals are better thought of as soft, pluralistic organizations generating a range of problems, some of which can be solved algorithmically, and others which need a different kind of more organic management approach.

Over the last decade, complexity theory has been increasingly used to describe how large healthcare organizations work. Complexity theory helps our understanding of the challenges inherent in managing such organizations, and why they frequently fail. The key ideas underpinning complexity in organizational theory are organic: organizations grow, they need to be fertilised with creative conversations, their roots lie in

Table 51.1 Characteristics of systems

Feature of the system	Comment
Hard	Expressed in a rigorous, usually numerical manner
Soft	More ambiguous, fluid and evolving, less easily defined numerically
Positivist	Permitting one undisputed interpretation of events
Pluralistic	Accepts that there are multiple views, each legitimately held within the system

the continuous interaction of all the people who work in them, and the pattern of their behaviour marks the 'culture' of the organization – in what is termed its emergent properties.

Complexity is one of four ways in which a system evolves dynamically (and here a 'system' means a set of agents, their interaction, and sense of purpose). A 'system' can be understood to evolve, dynamically, in four ways.

Systems can be:

1. **Static** – there is no dynamic evolution

2. **Ordered** – exhibiting rhythmic predictable dynamic movement, like a combustion engine

3. **Chaotic** – appearing to change randomly, but predicated on hidden rhythms and patterns, which can be computed mathematically, like the weather.

4. **Complex** – complex systems operate in the state of dynamic evolution between order and chaos, like the tube of the surfer's wave, before it crashes (chaotically) onto the beach.

A complex adaptive system (CAS) has five stages, or activities:

1. Receptive context

2. Complex responsive processes

3. Self-organization

4. Adaption or co-evolution

5. Emergent properties

For a system to evolve creatively, the agents in it needs to have first a *receptive context* – a general set of values the agents understand and accept. Then, the agents need to interact continuously in both predictable and unpredictable ways, in what is termed a series of *complex responsive processes*. The patterning of these processes gives rise to self-organization, essentially the patterns of behaviour by which the organization can recognize itself. The most often quoted example of self-organizing behaviour is when birds form a flock – flocking is self-organizing behaviour. Clearly, organizations don't just self-organize within their own boundaries, they will interact with other organizations in their environment, and change some of their activities accordingly. In complexity theory, this is called *adaption or co-evolution*, the fourth principle of complexity. In turn, the patterning of these self-organizing and adaptive activities gives rise to the 'feel' or 'culture' of the organization, called the organization's *emergent properties*; if flocking is the self-organizing behaviour, then the flock is the emergent property. By the same token, a wave is an emergent property of water. Emergence is a higher order feature of complex adaptive systems, and has been defined as

'*the arising of novel and coherent structures, patterns and properties during the process of self-organization in complex systems*'.

It therefore refers to the potential within such systems to create properties that could not have been predicted by understanding the nature of each separate element in the system.

It is proposed that, in thinking about safety, errors, near misses, or beneficial patient outcomes in a hospital, it is helpful to see that organization as a complex adaptive system (CAS). A blame culture often fails to see an NHS organization as complex; individuals are not isolated free-standing agents who just slot into a system somewhere. They are embedded in one system, for example their ward nursing group, which in turn forms part of a larger group, the intensive care department, which again exists within a particular directorate of the hospital, and so on. These units in the organization are interconnected, the agents engage in a complex responsive process continuously, and in so doing self-organize themselves (into rotas, for example), and interact with others (e.g. managers in the system). The output of all the interaction, within and between all the levels of the system, will be the emergent property of the system. This could be called the 'feel' or 'culture' of the hospital – what it feels like to work there.

Safety, safety culture, and high-reliability organizations (HRO)

Safety culture is hard to define. Safety expert Charles Vincent suggests we summon up our own experience in organizations, like hospitals, and remember wards in which the atmosphere was relaxed, but where the staff were conscientious, and standards uniformly high. Equally, we can recall more slapdash wards, where risks were run, and potentially dangerous practices might have been developing beneath the surface. Vincent asks us to consider the 'culture' of such wards, and suggests;

> 'culture points to the powerful influence of social forces in moulding our behaviour; we are all more malleable than we like to think and to some extent we develop good or bad habits according to the prevailing ethos around us.'

From the explanation of CAS above, it should be clear that the 'moulding of our behaviour' will take place via the complex responsive processes, and that the 'ethos' of the organization will be one of its emergent properties.

Ever since the 1940s high-reliability organizations (HROs), like aviation or the nuclear industry, have developed a systems approach to error. HROs accept that errors are inevitable, and are likely to be the outcome of a systematic failure within the wider organization, rather than the blameworthy behaviour of a single person. Many of the lessons learned in the aviation industry, where most accidents are attributable to human factors, have been usefully transferred to clinical practice. Although Vincent himself warns against seeing the parallels too pervasively, there is no doubt that looking at how HROs learn from errors has been helpful to some key areas of medical practice. This is especially important where clinical professionals work in close-knit teams, as in operating theatres. Teams, like individuals can create or erode safety. A landmark study by Lingard in 2004 concluded that about 25% of all communications in an operating theatre could be classified as communication failures, either unclear, incomplete, or just plain wrong. Working poorly, a team multiplies the possibility of error; working well, the team creates an environment which is safer than the combined efforts of the individuals; safety becomes, in those circumstances, a defining property of the system.

Error detection and management have always been central features of training programmes for cockpit crews in civil aviation. Human vulnerability to stressors, the nature of error, and how to respond to it are studied to achieve three aims:

1. Good teamwork

2. A culture of problem solving through good communication

3. Reducing the possibility that the crew will make errors

Key to this is that the aviation industry has a culture, which accepts that:

♦ errors are inevitable,

♦ systems failures or weaknesses often contribute to them, and

♦ being open about the proneness to error, by fostering good communication, is an essential way of reducing their incidence.

Unfortunately this contrasts with the culture within medical practice. This difference between the cultures of the two industries was highlighted in a study by Helmreich in 2000. Junior cockpit crew were asked if they should be able to question decisions made by senior colleagues; unanimously they said yes, and that this was, quite simply, another defence against error. When posed the same question, one quarter of senior consultant surgeons said that junior surgeons should not question their seniors.

The issue of a hierarchy of communication is not simply of theoretical or academic importance. In 2001, Wayne Jowett died after he had been given an intrathecal injection of vincristine, a drug that should only be given intravenously. The subsequent investigation showed a myriad of tacit assumptions about the roles of the two junior doctors involved, which, while not completely unreasonable, led to an interaction between the two which was literally fatal. In particular, when the more junior doctor was asked why he did not challenge the registrar about the second, fatal syringe, which contained vincristine, but was referred to as methotrexate by the registrar, he said, 'I was a junior doctor, and did what I was told by the registrar ... I assumed he had the knowledge ... and I did not intend to challenge him.' When sentenced to 8 months imprisonment, the registrar said, 'I know it's a lame excuse, but I am a human being'. Everybody is, which is precisely why solid systems, good teamwork, and open communication are needed to protect us from our own fallibility.

Resilience

The idea of resilience is a key element in understanding why NHS organizations have a poor patient safety record, and understanding how that situation might improve.

Resilience is a proactive concept of safety. In healthcare, it refers to an organization's ability to absorb and adapt to increasing pressure, to prevent adverse patient outcomes in the face of near disruption. In resilience, an operating envelope is imagined, within which the system is designed to be competent. Speculation then occurs as to how the system can maintain such competence in the face of pressures, such as rising demand for emergency care, which move it away from this safe operating envelope. Four boundaries to the operating envelope have been proposed:

1. Financial failure

2. Target failure

3. Unacceptable working conditions

4. Failure of safety.

There are obvious managerial and political pressures on healthcare organizations to achieve financial balance, and at the same time reduce waiting times. This promotes a strong productivity culture, which has to be balanced against proper working arrangements for key staff, like junior doctors. These three influences act interdependently, continuously challenging the fourth, safety boundary.

To promote and maintain an acceptable safety culture, and to manage risk appropriately, healthcare organizations have to know where their operating point lies in relation to the boundaries of this safe operating envelope. Recent work demonstrates that NHS organizations are predominantly influenced by the first two of the four boundaries described; financial and target failure. When organizations are seen as organic, flexible and adaptive, it is clear that in order to 'protect' these two boundaries, the other two (working practices and safety) may come under increasing pressure. Work is currently underway to develop more robust metrics to describe all four boundaries to help balance the dominant influence of the measures used to monitor the finance and targets boundaries.

Summary

Humans are fallible, and error is inevitable. Safe organizations accept that errors will occur, and try to reduce their number and effect by building systems to protect the people working within them.

Complexity theory helps us to understand how organizations operate, how they are simultaneously predictable and unpredictable, and how the interaction of the people working within them is fundamental to constructing the ethos, or culture of the organization.

The notion of resilience allows us to imagine how organizations evolve within a safe operating envelope, and what pressures impact on such organizations to move it out of this safe buffer zone. Clinicians need clear communication, good teamwork, and a supportive infrastructure to work safely.

Further reading

Vincent, C. (2006). *Patient Safety*. London: Churchill Livingstone.

Flin, R., O'Connor, P., Crichton, M. (2008). *Safety at the Sharp End: A Guide to Non-Technical Skills*. Aldershot: Ashgate.

Sweeney, K. (2006). *Complexity in Primary Care: Understanding its Value*. Abingdon: Radcliffe Medical Press.

Williams, M. (2008). *A Descriptive Model of Resilience in NHS Hospitals*. Proceedings of Euroma Conference, 16–18 May, Groningen, Holland.

Kernick, D. (ed) (2004). *Complexity and Healthcare Organisations*. Abingdon: Radcliffe Medical Press.

Index